MEDICAL RADIOLOGY

Diagnostic Imaging and Radiation Oncology

Non-Disseminated Breast Cancer

Controversial Issues in Management

Contributors

R. P. A'Hern · M. Baum · L. M. Douville · T. J. Eberlein · R. J. Epstein
G. H. Fletcher · R. M. Goldwyn · J. R. Harris · I. C. Henderson
J. N. Ingle · W. Lawrence, Jr. · S. H. Levitt · T. I. Lingos · M. D. McNeese
R. T. Osteen · A. Recht · L. E. Rutqvist · N. P. M. Sacks · S. J. Schnitt
E. A. Strom · M. Tubiana

Edited by

Gilbert H. Fletcher and Seymour H. Levitt

Foreword by

Luther W. Brady and Hans-Peter Heilmann

With 42 Figures and 32 Tables

Springer-Verlag
Berlin Heidelberg New York
London Paris Tokyo
Hong Kong Barcelona
Budapest

Gilbert H. Fletcher†, M. D.
Professor

Department of Radiotherapy
M. D. Anderson Cancer Center
1515 Holcombe Boulevard
Houston, TX 77030
USA

Seymour H. Levitt, M. D.
Head and Professor

Department of Therapeutic Radiology – Radiation Oncology
University of Minnesota
Box 494, UMHC
Harvard Street at East River Parkway
Minneapolis, MN 55455-0110
USA

MEDICAL RADIOLOGY · Diagnostic Imaging and Radiation Oncology

Continuation of
Handbuch der medizinischen Radiologie
Encyclopedia of Medical Radiology

ISBN-13: 978-3-642-84595-6 e-ISBN-13: 978-3-642-84593-2
DOI: 10.1007/978-3-642-84593-2

Library of Congress Cataloging-in-Publication Data
Non-disseminated breast cancer: controversial issues in management/contributors, R. P. A'Hern ... [et al.]; edited by Gilbert H. Fletcher and Seymour H. Levitt; foreword by Luther W. Brady and Hans-Peter Heilmann. p. cm. – (Medical radiology) Includes bibliographical references and index.
ISBN-13: 978-3-642-84595-6
1. Breast – Cancer – Treatment. I. A'Hern, R. P. (Roger P.) II. Fletcher, Gilbert H. (Gilbert Hungerford), 1911–1992. III. Levitt, Seymour H. IV. Series. [DNLM: 1. Breast Neoplasms – therapy. 2. Combined Modality Therapy. Wp 870 N812 1993] RC280.88N63 1993 616.99'44906-dc20 DNLM/DLC for Library of Congress 93-20548

Typesetting by Macmillan India Ltd., Bangalore 25
21/3130 SPS-5 4 3 2 1 0 – Printed on acid-free paper

This book is dedicated to
Dr. GILBERT H. FLETCHER,
mentor, colleague, and friend,
who will be missed by all of us
and to whom the entire oncology world
owes a great debt.

List of Contributors

Roger P. A'Hern, M.Sc.
Statistician in Computing
The Royal Marsden Hospital
Fulham Road
London SW3 6JJ
UK

Michael Baum, M.D.
Professor of Surgery
The Royal Marsden Hospital
Fulham Road
London SW3 6JJ
UK

Linda M. Douville, R.N.
Clinical Coordinator
Biological Cancer Therapy Program
Division of Surgical Oncology
Brigham and Women's Hospital
75 Francis Street
Boston, MA 02115
USA

Timothy J. Eberlein, M.D.
Associate Professor of Medicine
Harvard Medical School
Chief, Division of Surgical Oncology
Brigham and Women's Hospital
75 Francis Street
Boston, MA 02115
USA

Richard J. Epstein, M.D.
Instructor in Medicine
Harvard Medical School
Attending Physician
Breast Evaluation Clinic
Dana-Farber Cancer Institute
44 Binney Street
Boston, MA 02115
USA

Gilbert H. Fletcher, M.D.
Professor
Department of Radiotherapy
M.D. Anderson Cancer Center
1515 Holcombe Boulevard
Houston, TX 77030
USA

Robert M. Goldwyn, M.D.
Head, Division of Plastic Surgery
Beth Israel Hospital
Clinical Professor of Surgery
Harvard Medical School
330 Brookline Avenue
Boston, MA 02215
USA

Jay R. Harris, M.D.
Professor of Radiation Oncology
Harvard Medical School
Clinical and Educational Director
Joint Center for Radiation Therapy
50 Binney Street
Boston, MA 02115
USA

I. Craig Henderson, M.D.
Professor of Medicine
Chief, Medical Oncology
Director, Clinical Oncology Program
UCSF Cancer Center, Mount Zion USF Medical Center
505 Parnassus Avenue
San Francisco, CA 94143
USA

James N. Ingle, M.D.
Consultant, Division of Medical Oncology
Mayo Clinic
Betty J. Foust, M.D., and Parents' Professor of Oncology
Mayo Medical School
200 1st Street SW
Rochester, MN 55905
USA

Walter Lawrence, Jr., M.D.
Professor, Surgical Oncology
Massey Cancer Center
Medical College of Virginia
Virginia Commonwealth University
1200 E Broad Street, Box 11
Richmond, VA 23298
USA

Seymour H. Levitt, M.D.
Head and Professor
Department of Therapeutic
Radiology – Radiation Oncology
University of Minnesota
Box 494, UMHC
Harvard Street at East River Parkway
Minneapolis, MN 55455-0110
USA

Tatiana I. Lingos, M.D.
Instructor of Radiation Oncology
Joint Center for Radiation Therapy
Harvard Medical School
50 Binney Street
Boston, MA 02115
USA

Marsha D. McNeese, M.D.
Associate Radiotherapist
Associate Professor of Radiotherapy
Department of Radiotherapy
Division of Radiotherapy
M.D. Anderson Cancer Center
1515 Holcombe Boulevard
Houston, TX 77030
USA

Robert T. Osteen, M.D.
Associate Professor of Surgery
Harvard Medical School
Department of Surgery
Brigham & Women's Hospital
75 Francis Street
Boston, MA 02115
USA

Abram Recht, M.D.
Associate Professor
Joint Center for Radiation Therapy
Department of Radiation Oncology
Harvard Medical School
330 Brookline Avenue
Boston, MA 02215
USA

Lars E. Rutqvist, M.D.
Director, Oncologic Center
Radiumhemmet
Karolinska Hospital
104-01 Stockholm
Sweden

Nigel P. M. Sacks, M.D.
Associate Professor
Department of Surgery
The Royal Marsden Hospital
Fulham Road
London SW3 6JJ
UK

Stuart J. Schnitt, M.D.
Associate Professor of Pathology
Harvard Medical School
Pathologist
Beth Israel Hospital
330 Brookline Avenue
Boston, MA 02215
USA

Eric A. Strom, M.D.
Assistant Radiotherapist
Assistant Professor of Radiotherapy
Department of Radiotherapy
Division of Radiotherapy
M.D. Anderson Cancer Center
1515 Holcombe Boulevard
Houston, TX 77030
USA

Maurice Tubiana, M.D.
Honorary Director
Institut Gustave-Roussy
39, rue Camille Desmoulin
94800 Villejuif
France

Foreword

In the last two decades, there has been a major increase in the actual numbers of women diagnosed with breast cancer (from 65000 new cases 20 years ago in the United States to 183000 in 1993). Concomitant with this has been a shift toward making the diagnosis earlier and toward diagnosing an earlier stage of the disease (more than 70% of diagnoses were of advanced-stage disease two decades ago, whereas more than 70% of diagnoses are now earlier-stage disease in 1992). These changes are clearly related to the woman's greater sensitivity to abnormalities in the breast and her seeking medical care, to the physician's greater awareness of the potential diagnosis of cancer, and to the major and important impact of mammographic screening.

These changes have had a major impact on the questions of appropriate treatment, thereby contributing to the controversies in the disease. What is the role of surgery? What are the respective advantages of radical mastectomy, modified radical mastectomy, and conservation surgery with and without supplementary treatment? What is the role of radiation therapy? When should radiation therapy be performed after mastectomy, and what volumes should be irradiated post mastectomy? Where is radiation therapy indicated after conservation surgery, and when is radiation therapy an effective palliative treatment measure? When should chemotherapy and/or hormonal therapy be used as an adjuvant to primary treatment and when as an effective palliative treatment?

This book by Levitt and Fletcher addresses these critical and important issues. Clearly, in primary management, combined integrated multimodal treatment regimens at diagnosis have the greatest opportunity for maximizing the potential for cure, while minimizing the complications of treatment.

Philadelphia/Hamburg, May 1993 LUTHER W. BRADY · HANS-PETER HEILMANN

Preface

The idea for *Non-Disseminated Breast Cancer: Controversial Issues in Management* was conceived about three years ago after much discussion between Dr. Gilbert H. Fletcher and me about the need to evaluate treatment of early breast cancer. Despite the remarkable progress made in the management of this disease, controversy over screening, diagnosis, and treatment exists, as evidenced by the chapters that follow in this book. Our intention in writing this book is to present areas of most concern to the physician directly involved in the treatment of early breast cancer patients. By recruiting leaders to write about their expertise in the treatment and management of early breast cancer, we hope to provide material that will help physicians in their treatment decisions.

The publication of this book is a landmark. It is the last academic effort by Dr. Gilbert H. Fletcher, a world-renowned giant in the field of oncology and medicine. Despite being ill for over a year prior to his death, he was actively involved nearly to his last breath in both writing and editing. He died on January 11, 1992. This book is dedicated to his memory, to the memory of a man with a wonderful searching and inquisitive mind and who engaged both mind and heart in his love for teaching, research, and clinical practice. He has contributed magnificently to our knowledge of oncology.

I would like to thank everyone who participated in bringing this project to fruition, especially the authors for their time, effort, and knowledge, Mary Beth Nierengarten at the University of Minnesota for her editorial assistance, Barbara Foremsky and Mary Jane Oswald at the M. D. Anderson Hospital, and the staff at Springer-Verlag.

Minneapolis, May 1993 SEYMOUR H. LEVITT

Contents

1 Is Breast Cancer Curable?
GILBERT H. FLETCHER (With 2 Figures) 1

2 Criteria of Operability in Advanced Breast Cancer
WALTER LAWRENCE, Jr. and GILBERT H. FLETCHER (With 3 Figures). 5

3 Postoperative Radiotherapy and the Pattern of Distant Spread in Breast Cancer
MAURICE TUBIANA (With 5 Figures) 11

4 How Much of the Axilla Should Be Dissected?
ROBERT T. OSTEEN 27

5 How Much of the Effect of Chemotherapy Is Due to Hormonal Manipulation?
NIGEL P. M. SACKS, ROGER P. A'HERN, and MICHAEL BAUM (With 1 Figure) 35

6 Chemotherapy for Node-Negative Breast Cancer
RICHARD J. EPSTEIN and I. CRAIG HENDERSON (With 1 Figure). 43

7 Treatment of the Peripheral Lymphatics: Rationale, Indications, and Techniques
ERIC A. STROM, MARSHA D. McNEESE, and GILBERT H. FLETCHER (With 12 Figures). 57

8 What Is the Value of Clinical Trials?
SEYMOUR H. LEVITT and LARS-ERIK RUTQVIST (With 1 Figure) 73

9 What Have We Learned from the Stockholm Trials on Adjuvant Radiation Therapy in Early-Stage Breast Cancer?
LARS-ERIK RUTQVIST (With 5 Figures) 83

10 Pathologic Factors Predictive of Local Recurrence in Patients with Invasive Breast Cancer Treated by Conservative Surgery and Radiation Therapy
STUART J. SCHNITT 93

11 What Is the Optimal Technique of Irradiation in Breast-Conserving Treatment?
TATIANA I. LINGOS and JAY R. HARRIS 105

12 Which Patients Should Be Treated by Breast Conservation Surgery and Which by Modified Radical Mastectomy
TIMOTHY J. EBERLEIN and LINDA M. DOUVILLE (With 11 Figures). 117

13 What Is the Role of Adjuvant Chemotherapy in Postmenopausal Women with Operable Breast Cancer?
JAMES N. INGLE (With 1 Figure) 129

14 How Should We Treat Ductal Carcinoma In Situ?
ABRAM RECHT 143

15 How Successful Is Breast Reconstruction?
ROBERT M. GOLDWYN 155

Subject Index 161

1 Is Breast Cancer Curable?

GILBERT H. FLETCHER

CONTENTS

1.1 Introduction 1
1.2 Methods and Materials 1
1.2.1 Techniques of Irradiation 1
1.3 Results 2
1.4 Discussion 3
References 3

1.1 Introduction

After investigating breast cancer mortality since 1900, some epidemiologists in the middle of this century reached the conclusion that survival rates (using a 5-year survival index) of patients with breast cancer were not affected by treatment at all (PARK and LEES 1951). Other authors concluded, by constructing mathematical models of the behavior of breast cancer, that the same proportion of patients at any time during follow-up experience failure, indicating that eventually all patients die from breast cancer (CUTLER and AXTELL 1963). Other studies indicate that less than 15% of breast cancer patients with positive axillary lymph nodes will be free of disseminated disease (BROSS and BLUMENSON 1971). These hypotheses support the predominant view that nearly all breast cancer patients with histologically positive axillary nodes die of disease, thereby raising the controversial question of whether breast cancer is curable (BRINKLEY and HAYBITTLE 1977; BROSS and BLUMENSON 1971; FLETCHER 1984; HARRIS and HELLMANN 1986; RUTQVIST et al. 1984). In this chapter, these hypotheses are tested on a series of 941 patients treated at the University of Texas M.D. Anderson Cancer Center (UTMDACC) between 1963 and 1979; follow-up was a minimum of 14 years to a maximum of 28 years.

GILBERT H. FLETCHER, M.D., Professor, Department of Radiotherapy, M.D. Anderson Cancer Center, 1515 Holocombe Boulevard, Houston, TX 77030, USA

1.2 Methods and Materials

The study period began in 1963, at which time electron beams of energies from 7 MeV to 18 MeV became available allowing local irradiation to the peripheral lymphatics and chest wall. From 1963 to 1977, 941 patients with breast cancer were treated at UTMDACC with irradiation following a radical or modified mastectomy (FLETCHER et al. 1989). None of the patients received adjuvant chemotherapy. The mastectomy was performed in an outside hospital in 62% of the patients. The outside pathology report was available to determine the status of the axillary contents, and the pathology slides for all patients referred after mastectomy were reviewed at UTMDACC. The incidence of patients with histologically positive axillary nodes was 70%. The mean number of nodes per patient with positive nodes was 6.7% and 9% in those with chest wall irradiation. Since patients were referred to UTMDACC for postoperative irradiation when the axillary nodes were positive, the incidence of patients with positive nodes was high. The techniques used to treat all patients is described below.

1.2.1 Techniques of Irradiation

Postoperative irradiation to the peripheral lymphatics and the chest wall was indicated based on the histologic status of the axilla, the location of the tumor in the breast, or both (FLETCHER 1976). The lymphatics of the apex of the axilla, the supraclavicular area, and the internal mammary chain were irradiated in patients with histologically positive axillary nodes and in patients with central or inner quadrant primaries, regardless of axillary status.

With the availability of an electron beam in 1963, chest wall irradiation was added to that of the peripheral lymphatics. Initially this was used when more than 50% of the axillary recovered nodes were positive. Later on, the indication was extended to patients with only 20% axillary positive nodes, with the presence of grave signs, or with a tumor greater than 5 cm (FLETCHER 1976).

Peripheral lymphatic irradiation to the apex of the axilla, the supraclavicular area, and the internal mammary chain was administered through straight-on portals with electron beams of appropriate energy. Internal mammary vessel opacification and lymphoscintography demonstrated that the ipsilateral internal mammary chain nodes were adequately covered. The entire axilla was irradiated with ^{60}CO when there was an indication for irradiating the entire axilla, that is, if few nodes were recovered or tumor had invaded the axillary fat. Only 122 patients had ^{60}CO local irradiation of the internal mammary chain nodes. Prior to 1965, a given dose of 5400–5650 cGy was delivered in 3.5–4 weeks, five fractions per week. After 1965, the given dose was reduced to 5000 cGy in 4 weeks; a boost to the first three interspaces to 5000 cGy at 3 cm depth was added to patients with a high risk of internal mammary chain involvement. The given dose for chest wall irradiation was initially 6000 cGy in 4 weeks and was later reduced to 5000 cGy in 4 weeks.

1.3 Results

An analysis made in 1987 showed that the disease-free survival rate curves for all patients tend to flatten out after 10 years, even more so after 15 years (FLETCHER et al. 1989). At 10 and 20 years, the respective disease-free survival rates are 55% and 50% for all patients, 44% and 40% for all patients with positive nodes, 56% and 48% for patients with one to three positive nodes, and 33% and 30% for patients with four or more positive nodes. The disease-free survival at 10 years for patients with at least ten positive nodes is 20%.

An update in 1991 of the analysis done in 1987 showed that the disease-free and overall survival rate curves for all patients had not changed shape (Figs. 1.1, 1.2), that two patients developed distant metastasis at 16 and 19 years, and that few patients developed cancer in the opposite breast. Between 15 and 20 years the curves became parallel to the mortality curves of the general population.

Table 1.1 shows the incidence of failures by 5-year intervals. The incidence of failures is highest between 0 and 5 years, and still significant between 5 and 10 years, but after 10 years it is relatively

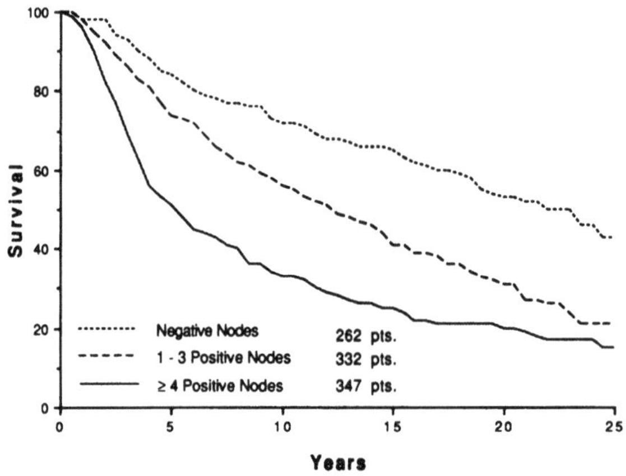

Fig. 1.1. Comparative overall survival rates among breast cancer patients with negative nodes, one to three positive nodes, and four or more positive nodes treated by radical mastectomy and postoperative radiotherapy, with no adjuvant chemotherapy, from 1963 to 1977 at the M. D. Anderson Hospital (analysis 1991)

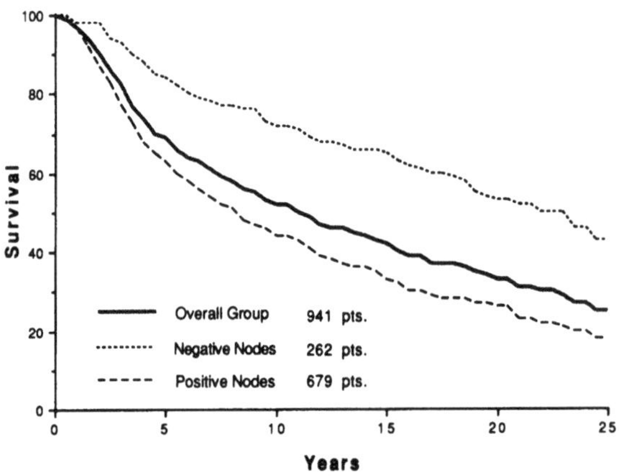

Fig. 1.2. Comparative survival rates among node-negative, node-positive and overall group of breast cancer patients treated by radical mastectomy and postoperative radiotherapy, with no adjuvant chemotherapy, from 1963 to 1966 at the M. D. Anderson Hospital (analysis 1991)

Table 1.1. Number of treatment failures by axillary node status at 5-year intervals after treatment 1963–1977 (analysis November 1987; from FLETCHER et al. 1989)[a]

Axillary node status	Number of years after treatment			
	≤ 5	5–10	10–15	≥ 15
Negative nodes (262)	50	10 (201)	3 (166)	2 (89)
Positive nodes (679)	302	51 (339)	12 (237)	7 (117)
1–3 nodes (332)	112	27 (206)	8 (149)	3 (68)
≥ 4 nodes (347)	190	24 (133)	4 (88)	4 (49)

[a] Numbers in parentheses indicate the number of patients alive and disease-free at beginning of the interval.

small. The majority of locoregional failures occurred on the chest wall with an incidence of 12% when four or more nodes were positive. A further analysis was done in 1991. Of the 331 patients alive in 1987, two experienced distant metastasis after 15 years. The survival curves stayed flat.

1.4 Discussion

Data from the present series of patients treated without adjuvant chemotherapy indicate that not all patients with histologically positive axillary nodes die from disease since at 15 years the curves flatten out, suggesting that the cure rate for patients with positive nodes is approximately 40% (Figs. 1.1, 1.2). These data conflict with a model that predicts that at most 15%, if any, of the patients with histologically positive axillary nodes will survive the disease.

The incidence of locoregional recurrences in the patients with chest wall irradiation was high, approximately 12% when four or more nodes were involved, but it must be viewed in comparison with the data of HAAGENSEN (1956) and of SPRATT and DONEGAN (1967); in their studies, the incidence of locoregional failures in patients with many positive nodes is between 40% and 50%. Because at the UTMDACC patients averaged nine positive nodes for patients with positive nodes, the density of clonogenic infestation of the chest wall was high, which has an impact on the recurrence rate. It would take more than 5000 cGy to bring the recurrence rate to a lower level, but irradiating such a large volume with high doses would lead to severe late sequelae.

The definition of a cured patient must be put in perspective. If a patient is alive without evidence of disease 20 or more years after mastectomy, she has had many disease-free years. If a patient dies without evidence of disease 20 years after the mastectomy, as far as the patient is concerned, she was cured. Asking whether breast cancer is a curable disease has conceptual merit, but the question can lead to therapeutic nihilism: if the disease is not curable, what good does it do to treat it, and particularly to prevent locoregional recurrences?

The second edition of Haagensen's book (1956) *Diseases of the Breast* contains a graph that compares the mortality of patients with breast cancer with the mortality of the general population. After 15 years, the curves became parallel, indicating that a portion of the patients are cured. In another series, a portion of patients was also shown to be cured by comparing the mortality of breast cancer patients with the mortality of the general population. Other models that try to approximate breast cancer survivals also suggest that a fraction is cured. In a series with a long-range follow-up from Memorial Sloan-Kettering Center, of 1458 patients treated in the years 1940–1943, 184 (60 of those with positive axillary nodes) are known to be alive after an average of 30.6 years (ADAIR et al. 1974).

The data presented confirm the reports noted above and demonstrate that a significant fraction of patients, even those with four or more positive nodes, can be cured of their disease even without adjuvant chemotherapy if they receive adequate, appropriate local treatment.

References

Adair F, Berg J, Jourbert L, Robbins GF (1974) Long-term follow-up of breast cancer patients: the 30-year report. Cancer 33: 1145–1150

Berkson J, Gage R (1950) Calculation of survival rates for cancer. Proc Mayo Clinic 25: 270

Brinkley D, Haybittle JL (1977) The curability of breast cancer. Lancet ii: 95–97

Bross IDJ, Blumenson LE (1971) Predictive design of experiments using deep mathematical models. Cancer 28: 1637–1646

Cutler SJ, Axtell SJ (1963) Partitioning of a patient population with respect to different mortality risks. Am Stat Ass J 701–712

Fletcher GH (1976) Reflections on breast cancer. Int J Radiat Oncol Biol Phys 1: 769–779

Fletcher GH (1984) The enigma of breast cancer. In: Ames FC, Blumenschein GR, Montague ED (eds) Current controversies in breast cancer. University of Texas Press, Austin, Texas, pp 139–147

Fletcher GH, McNeese MD, Owald MJ (1989) Long-range results for breast cancer patients treated by radical mastectomy and postoperative radiation without adjuvant chemotherapy: an update. Int J Radiat Oncol Biol Phys 17: 11–14

Haagensen CD (1956) Diseases of the breast, 2nd edn. Saunders, Philadelphia

Harris JR, Hellman S (1986) Observations on survival curve analysis and particular reference to breast cancer treatment. Cancer 67: 925–928

Park WW, Lees JD (1951) The absolute curability of cancer of the breast. Surg Gyn Obstet 93: 129–152

Rutqvist LE, Wallgren A, Nilsson B (1984) Is breast cancer a curable disease? A study of 14,731 women with breast cancer from the cancer registry of Norway. Cancer 63: 1793–1800

Spratt JS, Donegan WL (1967) Cancer of the breast. Saunders, Philadelphia

2 Criteria of Operability in Advanced Breast Cancer

WALTER LAWRENCE, Jr. and GILBERT H. FLETCHER

CONTENTS

2.1 Introduction 5
2.2 Staging 6
2.3 Mastectomy and Irradiation 7
2.4 Combined Treatment Using Chemotherapy . . . 8
2.5 Conclusion 8
References 9

2.1 Introduction

Radical resection of the breast, pectoral muscles, and regional lymph nodes for breast cancer was popularized by William S. Halsted late in the nineteenth century, and became the mainstay for treatment. The lack of benefit from this operation for some patients was first appreciated by Haagensen who, in classic publications with STOUT in 1942 and 1943, described clinical features that were predictors of a shortened life expectancy after radical mastectomy (HAAGENSEN and STOUT 1942, 1943). Based on a series of 640 patients treated by radical mastectomy, they defined what they called "specific criteria of clinical inoperability" in patients who were considered technically resectable at the time of initial clinical presentation but who experienced early recurrence after surgery. Haagensen and Stout concluded from their thoughtful analysis that other treatment strategies for the management of these patients with locally more advanced breast cancer had to be found.

In the almost 50 years that have elapsed since this classic study, both the locoregional and systemic therapy of breast cancer have undergone dramatic change in technical as well as philosophic terms. Because of major improvements in radiation therapy and the impact of systemic chemotherapy on both local and distant disease, the prognosis for these patients has improved such that surgery may again have a role to play in their management. Therefore, it seems appropriate now to re-examine these earlier criteria of operability. Specifically, the question is – what is the current role of surgery in patients presenting with locally advanced breast cancer, and which of these patients receive clear-cut benefit from mastectomy?

Haagensen's and Stout's criteria of inoperability were formulated against a setting in which radical mastectomy was the primary and only treatment for breast cancer. The criteria included the following:

1. Carcinomas developing during pregnancy or lactation (this criterion was later removed by Haagensen);
2. carcinomas associated with extensive edema of the skin over the breast (peau d'orange involving more than one-third of the breast);
3. satellite nodules of cancer in the skin of the breast;
4. gross intercostal or parasternal tumor nodules (actually large metastatic nodes in the internal mammary chain);
5. edema of the arm;
6. proven supraclavicular node metastases;
7. "inflammatory" breast cancer;
8. demonstrated distant metastases;
9. the presence of two or more of the following: ulceration of the skin, edema of the skin of limited extent (less than one-third of the breast), fixation of the tumor to the chest wall, axillary lymph nodes measuring 2.5 cm or more in transverse diameter and proven to contain metastases, and fixation of axillary lymph nodes to the skin or the deep structures of the axilla and proven to contain metastases.

One hundred and nine of the 640 patients undergoing radical mastectomy in Haagensen's and Stout's total series fulfilled these criteria of inoperability. Three of these patients did experience

WALTER LAWRENCE, Jr., M.D., Professor, Surgical Oncology, Medical College of Virginia, Virginia Commonwealth University, 1200 E, Broad St. Box 11, Richmond, VA 23298, USA; GILBERT H. FLETCHER, M.D., Professor; Department of Radiotherapy, M.D. Anderson, Cancer Center, 1515 Holocombe Boulevard, Houston, TX 77030, USA

5-year survival but, shortly thereafter, developed local recurrence with distant metastases and promptly died. Virtually one-half of these patients (48%) developed local treatment failure. This implied that incomplete surgical removal of the loco-regional disease was not only without benefit, but might actually be harmful. It is conceivable, however, that any potentially adverse affect of mastectomy on survival might not occur when operative treatment is combined with other modalities. Although survival is an important measure of success, we must also consider the importance of local disease control since this significantly impacts the quality of life.

2.2 Staging

The issue of clinical operability versus technical resectability relates to the TNM staging system (Table 2.1) (AMERICAN JOINT COMMISSION on CANCER, AJC, STAGING 1983). In the latest update of the TNM staging system, some of the elements of Haagensen's criteria of inoperability relegate patients to stage IV, while other elements lead to the classification of patients as stage IIIA or IIIB. Stage IV patients have disease clearly beyond the confines of resection and, with rare exceptions, should continue to be considered inoperable. Stage III patients are the ones in question regarding operability. To assess the relationship of criteria for clinical operability for these patients in terms of current treatment strategies we need to observe the outcome of stage III patients who have had an operation as part of a multimodal treatment program. This will help us answer questions regarding the possible selection of patients who might benefit from resection. Despite many randomized clinical treatment trials of stage I and II breast cancer, there are few such randomized data available for stage III breast cancer. We must examine nonrandomized series of stage III patients for comparisons of treatment results in patients managed by combinations of radiation and/or chemotherapy with mastectomy or mastectomy alone.

Table 2.1. AJC staging

	1983	1988
T Stage	Criteria	
Tx tumor	Size unknown	No evidence of primary
T1	Size < 2 cm	Subsets in T1s and from 0.5 cm to 2 cm
T2	Size > 2 cm but < 5 cm	
T3	Size > 5 cm	
T4	Any tumor with the following: inflammatory signs edema ulceration peau d'orange ridging peripheral satellite nodules central satellite nodules chest wall fixation	T4a direct extension to chest wall T4b-T4c grave signs T4d inflammatory
N Stage		
Nx	Status of axillary or supraclavicular nodes unknown	
N0	Normal	
N1	Axillary nodes: single or multiple	
N2	Matted or fixed axillary nodes or nodes > 3 cm	
N3	Arm edema or supraclavicular/infraclavicular nodes	M1 supraclavicular node
Clinical stage groups		
Stage IIIA	T3, N0-2, M0 or T0-3, N2, M0	T3, N0 stage IIB
Stage IIIB	T4, Any N, M0 or N3, Any T, M0	TM1, stage IV

2.3 Mastectomy and Irradiation

Between 1955 and 1984, 376 patients registered with stage III (AJC STAGING 1983) cancer of the breast at the M. D. Anderson Hospital were treated with some form of mastectomy followed by postoperative irradiation (202 stage IIIA and 174 stage IIIB) (STROM et al. 1991). The operative procedures chosen ranged from total mastectomy without axillary node dissection to standard radical mastectomy, and the radiation dose generally was 50 Gy delivered in 25 fractions over 5 weeks. Variations included a boost of 10–20 Gy to the areas of gross disease and to the area around the surgical scar, while a dose reduction occurred in the axilla after axillary dissection. The locoregional control at 10 years was 88% for stage IIIA and 74% for stage IIIB (Fig. 2.1). Disease-free survival rates at 10 years for IIIA and IIIB were 48% and 30%, respectively (Fig. 2.2). The 10-year disease-free survival rates were 64%, 47%, and 33% for patients with negative nodes, one to three positive nodes, and four or more positive nodes, respectively (Fig. 2.3). This appears to be a better local response rate than after surgical resection or radiation used as a single modality of treatment and appears to demonstrate a benefit from this combined treatment in some of the patients that were considered inappropriate resection candidates by Haagensen and Stout. This is a factor of some importance in terms of the concept of "quality of life."

A similar small group of 35 patients with selected technically resectable stage III breast cancers were treated at the Medical College of Virginia (MCV) during an 8-year period (1967–1975) by preoperative irradiation and radical mastectomy (TERZ et al. 1978). Some of Haagensen and Stout's criteria of inoperability were employed as eligibility criteria for entry into this pilot study, while some of the more adverse features (including clinically positive ipsilateral supraclavicular nodes, edema of the ipsilateral arm, edema involving the entire breast and satellite skin nodules) were indications for exclusion. However, lesions 5 cm or more in diameter, ulceration, edema of a significant portion of the breast and large matted or fixed axillary nodes were all stage III characteristics that were specific indicators for inclusion in this combined treatment program of preoperative radiotherapy and mastectomy. This approach did not significantly improve disease-free 5-year survival (17%), but local control was achieved in a large proportion of patients (29/35 or 83%), suggesting some improvement in the quality of life.

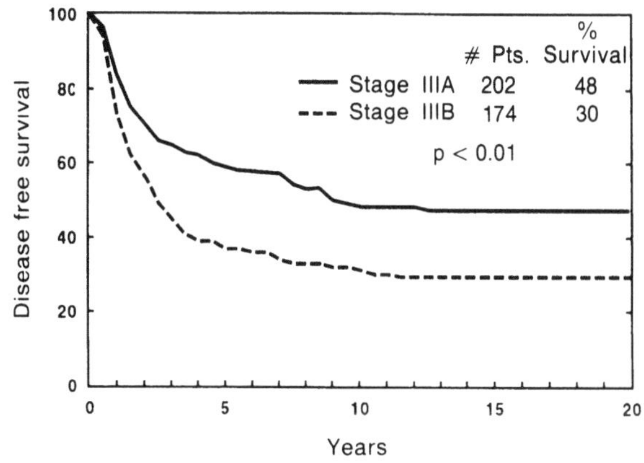

Fig. 2.2. Disease-free survival rates in stage IIIA and stage IIIB patients at 10 years (From AJC STAGING 1983 and BERKSON and GAGE 1950)

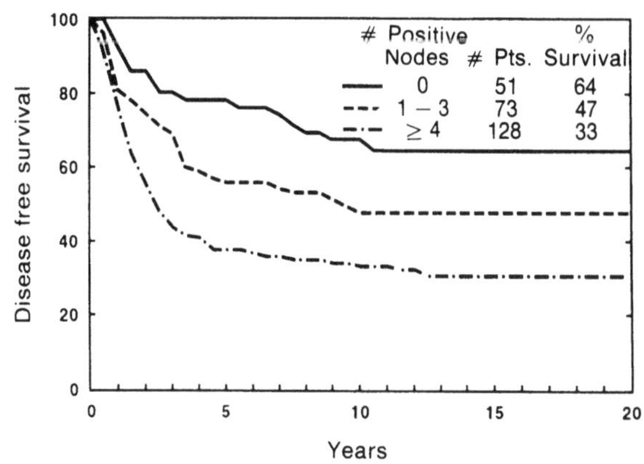

Fig. 2.3. Disease-free survival rates in stage III patients at 10 years in terms of nodal spreads (From AJC STAGING 1983 and BERKSON and GAGE 1950)

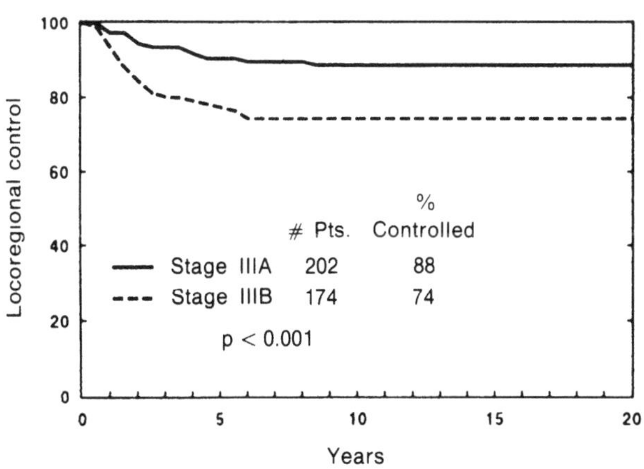

Fig. 2.1. Local regional control in stage IIIA and stage IIIB patients at 10 years. (From AJC STAGING 1983 and BERKSON and GAGE 1950)

In a series of 488 stage III breast cancer patients at Memorial Sloan-Kettering Cancer Center, some patients, but not all, demonstrating the criteria of inoperability were treated by standard radical mastectomy with some patients receiving postoperative radiation only to nodal areas (FRACCHIA et al. 1980). It is difficult to evaluate the combined locoregional therapy of this large series treated over a 10-year period since the radiation was not uniformly applied and, when used, it was limited to the node bearing areas. The locoregional recurrence rate was 25% in the patients with positive nodes, and the 10-year survival rate was 72% for those with negative nodes and 20% for patients with positive nodes.

In another nonrandomized series, the addition of well-administered radiation before or after mastectomy for advanced stage III lesions appeared to be somewhat more effective than radiation alone, or mastectomy alone, when locoregional control was the criterion of success (BEDWINEK et al. 1981). Although survival benefits from the combination are suggested but not proven, improved locoregional control does add to achieving "quality of life" goals in this group of patients. This may justify resection as part of a treatment strategy in these patients and may override some of the prior criteria of inoperability.

2.4 Combined Treatment Using Chemotherapy

Based on large prospective randomized trials, the beneficial effect of systemic chemotherapy as an adjuvant to the locoregional treatment of stage I and II breast cancer has become well-established in the last decade for some subsets of patients. Systemic chemotherapy has become commonplace in the treatment of stage III breast cancer despite a lack of comparable prospective trials. In fact, the major questions in terms of systemic chemotherapy of stage III breast cancer relate to the order of nonoperative therapies in relation to the surgical resection. Another reasonable question regarding systemic chemotherapy, before or after locoregional treatment, is whether this added treatment changes our concepts of inoperability for advanced lesions. Our criteria for inoperability have been "liberalized" as a result of combining mastectomy and radiation therapy, and now the question is whether they will be further modified by the addition of systemic pre- or postoperative chemotherapy. Furthermore, in the setting of effective chemotherapy, the question of the optimal extent of local surgery is raised.

The M.D. Anderson series of 174 noninflammatory stage III patients treated by combination chemotherapy, mastectomy and axillary dissection and/or radiation therapy between 1974 and 1985 is helpful in answering this question (HORTOBAGYI et al. 1988). Although this series included both clinically resectable and nonresectable lesions by their criteria, both local control and survival data were similar at 10 years to the series with mastectomy and radiation without chemotherapy (STROM et al. 1991). The disease-free 5- and 10-year survival for stage IIIA patients was 71% and 40%, and for those with stage IIIB it was 33% and 29%, respectively. Only 26 stage IIIB patients (22%) experienced a locoregional recurrence. This study does not clearly establish resectability guidelines, but it is interesting that only 6% of stage IIIA patients and 20% of stage IIIB patients were managed without mastectomy as a part of the combination treatment.

In a similar series of stage III breast cancers at MCV managed by surgery with or without radiation and with postoperative systemic chemotherapy in the years 1978 to 1987, data regarding locoregional and distant treatment failure are similar to those obtained by preoperative chemotherapy in the M.D. Anderson series (FRANK et al. 1992). As in other reports, this series fails to demonstrate an absolute need for mastectomy (as opposed to conservative breast resection) in addition to radiation and chemotherapy, even though these treatment protocols were developed on this premise. It is clear that radiation continues to provide added benefit to mastectomy even when patients receive aggressive chemotherapy. The optimal order of administration of these various modalities needs to be established. This is discussed elsewhere in this book.

2.5 Conclusion

Given this background of information from nonrandomized studies, along with the general acceptance that it is detrimental to cut through gross cancer tissue (and thereby leave gross cancer in situ), what are useful guidelines for determining operability of locally advanced cancer?

Clinical findings from Haagensen's and Stout's original list that still must indicate inoperability in most instances are the following:

1. Edema of the arm (demonstrating our inability to completely resect gross regional lymphatic spread in the axilla)
2. Proven supraclavicular metastases (demonstrating spread that is analogous to distant metastases)
3. Demonstrable distant metastases, unless a locally advanced breast cancer is extremely symptomatic, incompletely controlled by systemic treatment and/or primary radiation therapy, and removable with clear gross margins
4. Extensive edema of the skin of the breast or extensive satellite nodules that are not grossly encompassable by a mastectomy after systemic treatment and/or preoperative radiation therapy.

Lesions that were once considered inoperable, but now might well be considered operable, include those that show the following:

1. Edema limited to the breast
2. Ulceration
3. Satellite nodules adjacent to the primary
4. Large axillary lymph nodes
5. Limited inflammatory change than can be encompassed by a mastectomy incision, particularly if there is a clinical response to neoadjuvant chemotherapy.

Proof is lacking that the addition of surgical resection to the other treatment modalities has clearly improved overall survival in many of the above situations once considered "inoperable." Nevertheless, the potential impact of improved locoregional control on survival expectations cannot be discounted.

Better understanding of the biology of breast cancer and the relationship of the extent of locoregional disease to frequency of distant micrometastases has frequently led some to downgrade the clinical importance of local control and its impact on both quality of life and on survival. The pendulum may have swung too far in this regard, now that we are effectively exploiting multimodality therapy. While mastectomy provides little benefit to patients whose survival is expected to be quite short, the prolongation of survival resulting from aggressive systemic treatment increases the clinical importance of local control. Continued efforts that often include mastectomy may well improve both the quality of life and the length of survival of patients presenting with locally advanced breast cancer.

References

American Joint Commission on Cancer Staging and End-Result Reporting (1983) Manual for staging of cancer, 2nd edn. Lippincott, Philadelphia, pp 127–133

Bedwinek J, Rao DV, Perez C et al (1981) Stage III and localized stage IV breast cancer: irradiation alone versus irradiation plus surgery. Int J Radiat Oncol Biol Phys 8: 31–36

Berkson J, Gage RP (1950) Calculation of survival rates for cancer. Mayo Clin Proc 25: 270–286

Fracchia AA, Evans JF, Eisenberg BL (1980) Stage III and localized stage IV breast cancer: irradiation alone versus irradiation plus surgery. Ann Surg 192: 705–710

Frank JL, McCllesh DK, Dawson KS, Bear HD (1992) Stage III Breast Cancer – Is neoadjuvant chemotherapy always necessary? J Surg Onc 49: 220–225

Haagensen CD, Stout AP (1942) Carcinoma of the breast. I. Results of treatment. Ann Surg 116: 801

Haagensen CD, Stout AP (1943) Carcinoma of the breast. II. Criteria of operability. Ann Surg 118: 859

Hortobagyi GN, Ames FC, Buzdar AU et al (1988) Management of stage III primary breast cancer with primary chemotherapy, surgery and radiation therapy. Cancer 62: 2507–2516

Strom EA, McNeese MD, Fletcher GH et al (1991) Results of mastectomy and postoperative irradiation in the management of locally advanced carcinoma of the breast. Int J Radiat Oncol Biol Phys 21: 319–323

Terz JJ, Romero CA, Kay S et al (1978) Preoperative radiotherapy for stage III carcinoma of the breast. Surg Gynec Obstet 147: 497–502

3 Postoperative Radiotherapy and the Pattern of Distant Spread in Breast Cancer

MAURICE TUBIANA

CONTENTS

3.1	Introduction	11
3.2	Natural History of Human Breast Cancer	13
3.2.1	The Pattern of Axillary Lymph Node Involvement	16
3.3	Radiotherapeutic Studies	19
3.4	Conclusion	24
	References	24

3.1 Introduction

Postoperative radiotherapy (RT) has been widely used in the treatment of breast cancer since the inception of RT, and a marked reduction in the incidence of local recurrences has been observed in all studies. This finding demonstrates the effect of irradiation on residual neoplastic tissue (TUBIANA and SARRAZIN 1987). However, the impact of this treatment on long-term survival remains controversial and there is a large discrepancy between the highly effective local treatment and the somewhat modest gain in total survival (TUBIANA et al. 1986).

The meta-analysis of randomized clinical trials carried out by CUZICK et al. (1987) did not find any delay in distant metastases, nor a reduction in mortality during the first 5–10 years of follow-up. This meta-analysis was questioned for several reasons (LEVITT 1988; LEVITT and FLETCHER 1991). The main criticism is that it pooled trials in which patients were treated either by orthovoltage or megavoltage radiation with different techniques and various doses. In order to prevent local recurrence, it has been shown that a sufficient dose of 40–50 Gy in 4–5 weeks should be delivered (TUBIANA and SARRAZIN 1987). A dose–effect relationship has been observed and after lower doses the incidence of local recurrence is appreciable (ARRIAGADA et al. 1986; FLETCHER 1980). For example, HELLE et al. (1984) reported the results of a prospective study that showed a significant higher rate of locoregional recurrence following doses of 20 Gy than after 40 Gy or 50 Gy (47% versus 27%). After conservative treatment of breast cancer there is a significant correlation between dose, expressed in nominal single dose, and the probability of local relapse (CLARKE et al. 1985). In this study the breast dose was 45 Gy in all patients and the variation in the nominal single dose value was related to variations in treatment duration (CLARKE et al. 1985). In studies in which irradiation was carried out with 200-kV RT, the doses were generally insufficient; they were heterogeneous in some studies performed later with high-energy radiation. Moreover, the target volumes have to be properly delineated (FLETCHER and MONTAGUE 1978). Progress has been accomplished in this respect. For example, the internal mammary lymph nodes have been more precisely located through the use of lymphoscintigraphy. Although the average lateral displacement from the midsternal line is 2.5 cm, the actual distances range from 0 cm to 5.3 cm (ROSE et al. 1977). Similarly, the depth from the skin ranges from 0.7 cm to 5 cm. With many of the former standard techniques, such as the opposed tangential chest wall fields, an appreciable proportion of patients had some of their internal mammary lymph nodes underdosed because they were located at the margin of or outside the field (FLETCHER and MONTAGUE 1978; TUBIANA and SARRAZIN 1987). Thus, the absence of a difference between the two treatment arms of the meta-analysis cannot exclude the possibility of a beneficial effect on the patients who were correctly irradiated – that is, with a sufficient dose and with an adequate target volume. However, the results of the meta-analysis suggest that the effect, if any, is probably not very large (CUZICK et al. 1987).

It has been claimed that postoperative RT has a detrimental effect implicating radiation-induced immunodepression, which could enhance distant spread (STJERNSWARD 1974). Clinical and experimental data do not substantiate this claim

MAURICE TUBIANA, M.D., Honorary Director, Institut Gustave-Roussy, 39, rue Camille Desmoulin, 94800 Villejuif, France

(Tubiana et al. 1986). Since death is generally caused by distant metastases in patients with breast cancers, the limited impact of postoperative RT on survival may have two other explanations (Tubiana et al. 1986). First, local control of the tumor may not influence the incidence of distant metastases. Second, subgroups of patients for which postoperative RT may be beneficial may be difficult to identify in meta-analyses. The following examines each possible explanation.

Supporting the view that local control of the tumor does not influence the incidence of distant metastases is the claim that in most patients breast cancer is a systemic disease from its inception (Fisher 1980; Fisher et al. 1991). In this concept, node status and local recurrence are markers rather than risk factors for distant metastases. If tumors metastasize very early in their evolution, long before diagnosis, local control will not reduce the incidence of distant metastases and earlier diagnosis will have little effect on the development of metastases.

However, two sets of data are not consistent with this assumption. First the percentage of tumors cured by local treatment without systemic therapy is much greater for small than for large tumors (Koscielny et al. 1984); furthermore, screening and earlier diagnosis lead to a substantial reduction in the incidence of metastases (Tabar et al. 1992). It has been argued that there are two different groups of breast cancer: those that have initiated metastases almost from the outset and those with late distant dissemination (Slack et al. 1969). As discussed below, we previously showed that this hypothesis is not consistent with the data (Koscielny et al. 1985).

Furthermore, several data evidenced that metastatic dissemination may result from a lack of control of the primary tumor and the regional lymph nodes. The role of local recurrence in the initiation of distant metastases has been shown for a large number of cancer types (Leibel et al. 1991a, b), for example, in cancers of the cervix (Anderson and Dische 1981), prostate (Fuks et al. 1991), head and neck (Leibel et al. 1991a, b), and breast (Tubiana et al. 1986). In the cooperative Gustave-Roussy-Princess Margaret study, a multivariate analysis demonstrated that a lack of control of the primary breast tumor and axillary nodes was correlated with a higher risk of distant metastases. Moreover, the existence of a dose–effect relationship was documented (Arriagada et al. 1986). In the Guy's Hospital Study, carried out in London, the patients were randomized to undergo radical mastectomy or lumpectomy plus irradiation (25–27 Gy in 10 days) at a dose that was insufficient to control all axillary disease (Atkins et al. 1972). Among stage II patients with clinically positive lymph nodes, the frequency of axillary failures and of distant metastases was significantly higher in the group treated without axillary dissection (Atkins et al. 1972). This strongly suggests that lymph node metastases can be important foci for distant spread and is in accordance with the so-called multi-step dissemination process. The role of local recurrence in the initiation of remote metastases is confirmed by several other data that show that local failure exerts a dominant effect on the probability of spread to remote sites. Hayward and Caleffi (1987) in an analysis of two controlled trials in which radical mastectomy was compared to lumpectomy plus an irradiation at a dose of 30 Gy, reported a significant increase in metastatic disease after local recurrence in patients with T1N0 breast cancer.

Kurtz et al. (1991) have compared the long-term survival in 134 patients treated by RT. The patients were subdivided in two subgroups according to overall dose and dose per week. The 20-year survival rate was 69% in those who received adequate RT versus 57% in inadequately treated patients. However the difference was not significant.

In patients who for various reasons were treated with biopsy and a delayed mastectomy, the presence of residual cancer tissues was found to be significantly associated with an increased incidence of metastases, in particular brain metastases (Kamby et al. 1991). Moreover a recent study of Stotter et al. (1990) found that locoregional recurrence is associated with an additional hazard survival similar to that of a second primary tumor with the same extent of local and regional disease. Their conclusion is based on the consistency of the predictions of a simple mathematical model with the actuarial survival rate of 499 patients, 49 of whom had developed locoregional recurrence. The model predicts a deficit in survival equal to 8% at 5 years after initial treatment and of 22% at 5 years after local recurrence.

In summary, the assertion that local control of the tumor does not affect distant dissemination is not consistent with most data. However, the model of cascade spread of blood-borne metastases was questioned by Fisher et al. (Fisher 1980; Fisher et al. 1991). In particular, in a National Surgical Adjuvant Breast and Bowel Project (NSABP) study, the group of patients with clinical node-negative tumors was randomized to undergo simple mastectomy alone, followed by subsequent removal of axillary nodes if the nodes became positive, or total mastectomy followed by regional irradiation (FISHER et al. 1981). No difference was found in the incidence of distant metastases or survival up to the 6 years after initial treatment, although the incidence of local failure was 8.5% higher in the group treated without postoperative RT and axillary dissection. Moreover, FISHER et al. calculated that approximately 40% of the patients treated by total mastectomy alone did not undergo removal or treatment of positive axillary lymph nodes. Thus, they concluded that a positive axillary lymph node is not a pivotal factor in the sequence of events leading to distant disease (FISHER et al. 1981). Although their data are valuable, they are not conclusive (TUBIANA and SARRAZIN 1987): The follow-up is relatively short, the growth rate of clinically node-negative tumors in patients with breast cancer is relatively slow, and most local recurrences and remote metastases are only expected to become clinically detectable after relatively long periods. From this point of view, it is noteworthy that only a small proportion of the expected axillary failures have been detected during the first 6 years. This observation challenges the estimation that 40% of the patients had occult involvement of axillary nodes. Also, if the patients are carefully followed up, the positive nodes could have been detected at a time when their size was relatively small (approximately 1–2 g); it is known that, in patients with breast cancer without clinically involved lymph nodes, most disseminations occur when the size of the primary tumor is much larger than 1–2 g (KOSCIELNY et al. 1984; STOTTER et al. 1990; TUBIANA et al. 1986; TUBIANA and KOSCIELNY 1991).

In a recent article, FISHER et al. (1991) reported that local recurrence is significantly associated with a higher rate of distant metastases, in accordance with the data discussed above. They still claim in this article that local recurrence is not a cause of distant spread, but only a marker for a risk already present at initial treatment. However, their arguments are not convincing and the most likely explanation is that local recurrence is a step on the path to metastatic spread. Among patients in whom distant dissemination from the primary tumor has not occurred at the time of initial treatment, only a relatively small proportion have regional occult disease present after surgery. Moreover, of these deposits, only a small proportion will have a chance to disseminate before becoming detectable and they will do so after a long time interval. Thus, a large number of patients and a long follow-up is necessary to document the impact of local failure on survival. Moreover, a comparison of the whole population of irradiated and nonirradiated patients is of limited significance and an effort should be made to identify those subsets of patients in whom RT might be useful (TUBIANA et al. 1986).

The second explanation for the limited impact of postoperative RT on survival may be because if postoperative RT is not equally effective for all patients, pooling all of them might interfere with the identification of the subgroup(s) in which RT is worthwhile. The analysis of the effects of RT should be carried out in the various subsets of patients according to the well-known factors that influence the probability of relapse, such as involvement of axillary nodes or histologic grade (CONTESSO et al. 1987; TUBIANA and SARRAZIN 1987).

Long ago it was reported that postoperative RT is not justified in node-negative patients and does not significantly reduce the probability of locoregional recurrence which, in any case, is small (TUBIANA and SARRAZIN 1987). This conclusion agrees with the results of the Guy's Hospital trial in which radical mastectomy and tumorectomy plus irradiation at an insufficient dose yielded a similar relapse-free and metastasis-free survival rate in stage I (ATKINS et al. 1972), while, as discussed above, there was a clear advantage in favor of radical mastectomy in stage II patients. This suggests that postoperative RT at a sufficient dose is mainly useful in stage II subset of patients. Conversely, in patients with tumors of more than 5 cm in diameter, several data suggest that postoperative RT is ineffective, probably because metastatic dissemination has already occurred at the time of initial treatment in most patients (AUQUIER et al. 1992).

This discussion shows that the interpretation of the results of local treatment should be based on a deep knowledge of the pattern of spread and progression of human breast cancer, that is, on its natural history.

3.2 Natural History of Human Breast Cancer

Postoperative RT can prevent metastatic spread only in patients without distant metastases at the time of initial treatment. Moreover, local treatment is only effective when a regional recurrence can be a nidus for distant dissemination before it is detected and treated. In order to introduce some quantitative data in the analysis of these prerequisites, a study was initiated in 1975 in Villejuif to estimate the size of the primary breast tumor at metastatic dissemination (Tubiana et al. 1975). Until recently, the description of the natural history of human cancers had remained purely qualitative. However, with the introduction of computerized cancer registries, we are now able to extract reliable quantitative information that otherwise could not have been obtained from the huge amount of data found in patient files (Atkinson et al. 1986; Carter et al. 1989; Kamby et al. 1991; Koscielny et al. 1984; Koscielny et al. 1985; Tubiana and Koscielny 1991).

The main event during the growth of a human tumor is metastatic dissemination (Tubiana 1986). Prior to its occurrence, the breast cancer is a locoregional disease which is easily cured by local treatment. Thus, an accurate estimation of the likelihood of distant spread is of great value to identify the subset of patients for whom more effective local treatment could improve the outcome. Several prognostic factors, such as axillary lymph node involvement or the hormonal receptor content of the tumor, are being used for that purpose; however, the role of the size of the primary tumor is often overlooked, although intuitively it is felt to be important and remains the main criterion in all clinical staging systems, such as the TNM system (Tubiana 1986).

The tumor size at metastatic dissemination varies widely. Dissemination has already occurred in some breast cancers of less than 5 mm in diameter, whereas it has not occurred in some bulky tumors of more than 8 cm in diameter cured by local treatment alone. A major goal of the study of the natural history of breast cancer is the analysis of the relationship between tumor size and the probability of metastatic dissemination as well as the influence of the various tumor characteristics on this relationship.

The study that we performed was based on the analysis of the data registered at the Institut Gustave-Roussy in Villejuif on approximately 3000 breast cancer patients treated prior to the use of adjuvant chemotherapy, with a follow-up ranging from 15 to 32 years (Koscielny et al. 1984). The data showed that the proportion of distant metastases appearing more than 25 years after treatment is negligible. The proportion after 25 years can therefore be assumed to be equal to the probability of distant dissemination before initial treatment in a group of patients. We subdivided the population of patients into eight classes according to tumor volume and the tumor diameter at surgery, and plotted for each class the actuarial cumulated proportion of patients with metastases as a function of time after treatment up to 25 years. The patients with distant metastasis at initial work-up were included in this cumulated proportion. The relationship between the volume at the time of diagnosis (in logarithmic coordinates) and the cumulative proportion of patients with distant metastases is sigmoid (Fig. 3.1). The curve becomes linear in PROBIT log coordinates, which indicates that the distribution of tumor volumes at initiation of first distant metastasis is log-normal in the whole population of patients (including patients with detectable distant metastases at the time of initial treatment). The median volume (termed V50) is 23.6 ml (diameter: 3.56 cm) with a 95% confidence range of individual values from 0.14 to 4000 ml (Koscielny et al. 1984). Thus, in clear contrast with experimental tumors in which most metastatic disseminations occur within a small range of tumor sizes, the range in human tumors is much wider (Fig. 3.1). This illustrates their heterogeneity. Figure 3.1 also shows that for tumors larger than 1 cm in diameter, a small decrease in the size of the tumor at initial treatment results in a marked reduction in the proportion of patients with occult metastases. This is the rationale of screening procedures (Koscielny et al. 1985).

Moreover, it was found that the average threshold volume at which dissemination occurs, is inversely correlated with the number of involved lymph nodes and the histologic grade of the tumor (Tubiana and Koscielny 1991). In order to quantify the influence of histologic grade on the probability of metastatic dissemination for tumors of all sizes, the patients were subdivided into three groups according to the histologic grade. In each subgroup there was a significant correlation between tumor size and the probability of distant spread; the distributions were log-normal and the median size was markedly larger for grade 1 tumors.

Figure 3.2 depicts the relationship between tumor size and the probability of distant spread in patients with a grade 1, 2, or 3, tumors confirming that metastases were initiated earlier during the growth of the tumor in high-grade tumors. The curves differ significantly; the earliest occurrence of

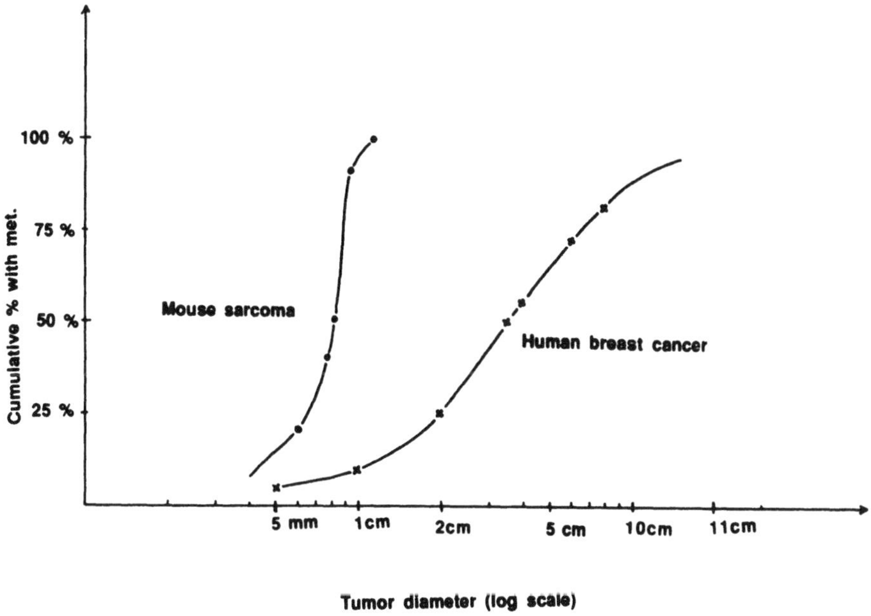

Fig. 3.1. Relationship between the diameter of human breast cancers and the probability of distant metastatic dissemination (*crosses*; from Koscielny et al. 1984). For comparison, on the left, relationship between the diameter of an experimental tumor and probability of distant dissemination (*circles*)

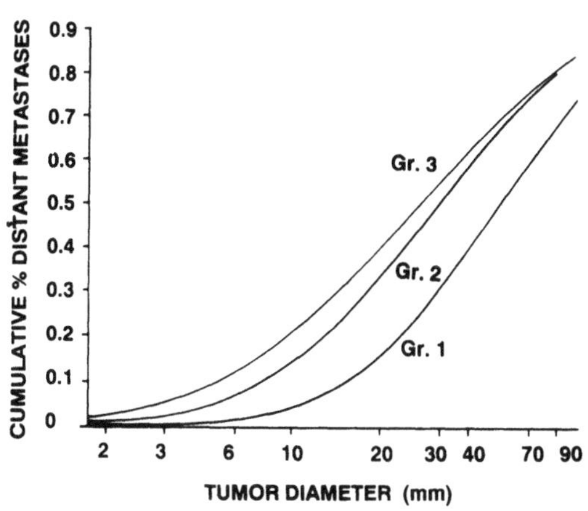

Fig. 3.2. Relationship between the diameter of breast cancers and the probability of metastatic dissemination in patients with histological grade (*Gr.*) 1, 2, or 3 tumors. (From Tubiana and Koscielny 1991)

metastatic spread in high-grade tumors provides quantitative data on the influence of grade on the prognosis. The difference between the three curves is greater for small tumors than for large ones. For large tumors the difference between the subsets with grade 2 or 3 vanishes. Among low-grade tumors, the cumulative probability does not reach 100% even for very large tumor sizes (Tubiana and Koscielny 1991). These data are consistent with the time intervals which have been observed between the treatment of the primary tumor and the clinical emergence of metastases. The delays are equal to 65, 44, and 21 months respectively for grade 1, 2, or 3 tumors confirming that in high-grade tumors, metastases were initiated earlier during the growth of the tumor.

An interesting observation made during the study is that the proportion of grade 1 tumors was higher in small tumors than in large ones while the reverse was observed for grade 3 tumors; these data suggest that, during their growth, tumors progress towards higher grades. In effect, by plotting the proportion of tumors with each of the three grades as a function of tumor size (Fig. 3.3), it can be seen that the percentage of grade 2 tumors is constant, that of grade 3 tumors increases gradually from 20% to 40%, and that of grade 1 tumors decreases from 30% to 12%. This confirms that some tumors with grade 1 progress towards grade 2 during their growth, while some grade 2 tumors progress to grade 3. The constancy in the proportion of grade 2 tumors is compatible with an equality between the inflow from grade 1 to grade 2 and the outflow from grade 2 to grade 3. This observation is in keeping with a slow but constant rate of progression of breast tumors during their growth (Tubiana and Koscielny 1991). The gradual increase in a tumor's malignant potential concurs with the concept of tumor progression, which postulates that tumors evolve from "bad to worse" (Tubiana 1986).

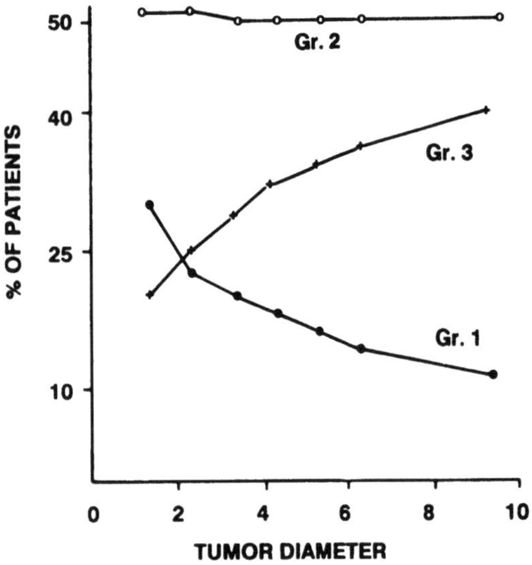

Fig. 3.3. Proportions of breast tumors with histological grade (*Gr.*) 1, 2, or 3 as a function of the diameter of the primary tumor. (From TUBIANA and KOSCIELNY 1991)

These data show that an early diagnosis has the advantage of detecting tumors that are not only smaller, but also, on average, of lower grades. This conclusion is supported by the data recently reported by TABAR et al. (1992). These authors compared tumors detected by screening with those of a control group. They found that tumors in the control group had higher malignancy grades than did incident tumors in the group invited to screening, i.e., advancing the time of diagnosis changed the grade distribution. These observations can be explained by the heterogeneity observed within human breast tumors, more rapid proliferation of the more malignant part would lead to a change in the tumor grade with time (MEYER and WITTLIFF 1991; TUBIANA 1986; TUBIANA and KOSCIELNY 1991).

3.2.1 The Pattern of Axillary Lymph Node Involvement

Axillary lymph node involvement is probably the best prognostic indicator in patients with breast carcinoma and is related to a considerable increase in the excess mortality rate during each follow-up period. Since distant metastases are the most frequent cause of death, the invasion of axillary nodes should be strongly correlated with the probability of distant hematogenous dissemination. However, the significance of the presence of a given number of involved axillary lymph nodes is probably different in a patient with a larger tumor of 5 cm in diameter than with a small tumor of 0.5 cm in diameter, and this difference deserved further investigation.

Previous data suggested that axillary lymph nodes are more frequently involved when the primary breast tumor is large than when it is small (CARTER et al. 1989; HANDLEY 1972). Other data showed that the likelihood of axillary node invasion is influenced by the histologic type of the cancer (PONTEN 1990). However, in order to fully assess the prognostic significance of the number of involved lymph nodes, the relationship between the primary tumor size and the probability of lymph node involvement had to be quantitatively studied in a large series of patients. We carried out this investigation on about 3000 patients in whom the size of the primary tumor and the number of involved lymph nodes had been prospectively measured on the surgical specimen. We found that the proportion of patients without lymph node involvement diminishes rapidly as a function of tumor size, and the proportion of patients with four or more involved nodes increases markedly (Fig. 3.4).

These observations are consistent with a model assuming the existence of a threshold volume for nodal invasion and gradual axillary node involvement during tumor growth (KOSCIELNY et al. 1989). The data support a model in which there is continuous progression from no lymph node involvement to involvement of one lymph node and subsequently of two lymph nodes and so on. Thus, the constancy in the proportion of patients with one involved lymph node means that the inflow (progression from 0 to 1) is equal to the outflow (progression 1 to 2). A classical statistical method was used to estimate the sizes at which 50% of the tumors have a number of involved lymph nodes equal to or greater than 1 node, 2 nodes and so on. The results are given in Table 3.1 and Fig. 3.4. They strongly suggest an orderly pattern of nodal involvement, which appears, is not a random process. Tumors involving one axillary node early on in their development are, on average, also those for which there is an early invasion of a second node and, subsequently, a third node and so on. Hence, there are tumors with high and low propensity for lymph node involvement. The data correspond to a unimodal distribution of the tumors, from those with the earliest to those with the latest nodal involvement, in clear contradiction with the model of SLACK et al. (1969) in which there are two subgroups of breast tumors. On the basis of these data, the prognostic significance of the number of in-

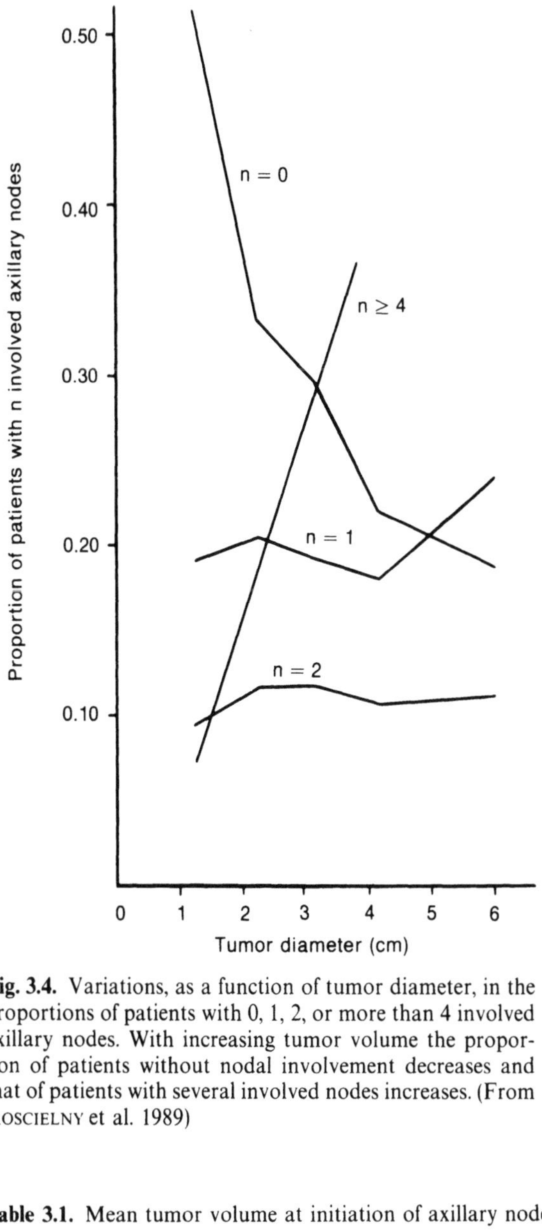

Fig. 3.4. Variations, as a function of tumor diameter, in the proportions of patients with 0, 1, 2, or more than 4 involved axillary nodes. With increasing tumor volume the proportion of patients without nodal involvement decreases and that of patients with several involved nodes increases. (From KOSCIELNY et al. 1989)

volved lymph nodes can be, in clinical practice, increased by taking into account the tumor's size (TUBIANA and KOSCIELNY 1991).

The orderly pattern of nodal involvement makes it possible to calculate the tumor size at invasion of the first axillary node in each subset of patients. Once the size of the tumor at initiation of distant metastasis and at invasion of the first lymph node was known, it was possible to show that a strong and highly significant correlation exists between these two sizes.

As a consequence of this study, the prognostic significance of axillary lymph node involvement can be more adequately interpreted and assessed. Intuitively, clinicians knew that the prognostic significance of a given number of involved lymph nodes was not the same for small and large tumors, but this concept was not quantified and could not be used in prognostic assessment. The relationship between the sizes of the tumor at first axillary node invasion and at distant dissemination makes it possible to compute the proportion of patients with occult metastases as a function of grade and number of involved lymph nodes for various tumor sizes. A good agreement was found between the values calculated with this method and the observed ones. Results are given in Table 3.2.

The present results also show that, on average, during tumor progression the capacity for lymphatic spread is acquired much earlier than the capacity for hematogenous spread (TUBIANA and KOSCIELNY 1991). Thus, the assumption that all patients with involved axillary nodes are at high risk of distant metastasis is overpessimistic. As can

Table 3.1. Mean tumor volume at initiation of axillary node involvement (from KOSCIELNY et al. 1989)

No. of nodes	All patients (n = 2408)			Outer quadrants (n = 1880)		Inner quadrants (n = 926)	
	Mean volume (ml)	Corresponding diameter (cm)	95% CI (ml)	Mean volume (ml)	Corresponding diameter (cm)	Mean volume (ml)	Corresponding diameter (cm)
0 < 1	1.21	1.32	0.97– 1.5	1.15	1.30	1.36	1.37
1 < 2	12.3	2.86	10.1 – 14.9	11.2	2.76	15.7	3.11
2 < 3	48.7	4.53	37.1 – 63.7	43.9	4.38	58.1	4.80
3 < 4	129	6.27	91.8 – 181	115	6.03	156	6.67
4 < 5	243	7.74	164 – 358	220	7.48	323	8.51
5 < 6	531	10	337 – 831	489	9.77	631	10.64
6 < 7	916	12	555 –1500	904	12	1050	12.6

95% CI, 95% confidence intervals of the mean

Table 3.2. Probability of metastatic dissemination as a function of histological grade and number of involved axillary nodes in patients with operable breast cancers of 1 or 2 cm in diameter (from TUBIANA and KOSCIELNY 1991)

Number of axillary nodes	Tumor diameter (cm)			
	1		2	
	Grade 1 (%)	Grades 2 + 3 (%)	Grade 1 (%)	Grades 2 + 3 (%)
0	4	12	8	19
1–3	11	36	17	44
4–9	16	51	24	59
≥10	19	58	29	67

be seen in Table 3.2 for low-grade tumors of 1 cm in diameter, the probability of distant spread remains small in patients with a small number of involved lymph nodes, while it is about twice as large in high-grade tumors of 2 cm in diameter without lymph node involvement. Even for low-grade tumors without lymph node involvement, the probability of metastatic dissemination becomes higher than 15% when their diameter is larger than 3 cm. If the boundary above which adjuvant chemotherapy is justified is put at a probability of distant spread of about 15%, some patients with a small number of involved lymph nodes will be in the no adjuvant chemotherapy group, while a sizeable proportion of patients without lymph node involvement will be in the adjuvant treatment group, in particular all patients with tumors of a diameter equal to or larger than 4 cm (TUBIANA and KOSCIELNY 1991). These predictions are consistent with the data of TABAR et al. (1992) which show that for small tumors of about 1 cm in diameter the probability of distant dissemination remains small, even when axillary nodes are involved.

Another problem investigated was the influence on nodal involvement of the location of the tumor in the breast. It has long been known that patients with inner quadrant tumors have a much higher probability of the internal mammary chain (IMC) involvement than patients with outer quadrant tumors (LACOUR et al. 1976). The proportion of lymph that takes the medial route is somewhat larger in the central and medial part of the breast compared to the lateral (KAMBY et al. 1991). The median volumes of the tumor at the initiation of the 1st, 2nd, etc. axillary nodes were calculated according to the method described above for subgroups of patients with tumor located in the inner or outer quadrants of the breast. The results are given in Table 3.1. Patients with outer quadrant tumors have earlier axillary node invasion. Tumor volumes at the invasion of the first axillary node are approximately 1.5 times larger in patients with a tumor located in the inner quadrants than in those with tumors located in the outer quadrants. This observation remains valid for the second and third axillary node and is consistent with what is known about the lymphatic pathways of the various quadrants of the breast. Conversely, for tumors located in the inner or the outer quadrants, the median size at first metastatic dissemination is not statistically different in the two subgroups, and if anything, is slightly smaller for the inner quadrant tumors (KOSCIELNY et al. 1989).

The discrepancy demonstrates that the correlation between node involvement and distant spread is not causal. Contrary to what has sometimes been assumed, distant dissemination is not a two-step process in most patients. Axillary involvement is a good index of the propensity of tumor cells to acquire the capacity for hematogenous spread, but it is not the cause of this spread. This conclusion is consistent with the concept developed by FISHER (1980). CARTER et al. (1989) observed a correlation between breast tumor size and the percentage of positive axillary nodes; they did not attempt to model their data, but they also suggested that nodal status reflected the ability of the tumor to spread. Furthermore, it is noteworthy that locoregional recurrence rates are much higher in patients with nodal involvement and are correlated with the number of invaded nodes (TUBIANA and SARRAZIN 1987). Hence lymphatic spread is also a pointer of tumor cell migration and seeding into surrounding tissues. KAMBY et al. (1991) reported a higher incidence of pleural and mediastinal recurrences in patients with inner quadrant tumors.

The relationship between the size of primary tumor and the proportion of patients with IMC involvement was established for the 646 patients with a tumor located in the inner quadrants who had undergone a dissection of this chain in controlled studies (TUBIANA and KOSCIELNY 1991). The median tumor volume at the initiation of the first internal mammary nodes was 243 ml (confidence interval, CI: 117–506), and the second node, 2031 ml (CI: 699–5900), the corresponding diameters being 7.9 cm and 15.8 cm respectively. Thus in 50% of patients, the volume of the primary tumor with involvement of the internal mammary nodes is approximately 100 times larger than the corresponding value for the axillary nodes. The average number of invaded axillary nodes is slightly greater than five when the first internal mammary node is invaded. The ratios between the volumes of the primary tumor at the initiation of the first and second nodes are similar for axillary and internal mammary nodes. Moreover, the slope of the curve relating the proportion of nodal involvement to the size of the tumor is identical for the two lymphatic areas.

Among patients with tumors located in the inner quadrants, there is a much higher propensity for axillary node involvement in patients with invaded internal mammary nodes than in patients without internal mammary invasion; only 9% of the patients with an invaded IMC are without axillary involvement compared to 32% without axillary involvement when the IMC is not involved. Thus there is a highly significant correlation between the propensity for axillary invasions and internal mammary node invasions. This confirms that the size of the tumor at first invasion of axillary nodes is a good index of the tumor's capacity to migrate and to seed in other tissues. The proportion of patients with involvement of the IMC and without distant metastasis is slightly higher for small tumors (of less than 2 cm in diameter) than for larger tumors. An involvement of the IMC was found in 18% of the 152 patients with a breast cancer of less than 2 cm in diameter, located anywhere in the breast; in patients with IMC involvement following a surgical dissection of IMC, the long-term metastasis-free survival was 70%. Only in those patients who represent about 13% of all patients with tumors of less than 2 cm in diameter is treatment of the IMC potentially useful. In 717 patients with tumor larger than 2 cm, the proportion of IMC involvement was 33% and the long-term metastasis free survival was 31%. Therefore, only 10% of patients with tumor larger than 2 cm could benefit for IMC treatment. These proportions are, of course, greater in patients with medial tumors than in patients with tumors located in the outer quadrants. Furthermore, the advantage of postoperative RT is not limited to the control of IMC. These predictions are consistent with the results of the IMC treatment reported by our group and by the other studies (ARRIAGADA et al. 1988; AUQUIER et al. 1992; TUBIANA et al. 1986) (see below).

3.3 Radiotherapeutic Studies

These studies on the natural history of breast cancer can help to interpret the results of postoperative RT; those studies carried out in Villejuif are particularly helpful as they attempt to identify the subgroup in which RT is effective.

In 1963, an international group initiated a cooperative study with Villejuif acting as the coordinating center. The aim of this trial was to find out whether the theoretical advantages of internal mammary dissection resulted in an increased survival rate. The 5-year results of 1580 breast cancer cases published by LACOUR et al. (1976) showed that an extended mastectomy, including internal mammary dissection, improved the results in only one small subgroup, namely, patients with T1 or T2 tumors in the medial quadrants and histologically positive axillary lymph nodes. This subset represented only 13% of the total group of patients, but within it, 31% of the patients had internal mammary node involvement, an incidence that was much higher than in other T1 and T2 subgroups. The 10-year published results showed that the overall comparison did not demonstrate increased survival in the arm treated with internal mammary dissection. However, there were major differences between cooperative centers in the number of axillary nodes examined – and therefore in the relative proportion of node-negative and node-positive patients – and in the prognostic value of axillary involvement. Hence, it was of interest to study the results of each center separately.

From 1963 to 1967, 243 patients were included in Villejuif as a part of this international trial. All patients have been followed for at least 15 years. The difference in survival between extended mastectomy or radical mastectomy varies with the site of the breast tumor (medial or lateral) and the lymph node involvement. A multivariate analysis showed that for patients with positive axillary nodes and medial tumors, the relative risk of death is 2.1 times higher in patients treated by radical mastectomy without internal mammary dissection than in patients treated by extended mastectomy (15-year survival rate: 28% versus 53%, $p = 0.01$). Thus, despite the relatively small number of cases, these surgical data strongly suggest that treatment of the IMC is beneficial for the small subset of patients with inner quadrant tumors and positive axillary nodes (LACOUR et al. 1987). This conclusion is supported by the results obtained in Villejuif for postoperative RT of the IMC, which were previously reported (SARRAZIN et al. 1982a, b; TUBIANA and SARRAZIN 1980; TUBIANA et al. 1986).

In this study, four groups of approximately 90 patients with involved axillary nodes were compared. Patients in group one were included in the IMC trial, but randomized to the arm treated by radical mastectomy (without IMC dissection). These patients did not receive postoperative RT. Patients in group two were included in the trial and randomized to the group treated by extended mastectomy (radical mastectomy plus internal mammmary chain dissection). No postoperative RT was performed. Patients in group three were not included in the trial and treated in Villejuif from 1958 to 1967. The surgical procedure was the same as that in group one – that is radical mastectomy – but surgery was followed by postoperative RT. Patients in group four were not included in the trial and treated as in group two by extended mastectomy, but followed by postoperative RT.

Adjuvant chemotherapy was not used in any of these patients. In the four groups of patients, radiotherapeutic castration was performed in premenopausal patients. It was statistically verified that these groups did not differ in the size of the primary tumor, the histologic type of cancer, nor the histologic grade. Adjustments were carried out for age and the number of metastasis-bearing lymph nodes.

When the groups are considered irrespective of the location of the tumor, no significant difference is observed for overall or relapse-free survival. When the location of the tumor is taken into account, no difference is observed for patients with tumors of the outer quadrants. However, for patients with tumors of the inner quadrants, the overall or relapse-free survival is significantly lower for the group treated by radical mastectomy alone than for the three other groups in which the IMC had been treated either by surgical dissection or RT. The difference remains significant after adjustment for age and the number of metastasis-bearing lymph nodes (log-rank test, $p < 0.05$).

Furthermore, the cumulative incidence of distant metastases is similar for tumors of the outer quadrants in the four therapeutic groups, whereas for tumors of the inner quadrants, the cumulative incidence is significantly higher in the group treated by radical mastectomy without postoperative RT than in the three other groups. Thus, similar results are obtained by treatment of the IMC either by RT or surgery (TUBIANA et al. 1986). No increase in the incidence of pleural or pulmonary metastases was observed in patients with tumors of the inner quadrants treated by radical mastectomy without postoperative RT or IMC dissection. Thus, the improvement in survival is due to a decrease in the incidence of blood-borne metastases. These data seem to indicate that the internal mammary nodes, when involved, are a likely nidus for further distant dissemination.

Why is there a difference between recurrence in the axilla and in the IMC? This is probably because axillary recurrences are generally detected early, whereas IMC recurrences are much more difficult to detect and are probably treated only when they reach a much larger size – above the threshold size for distant dissemination. In effect, the risk involved in a local recurrence varies with the type of tumors and depends upon at least two factors: (a) the detectability of the local recurrence, and (b) the relationship between the size of the primary tumor and the probability of metastatic dissemination.

However, these conclusions were based on a relatively limited number of patients. That is why we undertook a retrospective analysis to evaluate the long-term effects of the treatment of the IMC on a larger series of patients. Included in the study were all women younger than 70 years of age treated at the Institut Gustave-Roussy for operable unilateral primary infiltrating adenocarcinoma of the breast between 1958 and 1978 who had the following: UICC stages M0, T1a, T2a, or T3a, N0 or N1; tumors less than 7 cm in greatest diameter; tumors not completely fixed to the pectoral muscle; and histologically involved axillary lymph nodes. All the 1195 eligible patients were treated by mastectomy with an axillary dissection (Halsted or Patey mastectomy). The IMC treatment was systematically performed for all patients during this period of 21 years. When the results of the frozen section examination of the axillary lymph nodes were positive, IMC dissection and irradiation of this chain were systematically undertaken, regardless of the site of the tumor, except in cases of major medical contraindications or patient refusal. When the results of the frozen section were negative, but those of the definitive examination positive, the IMC was only treated by RT. When only microinvasion of axillary lymph nodes was found, the IMC was not treated at all (ARRIAGADA et al. 1988).

During that period, only 135 patients had no IMC treatment. Most of them had been included in the previously described therapeutic trials comparing postoperative treatment with no treatment. Thus the aim of this analysis was to compare the 135 patients with IMC treatment to the other 1060 patients (ARRIAGADA et al. 1988). The results confirmed that the risk of death was decreased when the IMC was treated by RT and/or surgery (Fig. 3.5). The effect was similar for each treatment modality and for the combination of the two modalities. The beneficial effect of IMC treatment on the total population was mainly observed in these patients with medial tumors ($p = 0.01$); treatment of the IMC did not decrease the risk of death or metastasis for patients with lateral tumors (ARRIAGADA et al. 1988). A multivariate analysis was performed, taking into account the age of patients at diagnosis, the largest diameter of the tumors, the histoprognostic grading (CONTESSO et al. 1987), the number of positive axillary nodes, and the location of the tumor in the breast (LE et al. 1990). Quantitative interaction tests were used to determine whether the effects of IMC treatment on each type of malignant event were significantly different for patients with a lateral tumor compared with those

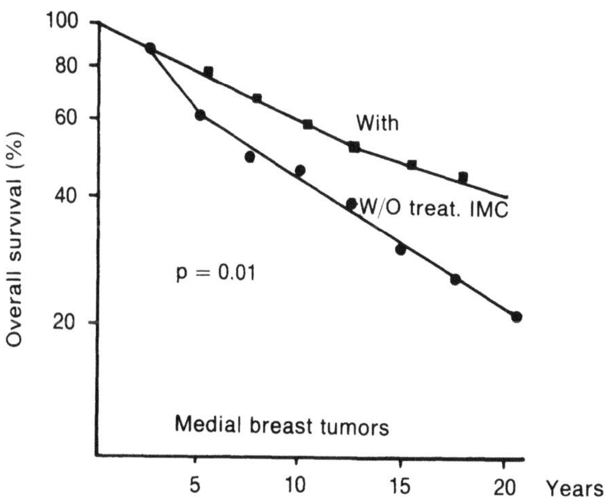

Fig. 3.5. Computed overall survival for patients with medial breast tumors with or without (*W/O*) treatment of the internal mammary chain (*IMC*) after adjustment for tumor size, histological grade, and number of involved lymph nodes (ARRIAGADA et al. 1988)

with a medial tumor. It was found that the effects of this treatment on the relative risks of distant metastases and of secondary breast cancer were not the same for the patients with a medial tumor as for those with a lateral tumor. For the untreated patients with a medial tumor, the risks of distant metastases and second breast cancer were 1.6 ($p = 0.02$) and 2.9 ($p = 0.02$), respectively, compared with the treated patients. Conversely, no difference was observed between the two treatment groups for women with lateral tumors. Thus, IMC treatment improved the long-term survival rate in patients with a medial tumor and positive axillary lymph nodes essentially by decreasing the risk of developing distant metastases (mainly brain, distant lymph nodes, multiple simultaneous metastases) and a secondary breast cancer (LE et al. 1990).

The lower incidence of secondary contralateral breast cancer in patients with medial tumors is remarkable since it was previously suspected that RT could increase this incidence due to contralateral breast irradiation by scattered radiation (STORM and JENSEN 1986). A possible explanation of this unexpected result is the propagation of malignant cells through the retrosternal lymphatic system when the mammary chain is not treated by surgery or RT (LE et al. 1990). Indeed, in the general population lymphatic connections between the two lateral lymphatic trunks in the first costal interspace were found in 30%–60% of cases.

The decrease in the incidence of remote metastases supported our previous findings, but was nevertheless open to criticism because the number of patients without IMC treatment was small and because IMC treatment was not allocated at random. However, three other studies have also shown a beneficial effect of postoperative RT, in particular in patients with medial tumors.

In a retrospective but informative study, Fletcher compared the 10-year survival rates for patients treated with radical mastectomy alone, radical mastectomy followed by postoperative peripheral lymphatic irradiation, or 40 Gy of preoperative irradiation followed by radical mastectomy (FLETCHER 1980; FLETCHER and MONTAGUE 1978). For those patients with histologically positive axillary lymph nodes, the 5-year survival rate is significantly higher for patients having received postoperative irradiation. This comparison is instructive because the patients treated by surgery were essentially only patients with tumors of the outer quadrants, whereas the patients treated by postoperative RT were essentially patients with tumors of the medial quadrants whose prognosis is normally poorer. This is probably due to the frequent involvement of the IMC.

In the Oslo randomized trial only a small subgroup of 38 node-positive patients with the medial and central tumors received postoperative cobalt therapy: their 10-year survival rate was higher than that of the 34 nonirradiated controls, but the difference was not statistically significant (Host and Brennhovd 1986).

In the Stockholm randomized trial, the 58 patients with inner quadrant tumors treated by postoperative RT had a higher 5-year survival rate than the 70 unirradiated patients, but the difference was not significant. In this study, most of the patients treated by postoperative RT received a relatively low dose to the IMC for technical reasons (Strender et al. 1981; Wallgren et al. 1986). A more recent analysis showed a significant beneficial effect of postoperative RT on the cumulative frequency of distant metastases of up to 10 years in patients with histologically involved axillary nodes (Einhorn 1991; Rutqvist et al. 1989).

A report from Fisher et al. (1985a, b) also analyzed the role of postoperative RT for the subset of patients with medial and central tumors and clinically involved axillary nodes (N1b). In this study, a subgroup of 85 patients treated by radical mastectomy alone was compared with 95 patients with similar characteristics treated by simple mastectomy plus RT. There was a slight (but nonsignificant) survival advantage for the radical mastectomy group. Two reasons may explain these divergent results: First, the technique of treatment of the axillary lymph nodes was not the same in the two groups of patients: axillary nodes were removed by surgery in the first group, and treated only by irradiation in the second. Further studies are needed to determine whether surgery and the type of RT used have a similar effect on clinically involved axillary nodes. Thus, the small advantage resulting from IMC RT is likely to be overshadowed by a lesser effectiveness in the treatment of the axilla. Second, in patients with histologically involved axillary nodes, the probability of distant dissemination is greater when the nodes are clinically positive than when they are not clinically involved. For example, among the 672 operable node-positive patients treated at the Institut Gustave-Roussy between 1954 and 1967 whose clinical axillary node status was recorded, the relative risk of distant metastasis was twofold higher in the 332 patients with clinically involved axillary nodes than in the 340 patients in whom the axillary nodes were pathologically invaded but not clinically suspicious ($p = 10^{-4}$) (Arriagada et al. 1988). This observation is in keeping with the data on the natural history of breast cancer, since the clinically positive nodes are larger than the clinically negative histologically involved nodes (Tubiana 1986). Thus, the proportion of patients with subclinical metastases at the time of initial treatment was probably higher in the first subset of patients than the second, which is consistent with several published reports. Therefore, the impact of locoregional treatment on survival is likely to be smaller as discussed previously (Tubiana et al. 1986).

A major criticism that can be made of all these studies is that in each trial the number of patients is relatively small. We therefore thought that a meta-analysis of all relevant trials would be useful. Only trials in which the IMC was adequately irradiated (dose 45 Gy) were considered. The NSABP trial was not included because in the mastectomy plus RT trial the axillary nodes were treated by RT only even when clinically involved, while in the other arm they were treated by surgical resection (Fisher et al. 1981). Similarly, we had to exclude the Villejuif trial in which treatment of the IMC differed: some patients were treated by surgery, some by surgery plus RT, and others by RT alone (Arriagada et al. 1988; Sarrazin et al. 1982b; Tubiana et al. 1986).

Only the two Oslo and Stockholm randomized trials fulfilled all the criteria. A meta-analysis was recently carried out with the help of Villejuif group, which compared postoperative megavoltage RT versus surgery alone. This joint analysis of long-term results (13–16 years of follow-up) evidenced a significant 37% relative reduction in distant metastasis with radiation among node-positive patients ($p = 0.01$) (Auquier et al. 1992). It is noteworthy that the effect was identical in both centers despite some differences in the therapeutic schedule. The reduction in the incidence of metastasis was much larger in the medial or central tumors than in the lateral ones. However, the difference between inner quadrant or outer quadrant tumors was not statistically significant, probably because of an insufficient number of patients (1185 patients with breast cancer but only 395 node-positive patients). The effect of RT on survival among node-positive patients was less pronounced than on distant metastasis. This was probably due to a dilution of the treatment effect from a significant number of intercurrent deaths and a rather long survival of patients after detection of their metastases. This possible beneficial effect on survival corresponded to a 22% relative reduction of deaths, which was only marginally significant ($p = 0.06$). No significant benefit was observed among node-negative patients with radiation for metastasis-free survival or overall survival (AUQUIER et al. 1992).

In node-positive patients the reduction in the incidence of metastases was related to tumor size and was greatest among patients with small tumors (less than 2 cm in diameter); the effect observed in tumors ranging from 2 cm to 5 cm in diameter was smaller and no effect, either beneficial or detrimental, was observed in tumors larger than 5 cm in diameter (AUQUIER et al. 1992). These results are consistent with the studies on the natural history of breast cancer, which show that the likelihood of subclinical distant metastasis at the time of initial treatment is lower in patients with small tumors and it is in these patients that a beneficial effect can be expected. Moreover, these data further confirm the observation made in the study of the natural history of breast cancer (TUBIANA and KOSCIELNY 1991), which shows that the mean tumor size at the time of distant dissemination is markedly larger than the mean size at the time of first axillary involvement

In summary, the data of the meta-analysis of the Stockholm and Oslo trials (AUQUIER et al. 1992) and of the Villejuif studies confirm that the control of local residual disease by postoperative RT can reduce the incidence of distant metastases and leave little doubt about the usefulness of postoperative RT. The divergent results that are reported by some other groups may be explained by the technique of treatment or of irradiation. The data produced by studies in which the IMC was properly irradiated strongly suggest that irradiation of this region of considerable value, at least in patients with medial moderate-sized breast tumors. However, several questions are still open to discussion. The first is the size of the target volume. Should it comprise both the axillary and the IMC chains or is it sufficient to irradiate the IMC when the axillary nodes have been properly resected?

Another question is related to chemotherapy. All the above data were obtained in patients who did not receive adjuvant chemotherapy and a major problem is whether postoperative RT remains useful in patients who are administered adjuvant chemotherapy.

There are no direct data regarding the long-term impact of postoperative RT in patients receiving adjuvant chemotherapy. However, the relative efficacy of RT and chemotherapy on the rate of locoregional recurrence has been assessed in several studies. The controlled clinical trials on adjuvant chemotherapy have shown that the cyclophosphamide, methotrexate, 5-fluorouracil (CMF) regimen reduces the incidence of distant metastases in premenopausal women with breast cancer by approximately 30%. An analysis with a simulation mathematical model of the metastasis appearance curve in treated and in controlled patients has shown that the maximum number of cells in the occult metastases controlled by the chemotherapy is approximately 10^6 (GUIGUET et al. 1986). Assuming that the proportion of clonogenic cells is 10^{-3}, it follows that the proportion of surviving tumor cells after completion of 6 cycles of CMF is 10^{-3} (GUIGUET et al. 1986). This corresponds to a radiation dose equal to $10D_{50}$ (approximately 25 Gy). This estimation is consistent with the data on the impact of chemotherapy on the control of residual tumor after surgery. FISHER et al. (1985a, b) reported that a local recurrence occurred in 36% of the patients with axillary lymph node involvement who were treated by conservative surgery plus chemotherapy, whereas in the arm treated by conservative surgery plus chemotherapy plus RT, this incidence was much lower, approximately equal to 2%.

Nevertheless, even though adjuvant chemotherapy after RT has been shown to further reduce local recurrence, its effectiveness is limited. In the Danish Breast Cancer controlled trials, the incidence of locoregional recurrence was slightly, but not significantly, lower in the arm treated by RT plus adjuvant chemotherapy than in the arm treated by RT alone (7% versus 12% in premenopausal patients, 12% versus 17% in postmenopausal patients) (OVERGAARD et al. 1988). In another Danish trial the local recurrence rate was significantly lower in patients treated by RT plus CMF than in those treated by chemotherapy alone (7% versus 24% in premenopausal patients, 5% versus 25% in postmenopausal patients) (OVERGAARD et al. 1988). This study has recently been updated (OVERGAARD et al. 1991). With a 7-year follow-up the actuarial rate of locoregional recurrence was 9% in 1992 premenopausal patients treated by postoperative RT plus chemotherapy by CMF and 32% in patients treated by CMF alone. Moreover, the overall survival rate at 7 years was significantly higher in patients treated by RT plus CMF than in those treated by CMF alone (63% versus 56%). Among 1994 post-menopausal patients three arms were compared: postoperative RT plus tamoxifen, tamoxifen alone, and tamoxifen plus CMF. At 7 years the actuarial locoregional recurrence rate was significantly lower in irradiated patients (9% versus 39% and 31%). However, the 7-year survival rate was identical in patients treated by RT plus tamoxifen or tamoxifen plus CMF and was slightly, but not significantly, lower in patients treated by tamoxifen alone (58% versus 52%). This study (OVERGAARD et al. 1991) indicates that optimal treatment of high-risk breast cancer can only be achieved if both locoregional and systemic tumor control is aimed for.

The second Stockholm trial (EINHORN 1991; RUTQVIST et al. 1989) compared 1020 patients with breast cancer chemotherapy with CMF versus postoperative RT. The incidence of local recurrence was lower in the group treated with RT; the overall survival was higher in the CMF arm among premenopausal patients, but higher in the postoperative RT arm among postmenopausal patients (EINHORN 1991).

Thus adjuvant chemotherapy and postoperative RT do not compete but are complementary for node-positive patients and the main problem is scheduling the two modalities. However, each treatment modality, in particular RT and chemotherapy, is associated with some early or late toxicity and therefore should be delivered only when its beneficial effect outweighs its possible detrimental consequences. Thus the late effects of RT alone or combined with chemotherapy should be carefully evaluated. Their impact on long-term survival has recently been a matter of debate (LEVITT and FLETCHER 1991), and can only be assessed in large series of patients who have been properly irradiated and followed-up for at least 15 years.

Another matter of debate is the radioresponsiveness and the chemosensitivity of local recurrences. In keeping with the concept of tumor progression (CLARKE et al. 1989; TUBIANA 1986; TUBIANA and KOSCIELNY 1991), some authors fear that relapses are more malignant than the primary tumor (LEIBEL et al. 1991a, b; SUIT and DUBOIS 1991; TUBIANA 1986). This view is still debated; if confirmed, it should constitute further reasons to avoid local recurrences.

3.4 Conclusion

Several data point out that locoregional residual neoplastic tissue is associated with a decrease in overall survival; however, this deficit is relatively small and is only observed in series of patients who have been followed-up for 15–20 years.

The Villejuif studies show that the benefit associated with treatment of the IMC is observed in node-positive patients with relatively small tumors located in the medial quadrants of the breast. This benefit was not observed in series in whom the dose of postoperative irradiation was insufficient or in whom the IMC was not properly irradiated. This beneficial effect of postoperative RT on metastasis-free survival was confirmed by a recent meta-analysis of the Oslo and Stockholm trials.

RT is more effective for the control of residual locoregional tumor than adjuvant chemotherapy. The combination of adjuvant chemotherapy and postoperative RT is well-tolerated and is justified when the likelihood of local residual neoplastic tissue and of occult distant metastases is significant.

References

Anderson P, Dische S (1981) Local tumor control and the subsequent incidence of distant metastatic disease. Int J Radiat Oncol Biol Phys 7: 1645–1648

Arriagada R, Mouriesse H, Sarrazin D et al (1986) Radiotherapy alone in breast cancer. I. Analysis of tumor parameters, tumor dose and local control: the experience of the Gustave-Roussy Institute and the Margaret Hospital. Int J Radiat Oncol Biol Phys 11: 1751–1757

Arriagada R, Le MG, Mouriesse H et al (1988) Long-term effect of internal mammary chain treatment: results of a multivariate analysis of 1195 patients with operable breast cancer and positive axillary nodes. Radiother Oncol 11: 213–222

Atkins H, Hayward JL, Klugman DJ, Wayte AB (1972) Treatment of early breast cancer: a report after ten years of a clinical trial. BMJ 2: 423–429

Atkinson EN, Brown BW, Montague ED (1986) Tumor volume, nodal status and metastasis in breast cancer women. J Nat Cancer Inst 76: 171–178

Auquier A, Rutqvist LE, Host H, Rotstein S, Arriagada R (1992) Post-mastectomy megavoltage radiotherapy: the Oslo and Stockholm trials. Eur J Cancer 28: 433–437

Carter CL, Allen C, Herson DE (1989) Relation of tumor size, lymph node status and survival in 24740 breast cancer cases. Cancer 63: 181–187

Clarke DH, Le MG, Sarrazin D et al (1985) Analysis of locoregional relapses in patients with early breast cancers treated by excision and radiotherapy: experience of the Institut Gustave-Roussy. Int J Radiat Oncol Biol Phys 11: 137–145

Clarke R, Brunner N, Thompson EW et al (1989) Progression of human breast cancer cells from hormonal dependent to independent growth both in vitro and in vivo. Proc Nat Acad Sci USA 86: 3649–3653

Contesso G, Mouriesse H, Friedman S et al (1987) The importance of histologic grade in long-term prognosis of breast cancer: a study of 1,010 patients, uniformly treated at the Institut Gustave-Roussy. J Clin Oncol 5: 1378–1386

Cuzick J, Stewart H, Peto R et al (1987) Overview of randomized trials of postoperative adjuvant radiotherapy in breast cancer. Cancer Treat Rep 71: 15–30

Einhorn J (1991) Locoregional therapy in breast cancer: the Stockholm trials – Update. Int J Radiat Oncol 21 [Suppl]: 107–108

Fisher B (1980) Laboratory and clinical research in breast cancer. A personal adventure. Cancer Res 40: 3863–3874

Fisher B, Wolmark N, Redmond C et al (1981) Findings from NSABP protocol no. B-04: comparison of radical mastectomy with alternative treatments. II. The clinical and biologic significance of medial-central breast cancers. Cancer 48: 1863–1872

Fisher B, Bauer M, Margolese R et al (1985a) Five-year results of a randomized clinical trial comparing total mastectomy and segmental mastectomy with or without radiation in the treatment of breast cancer. N Engl J Med 312: 665–673

Fisher B, Redmond C, Fisher E et al (1985b) Ten-year results of a randomized clinical trial comparing radical mastectomy and total mastectomy with or without radiation. N Engl J Med 312: 674–681

Fisher B, Anderson S, Fisher ER et al (1991) Significance of ipsilateral breast tumour recurrence after lumpectomy. Lancet 338: 327–331

Fletcher GH (1980) Textbook of radiotherapy, 3rd edn. Lea and Febiger, Philadelphia, pp 527–571

Fletcher GH, Montague ED (1978) Does adequate irradiation of the internal mammary chain and supraclavicular nodes improve survival rates? Int J Radiat Oncol Biol Phys 4: 481–492

Fuks Z, Leibel SA, Wallner KE et al (1991) The effect of local control on metastatic dissemination in carcinoma of the prostate: long term results in patients treated with I 125 implantation. Int J Radiat Oncol 21: 537–547

Guiguet M, Koscielny S, Valleron AJ, Tubiana M (1986) Estimation par un modèle de simulation de la taille maximale des nodules métastatiques guéris par une thérapie adjuvante. In: Jacquillat C (ed) Congress on neo-adjuvant chemotherapy, vol 137. John Libbey Eurotext, Paris, pp 825–833

Handley RS (1972) Observations and thoughts on cancer of the breast. Proc R Soc Med 65: 437–444

Hayward J, Caleffi M (1987) The significance of local control in the primary treatment of breast cancer. Arch Surg 122: 1244–1247

Helle PA, Treurmet-Donker AD, Van Putten WLJ (1984) Effect of post-operative radiotherapy on local and regional recurrence rate and survival in mammary carcinoma. An intercomparison of three different radiotherapy schedules. Proceedings of the Third Meeting European Society Therapeutic Radiology and Oncology, Jerusalem, pp 185

Host H, Brennhovd IO (1986) Post-operative radiotherapy in breast cancer. Long-term results from the Oslo study. Int J Radiat Oncol Biol Phys 12: 727–732

Kamby C, Andersen J, Ejlertsen B et al (1991) Pattern of spread and progression in relation to the characteristics of the primary tumour in human breast cancer. Acta Oncol 30: 301–308

Koscielny S, Tubiana M, Le MG et al (1984) Breast cancer: relationship between the size of the primary tumour and the probability of metastatic dissemination. Br J Cancer 49: 709–715

Koscielny S, Tubiana M, Valleron AJ (1985) A simulation model of the natural history of human breast cancer. Br J Cancer 52: 515–524

Koscielny S, Le MG, Tubiana M (1989) The natural history of breast cancer: the relationship between involvement of axillary lymph nodes and the initiation of distant metastases. Br J Cancer 59: 775–782

Kurtz JM, Amalric R, Brandone H et al (1991) How important is adequate radiotherapy for the long term results of breast-conserving treatment. Radiother Oncol 20: 84–90

Lacour J, Bucalossi P, Caceres E et al (1976) Radical mastectomy versus radical mastectomy plus internal mammary dissection: five-year results of an international cooperative study. Cancer 37: 206–214

Lacour J, Le MG, Mouriesse H et al (1987) It is useful to remove internal mammary nodes in operable breast cancer patients. Eur J Surg Oncol 13: 309–314

Le MG, Arriagada R, de Vathaire F et al (1990) Can internal mammary chain treatment decrease the risk of death for patients with medial breast cancers and positive axillary nodes. Cancer 66: 2313–2318

Leibel SA, Ling CC, Kutcher GJ et al (1991a) The biological basis for conformal three dimensional radiation therapy. Int J Radiat Oncol 21: 805–811

Leibel SA, Scott CB, Mohinddin M et al (1991b) The effect of locoregional control on distant metastatic dissemination in carcinoma of the head and neck: results of an analysis from the RTOG database. Int J Radiat Oncol 21: 549–556

Levitt SH (1988) Is there a role for post-operative adjuvant radiation in breast cancer? Beautiful hypothesis versus ugly facts. Int J Radiat Oncol 14: 787–796

Levitt SH, Fletcher GH (1991) Trials and tribulations: do clinical trials prove that irradiation increases cardiac and secondary cancer mortality in the breast cancer patient? Int J Radiat Oncol 20: 523–527

Meyer JS, Wittliff JL (1991) Regional heterogeneity in breast carcinoma: thymidine labelling index, steroid hormone receptors. Int J Cancer 47: 213–220

Overgaard M, Christensen JJ, Johansen H et al (1988) Postmastectomy irradiation in high risk breast cancer. Acta Oncol 27: 707–714

Overgaard M, Christensen JJ, Rose C et al (1991) Importance of locoregional tumor control in high-risk breast cancer patients given adjuvant systemic treatment with or without radiotherapy. DB C G protocol 82 and 82c (Abstract)

Ponten J (1990) Natural history of breast cancer. Acta Oncol 29: 325–334

Rose CM, Kaplan WD, Marck A (1977) Lymphoscintigraphy of the internal mammary lymph nodes. Int J Radiat Oncol Biol Phys 2 [suppl. 2]: 102

Rutqvist LE, Cenark B, Glas U et al (1989) Radiotherapy, chemotherapy, tamoxifen as adjuncts to surgery in early breast cancer: a summary of three randomized trials. Int J Radiat Oncol 16: 629–639

Sarrazin D, Le M, Lacour J, Tubiana M (1982a) Die postoperative strahlentherapie beim mammarkarzinom. Die Erkrankungen der weiblichen Brustdrüse. Thieme, Stuttgart, pp 196–201

Sarrazin D, Le M, Mouriesse H et al (1982b) Radiotherapeutic studies on breast cancer at Villejuif. Cancer Bull 34: 242–249

Slack NH, Blumenson LE, Bross IDJ (1969) Therapeutic implications of a mathematical model characterizing the course of breast cancer. Cancer 24: 960–971

Stjernsward J (1974) Decreased survival related to irradiation post-operatively in early operable breast cancer. Lancet 2: 1285–1286

Storm HH, Jensen OM (1986) Risk of contralateral breast cancer in Denmark 1943–80. Br J Cancer 54: 483–492

Stotter A, Atkinson EN, Fairston BA et al (1990) Survival following locoregional recurrence after breast conservation therapy for cancer. Ann Surg 212: 166–172
Strender LE, Wallgran A, Arndt J et al (1981) Adjuvant radiotherapy in operable breast cancer: correlation between dose in internal mammary nodes and prognosis. Int J Radiat Oncol Biol Phys 7: 1319–1325
Suit H, Dubois W (1991) The importance of optimal treatment planning in radiation therapy. Int J Radiat Oncol 21: 1471–1478
Tabar L, Fagerberg G, Day NE et al (1992) Breast cancer treatment and natural history: new insights from results of screening. Lancet 339: 412–414
Tubiana M (1986) The growth and progression of human tumors. Implications for management strategy. Radiother Oncol 6: 167–184
Tubiana M, Koscielny S (1991) Natural history of human breast cancer: recent data and clinical implications. Breast Cancer Res 18: 125–140
Tubiana M, Sarrazin D (1980) A reappraisal of radiotherapy in the treatment of operable breast cancer: The new light on the internal mammary chain role. In: Mouridsen HT, Palshof T (eds) Breast cancer: experimental and clinical aspects. Pergamon, Oxford, pp 243–249
Tubiana M, Sarrazin D (1987) The role of post-operative radiotherapy in breast cancer. In: Ariel JM, Cleary JB (eds) Breast cancer: diagnosis and treatment. McGraw Hill, New York, pp 280–299
Tubiana M, Chauvel P, Renaud A, Malaise EP (1975) Vitesse de croissance et histoire naturelle du cancer du sein. Bull Cancer (Paris) 62: 341–358
Tubiana M, Arriagada R, Sarrazin D (1986) Human cancer natural history, radiation induced immunodepression and post-operative radiation therapy. Int J Radiat Oncol Biol Phys 12: 477–485
Wallgren A, Arner O, Bergstrom J et al (1986) Radiation therapy in operable breast cancer. Results from the Stockholm trial on adjuvant radiotherapy. Int J Radiat Oncol Biol Phys 12: 533–537

4 How Much of the Axilla Should Be Dissected?

Robert T. Osteen

CONTENTS

4.1 Introduction 27
4.2 Axillary Node Status as a Prognostic Indicator and Its Relationship to Other Indicators 27
4.3 Clinical Assessment of Axillary Status 29
4.4 Pathologic Assessment of Axillary Status 29
4.5 Local Recurrence in the Untreated Axilla 30
4.6 Irradiation of the Undissected, Clinical N0 or N1a Axilla 30
4.7 Irradiation of the Undissected, Clinical N1b Axilla 31
4.8 Conservative Breast Surgery and Axillary Dissection with Breast and Axillary Irradiation 31
4.9 Conservative Breast Surgery and Axillary Dissection with Breast Irradiation but No Axillary Irradiation 31
4.10 Effect of Chemotherapy on Axillary Node Recurrence 31
4.11 Carcinoma In Situ and Axillary Lymph Nodes 32
4.12 Complications of Axillary Dissection 32
4.13 Conclusion 33
References 33

4.1 Introduction

The spread of breast cancer from the primary tumor in the breast to regional lymph nodes is an indication of the capacity of cancer cells to implant and grow, as well as a comment on the host–tumor relationship; it also is a potential source of morbidity. Despite the clear impact of axillary nodal metastases on prognosis, there is no evidence that axillary treatments significantly affect survival. Although the possibility of a small therapeutic benefit cannot be excluded by the studies to date, the primary benefits of removing axillary lymph nodes are to gather information on staging and to prevent complications arising from uncontrolled tumor growth in the axilla. Information on axillary staging is vital when the axillary node status is a major determinant of the use of systemic therapy. The need to prevent axillary tumor progression depends on the risk of the event, the morbidity rate incurred if treatment is delayed, and the morbidity of the treatment.

As the use of cytotoxic chemotherapy for all premenopausal patients and the use of tamoxifen for many postmenopausal patients has become widespread, the value of information regarding axillary nodal status has been questioned. Also, the surgical management of the axilla has changed as treatments of the breast have evolved from radical mastectomy to more conservative operations. It seems likely that in the future the extent of axillary node dissection will vary with different circumstances. Currently in the United States, many surgeons recommend no axillary dissection for patients with a small area of ductal carcinoma in situ (DCIS), a low axillary dissection for larger areas of DCIS, and a more extensive dissection for invasive cancers. Further modifications of these indications can be anticipated.

This chapter describes the results obtained from different types of surgical procedures by addressing the following questions. How good is the staging information from the various procedures? How effective is a procedure or policy in preventing axillary recurrence? What is the danger of uncontrolled axillary disease with different treatment policies? What is the morbidity of different axillary treatments?

4.2 Axillary Node Status as a Prognostic Indicator and Its Relationship to Other Indicators

In virtually every report of breast cancer prognosis, the extent of axillary involvement has been an important predictor of systemic metastases and survival. Along with tumor size, lymph node status forms the basis for the accepted TNM staging system. In a recent review of 24 740 breast cancer cases, tumor diameter and lymph node status acted as independent but additive prognostic indicators (Carter et al. 1989). Although there was a linear

Robert T. Osteen, M. D., Associate Professor, Brigham and Women's Hospital, 75 Francis Street, Boston, MA, USA increase in the risk of lymph node positivity with increasing tumor size, patients with the smallest tumors (5 mm or less) still had a 20% risk of having positive axillary lymph nodes. Most studies correlated prognosis with nodal status prior to chemotherapy, but McCready et al. (1989) reported that prognosis is still related to nodal status even when the dissection is performed after chemotherapy is used preoperatively for locally advanced (T3–4 and/or N2–3) breast cancer.

Based on an average follow-up of 49 months after mastectomy, Fisher et al. (1978) reported that the survival of patients with axillary micrometastases (< 2 mm) was comparable to the survival of patients without nodal metastases. With 10-year follow-up data, Rosen et al. (1981) showed that patients with T1 tumors and micrometastases had survival curves similar to node-negative patients for the first 6 years. After 6 years the curves for micro- and macrometastases begin to converge, becoming nearly identical at 12 years. Women with T2 tumors and negative lymph nodes or single micrometastases had survival curves that were similar throughout the period of observation.

The risk of axillary metastases has been correlated with the size of the primary tumor as well as nonanatomic indicators such as the degree of differentiation of the tumor assessed histologically, the presence of estrogen receptors (ER), ploidy, s-phase fraction, enzyme production, thymidine incorporation or gene overexpression. These prognostic variables have not been collected in a way that allows for prediction of outcome independent of knowledge of the axillary nodal status. In general, the information that lymph nodes are positive has taken precedence over the nonanatomic prognostic indicators which are invoked primarily to discriminate high- and low-risk patients when the lymph nodes are known to be negative (Winchester 1991). Parl et al. (1984) noted a synergistic effect of ER status on the risk associated with lymph node metastases, but no large series has yet adequately correlated anatomic and nonanatomic variables. Therefore, it appears that prognosis is still highly dependent on knowledge of lymph node status.

In the past, adjuvant systemic therapy was recommended only to patients with a relatively poor prognosis as indicated by positive lymph nodes. However, evidence that even node-negative patients may benefit from systemic therapy resulted in a controversial Clinical Alert from the National Cancer Institute and a tendency to treat all patients with adjuvant systemic therapy (National Cancer Institute 1988). If everyone receives adjuvant therapy, then staging for that purpose becomes unnecessary. However, staging is important if more intensive systemic therapies are selected for patients with worse prognoses, such as those with more than ten positive lymph nodes.

Finally, there are some patients who have such a good prognosis that systemic therapy is of dubious value. In the surveillance, epidemiology, and end results (SEER) data reported by Carter et al. (1989), the 5-year survival for patients with tumors less than 2 cm and negative nodes was 96.3%. At a median follow-up of 18 years, Rosner and Lane (1991) reported that 89% of patients with tumors less than 1 cm in diameter and negative lymph nodes were "cured". With screening mammography, these types of cases of small node-negative tumors are now common. Rosner and Lane described four low-risk groups which together comprised 35% of their node-negative population. Patients with well- or moderately well-differentiated tumors and negative axillary nodes had a 7-year disease-free rate (DFR) of 100%. Patients older than 50 years of age with poorly differentiated or anaplastic tumors less than 1 cm and negative lymph nodes had a DFR of 97%. Patients older than 50 years of age with a well- or moderately well-differentiated tumor 1.1–2 cm and negative nodes had a DFR of 94%. Patients with DCIS and microinvasion and negative nodes had a DFR of 100%. Trials are currently underway investigating the utility of systemic therapy in various categories of patients with T1, node-negative tumors. Information regarding those studies will bear on the question of the need for axillary staging. Until it is established that all patients need systemic therapy and nonanatomic indicators yield information that can substitute for histologic proof of lymph node metastasis, staging by axillary dissection will be valuable.

Although selection of treatment is the primary purpose of staging, there are several other reasons to group patients into prognostic categories. For clinical studies it is helpful to be able to understand the stage of disease for comparison with other studies. Patient counselling also requires prognostic information. When informing a premenopausal patient of the risk factors of pregnancy or when advising the postmenopausal patient who wants to take supplemental estrogens, precise staging information is helpful.

4.3 Clinical Assessment of Axillary Status

In the TNM staging system, lymph node status is described as follows: N0, not abnormal; N1a, palpable but not abnormal; N1b, suspected to contain cancer; and N2, matted or fixed. The accuracy of clinical assessment probably varies with the size of the primary tumor, the weight of the patient, and the amount of tumor in the axilla. In a multi-institutional trial (National Surgical Adjuvant Breast and Bowel Project, NSABP, B-04), 40% of patients with clinically negative lymph nodes had pathologically positive nodes upon examination of the specimen from an axillary dissection (FISHER et al. 1985). Thus the false-negative error rate appears to be substantial, although some single institution studies have reported lower rates than the NSABP. In a series reported by SENOFSKY et al. (1991) the false-negative rate was 21%, and in the Milan trial of conservative surgery and radiation therapy versus mastectomy the false-negative rate was only 26% (VERONESI et al. 1981). The false-negative rate was 38% in the series reported by DANFORTH et al. (1986). In a report from the Breast Adjuvant Chemotherapy study of the Anti-Cancer Council of Victoria (Australia), 47% of pathologically positive nodes were not palpable (KITCHEN et al. 1980). Although lymphoscintigraphy has been used to identify the internal mammary lymph node chain for purposes of planning radiation fields, the diagnostic use of lymphoscintigraphy for assessment of a status of the axilla has not been widely accepted.

The assessment of clinically positive lymph nodes (N1b and N2) is more accurate. DANFORTH et al. (1986) reported a false-positive rate of 11.1%.

4.4 Pathologic Assessment of Axillary Status

Several different objectives may be sought through evaluation of the axillary lymph node status and the accuracy of that assessment varies with both the extent of the dissection and the objective. Assessing the axilla as positive or negative may require only a limited dissection to yield an acceptably accurate answer, whereas determining the extent of lymph node involvement may require a more thorough dissection.

It is important to understand the anatomy of the axilla and the choices or limitations for the surgeon. The lymph nodes of the axilla are a network of filters receiving drainage from the breast, arm, skin, and chest wall. Although some nodes (such as the central group) predominantly drain the breast, it is not possible for the surgeon to select exclusively breast-draining nodes and avoid arm-draining nodes. Although the axilla is arbitrarily divided into three levels based on the relationship to the pectoralis minor muscle, the lymph nodes are not separated into packets and the levels blend imperceptibly. Level I lymph nodes are lateral and inferior to the pectoralis minor muscle. Level II nodes are posterior to the pectoralis minor muscle. Level III nodes are medial to the pectoralis minor muscle. When axillary lymph nodes are removed as part of a radical mastectomy specimen or when the pectoralis minor muscle is removed as part of a modified radical mastectomy, the pathologist can accurately evaluate the level of lymph nodes removed and involved. Otherwise, the level of lymph nodes dissected or involved by tumor must be marked by the surgeon intraoperatively, which is not a common practice outside of a protocol. Interpectoral nodes (Rotter's nodes) are removed as part of a radical mastectomy specimen but are not routinely removed when a modified radical mastectomy or as part of an axillary sampling. CODY et al. (1984) reported positive Rotter's nodes in 8.2% of axillary node-positive patients and 0.5% of node-negative patients.

Along with understanding the anatomy of the axilla, it is important to understand the terms used to define surgical procedures involving the axilla. A "full axillary dissection" usually means dissection of levels I, II, and III and usually requires the division or resection of the pectoralis minor muscle. The morbidity from a full axillary dissection is appreciable with atrophy of the pectoralis major muscle secondary to division of the lateral pectoral nerve, numbness of the posterior skin of the upper arm caused by division of the intercostobrachial nerve, and a risk of significant arm edema of about 5%–8% (DANFORTH et al. 1986; KISSIN et al. 1982; OSTEEN and SMITH 1990). Less extensive dissections seek to decrease morbidity while providing staging information and prophylaxis against axillary recurrence. "Axillary sampling" is a vague term implying a procedure that is less than a "full dissection", but it is usually not clear whether it means a dissection of levels I and II or only level I (or less) (ROSE et al. 1983). "Pectoral node biopsy" is a term invented to describe the removal of nodes around the axillary tail, probably level I (FORREST et al.

1976). Even "no dissection" can be a surprisingly vague term since approximately one-third of the simple mastectomy specimens of the NSABP B-04 trial contained lymph nodes (WOLMARK and FISHER 1982).

Although it would be a mistake to envision an orderly progression of lymph node metastases from level I to level II to level III, it is unusual to find skip metastases to level III. The chance of mistakenly declaring an axilla negative on the basis of a level I and II dissection appears to be less than 2% (ROSEN et al. 1983). On the other hand, dissection of only level I may have a high false-negative rate. DAVIES et al. (1980) found that when a radical mastectomy was performed immediately after node sampling, 42% of the patients with positive axillas went undetected by the sampling procedure. If examination had been limited to lymph nodes around the axillary tail (pectoral nodes) 14% of node-negative patients would have gone undetected. CLARKE et al. (1985) reported a stepwise approach to the axilla in which initially level I lymph nodes were biopsied, and a full dissection was performed only if the frozen section showed pathologic involvement of the level I nodes. Only eight of 436 patients suffered axillary relapse. Similar results from a smaller series were reported by ADAMI et al. (1978).

Few studies have addressed the issue of how many lymph nodes are needed in order to make accurate statements regarding the extent of axillary involvement and to decrease the risk of axillary recurrence. GRAVERSEN et al. (1988) noted that the risk of relapse in the axilla was inversely related to the number of lymph nodes removed, ranging from a 3% risk of recurrence, if three to ten lymph nodes were removed to 19% when no lymph nodes were removed. Analysis of the data from the NSABP B-04 trial showed that accurate statements can be made about whether four or more nodes are positive if approximately ten lymph nodes are removed in the specimen (FISHER et al. 1985). A dissection of level I and II lymph nodes generally assures that ten lymph nodes or more are removed.

In summary, staging information may be helpful for electing and selecting systemic therapy and may influence overall patient management. Evaluation of the clinically negative axilla by physical examination is highly inaccurate, whereas few false positives are seen among patients who have clinically suspicious axillas. Although some information can be gained regarding the status of axillary lymph nodes from a minimal sample such as a level I dissection or pectoral node biopsy, dissection of level II lymph nodes with removal of approximately ten or more lymph nodes permits further refinement of the prognosis.

4.5 Local Recurrence in the Untreated Axilla

Part of the rationale offered for prophylactic axillary dissection is the prevention of axillary recurrence and progression of uncontrolled axillary disease. Few modern studies have examined the risk of recurrence in the untreated axilla. The Cancer Research Campaign Trial in the United Kingdom reported a 5-year local recurrence rate of 11% for patients treated by simple mastectomy and axillary irradiation compared to 30% local recurrence in patients treated by simple mastectomy alone (CANCER RESEARCH CAMPAIGN WORK PARTY 1980). The incidence of uncontrolled axillary disease was not given. In the NSABP B-04 trial, 17.8% of patients who received neither an axillary dissection nor irradiation manifested axillary metastases (FISHER et al. 1985). Interestingly, 40% of patients with clinically negative axillas randomized to axillary dissection had positive lymph nodes. This finding suggests that at a median follow-up of over 5 years, more than half of the patients with positive axillary lymph nodes will not have a clinically relevant recurrence in their axilla. Only 4 of 365 patients experienced progression to uncontrolled axillary disease. In neither of the two studies cited above was overall survival affected in the group with untreated axillas. Unfortunately, not all nodal relapse can be controlled. In the series from the Joint Center for Radiation Therapy (JCRT) at Harvard, uncontrolled disease occurred in 18 of 38 (47%) patients who developed axillary recurrences (RECHT et al. 1991).

4.6 Irradiation of the Undissected, Clinical N0 or N1a Axilla

Two trials reported by Hayward utilized low doses of radiation to the undissected axilla and were associated with a 16% rate of axillary recurrence (HAYWARD 1984; HAYWARD and CALEFFI 1987). With long (15-year) follow-up, there was a statistically significant difference in survival for T1, N0 patients who were treated by radical mastectomy compared to patients treated by wide excision and inadequate doses of radiation. This study raises a cautionary note against any treatment plan that does not include adequate local therapy. With adequate doses of radiation the recurrence rate in the clinically negative, undissected axilla is quite low. RECHT et al. (1991) reported axillary recurrences in only 3 of 355 patients whose clinically negative, undissected axillas were irradiated. The failure rate was 3% (1/35) for N1a patients who were irradiated without axillary dissection. These patients were probably highly selected since most N1 patients underwent axillary dissections. Similar low recurrence rates were reported by ALMARICK et al. (1982) and OSBORNE et al. (1984).

4.7 Irradiation of the Undissected, Clinical N1b Axilla

Clinically suspicious axillary lymph nodes are usually removed to confirm the diagnosis and because of the high dose of radiation required to control gross disease. Axillary recurrence was reported in 15 of 52 patients (29%) in whom N1b axillas were irradiated without dissection (OSBORNE et al. 1984). Hayward reported axillary recurrence in 13 of 63 patients (21%) in whom N1 axillas were treated with doses of radiation currently felt to be too low for adequate control (HAYWARD 1984).

4.8 Conservative Breast Surgery and Axillary Dissection with Breast and Axillary Irradiation

The JCRT reported two axillary recurrences among 289 patients (0.78%) with positive axillary nodes who had less-than-complete axillary lymph node dissections and an axillary radiation field (RECHT et al. 1991). No axillary recurrences were noted among 125 patients in a series from the Institut Gustave-Roussy who were treated with level I or level I–II dissection and 4500 cGy (DEWAR et al. 1987).

4.9 Conservative Breast Surgery and Axillary Dissection with Breast Irradiation but No Axillary Irradiation

The upper portion of the axilla (level III) is usually within the field of breast radiation, therefore axillary recurrence rates are probably reduced in patients having breast irradiation even without an axillary field. Patients in the lumpectomy plus axillary dissection and radiation arm of the NSABP B0-6 protocol had a 4.5% rate of regional recurrences compared to a 7.2% regional recurrence rate among patients who had no breast irradiation (FISHER et al. 1985). Neither group had an axillary field. SARRAZIN et al. (1989), reporting a randomized trial at the Institut Gustave-Roussy, were unable to demonstrate a difference for adding axillary irradiation to node-positive patients who had undergone a complete dissection. RECHT et al. (1991) reported only a 2.1% axillary recurrence rate in pathologically node-negative patients receiving breast irradiation only. An identical axillary recurrence rate (2.1%) was seen among the 47 patients with one to three positive nodes who did not receive axillary irradiation. In the Milan trial of quadrantectomy, complete axillary dissection and radiation therapy versus radical mastectomy, there were no axillary recurrences (VERONESI et al. 1981). All patients had supraclavicular irradiation, but no axillary irradiation. Therefore, it would appear that axillary irradiation can safely be omitted when the axilla is proven to be negative by dissection. The data from RECHT et al. (1991) suggests that after a level I–II dissection, radiation therapy can be omitted safely if the patient has less than four positive lymph nodes.

4.10 Effect of Chemotherapy on Axillary Node Recurrence

Chemotherapy appears to have a positive effect on decreasing breast recurrence in patients treated conservatively with lumpectomy and radiation. The axillary recurrence rates in patients selected for conservative therapy is low, probably too low to see an impact from systemic therapy (ROSE et al. 1989; HAFFTY et al. 1991).

GRIEM et al. (1987) noted that recurrences on the chest wall or draining lymphatic areas were significantly reduced in high-risk (four or more positive nodes) patients randomized to receive both radiation therapy and chemotherapy compared to chemotherapy alone after a mastectomy and axillary node dissection. Despite the difference in local recurrence rates, disease-free and overall survival were not affected. In that report, axillary recurrences were not distinguished from the overall local regional recurrences.

Reporting the Eastern Cooperative Oncology Group (ECOG) adjuvant trial results, FOWBLE et al. (1988) noted an 11% incidence of local regional recurrence despite chemotherapy when four to seven nodes were positive or the tumor was at least 2.5 cm in size.

Therefore, even though chemotherapy may contribute to decreasing the risk of recurrence in the breast in patients with early-staged disease, its contribution to axillary control is probably minimal because radiation therapy and surgery control axillary disease so well. In patients with advanced disease (more than four positive lymph nodes), axillary disease may not be adequately controlled by surgery and chemotherapy in upwards of 20% of patients, and radiation appears to increase local control without significantly effecting survival.

4.11 Carcinoma In Situ and Axillary Lymph Nodes

The risk of lymph node metastases from in situ carcinoma appears to be very low. Rosen (1980) found that 1% of patients undergoing axillary dissections for intraductal or lobular carcinoma in situ had lymph node metastases. Silverstein et al. (1987) noted axillary nodal metastases in only 1 of 175 dissections and recommended reservation of dissection for those cases demonstrating microinvasion. No lymph node involvement was seen in any of the 226 patients with in situ breast cancer dissected or followed by Temple et al. (1989). The risk of microinvasion in in situ carcinoma is related to the size of the in situ component and the type of disease.

In a detailed study of DCIS using the serial subgross radiographic examination of tissue specimens, Lagios found microinvasion in 11 of 25 specimens larger than 25 mm and no occult invasion in 29 specimens with DCIS less than 25 mm (Lagios et al. 1982). In a study utilizing several clinical and pathologic findings, Kinne et al. (1989) reported that gross DCIS presenting as a mass, Paget's disease, or nipple discharge was associated with a 13% incidence of microinvasion and 1 out of 52 patients had positive nodes. Patients with mammographically detected DCIS had no microinvasion and no positive nodes. Rosen (1980) cautioned that in situ carcinoma by light microscopy may be associated with electron microscopic evidence of breaks in the basement membrane and that axillary metastases could occur without invasion. However, the association of microinvasion with increasing size of the tumor suggests that sampling error is a likely explanation for those few incidences of axillary metastases from "in situ" carcinoma. Silverstein et al. (1990) reported a rate of microinvasion of 20% in comedo-type DCIS compared to 6% in noncomedo DCIS. Of the 28 patients with microinvasion, only 1 (5%) had positive lymph nodes.

The risk of lymph node metastases from in situ carcinoma is low and does not appear to justify lymph node dissection except possibly when microinvasion is identified or the extent of the in situ carcinoma is such that microinvasion is likely.

4.12 Complications of Axillary Dissection

If the pectoralis major and minor muscles are not removed, mobilization of the shoulder is limited only be scarring of the incision. Limitation of shoulder motion is usually overcome by simple exercises starting within a week of surgery. The risk of other complications is related to the aggressiveness of the dissection. Partial paralysis of the pectoralis major muscle can result from damage to the lateral pectoral nerve. The intercostobrachial nerve traverses the axilla passing through the central group of lymph nodes and supplies sensation to the skin of the axilla and posterior upper arm. The intercostobrachial nerve is usually cut deliberately in order to put traction on the lymph node bearing axillary fat. The intercostobrachial nerve can be preserved but may result in paresthesias. After approximately 1 year the numbness on the upper posterior arm is no longer noticeable to most patients. Decreased sensation of the skin of the axilla and distortion of the skin folds can cause problems for shaving axillary hair. The long thoracic and thorocodorsal nerves are no longer routinely divided and weakness of the latissimus dorsi and serratus anterior muscle should not occur.

Edema of the arm is also a potential problem. Even full axillary dissections generally avoid the perivenous lymphatic channels and arm edema is less of a problem than it was in the past when elimination of all lymphatic tissue was considered desirable. The risk of a swollen arm from axillary dissection alone is generally quoted as less than 10% (Larson et al. 1988). Combining radiation and axillary dissection increases the risk of both arm edema and breast edema. Clarke et al. (1982) related edema of the breast after radiation therapy to the extent of the axillary dissection. A total of 26 of 33 patients (79%) had breast edema after a more thorough axillary node dissection compared with 25% for axillary sampling and 6% for no axillary surgery. The edema usually resolved within 3 years. Rose et al. (1989) reported that chemotherapy given concomitantly with radiation contributed to a poor cosmetic outcome including breast edema. Arm edema is clearly related to the extent of axillary dissection and to radiation therapy. Kissin et al. (1986) reported only a 7.4% incidence of lymphedema after complete axillary dissection, but the incidence of edema rose to 38.8% when the patient was treated with both axillary clearance and radiotherapy. Similar findings have been reported from the JCRT (Larson et al. 1988; Osteen and Smith 1990).

4.13 Conclusion

The prognostic information that can be obtained from a dissection of level I and II axillary lymph nodes currently cannot be duplicated by nonanatomic prognostic indicators. The value of that prognostic information varies with the circumstance. Patients with small, noncomedo carcinomas in situ have a very low risk for axillary metastases making dissection unjustifiable; while small invasive carcinomas have an appreciable risk of lymph node metastases and axillary dissection may be helpful for treatment planning, overall patient management, and to avoid the use of axillary irradiation.

Axillary treatment probably has little effect on survival. Uncontrolled progression of tumor in the axilla can be a major problem, but it is uncommon with patients treated by axillary dissection or axillary irradiation. Close follow-up of patients with clinically negative axillas usually allows detection of early axillary recurrences and prevention of serious morbidity. Combined dissection and radiation is justifiable only for the extensively involved axilla. Strategies of prophylactic irradiation or close follow-up only of patients with clinically negative axillas will result in an understaging of approximately 20%–40% of patients. Axillary sampling procedures with a dissection of level I nodes reduce that rate of error by approximately half. A dissection of level I and II lymph nodes has a very low false-negative rate, allows the division of node-positive patients into low- and high-risk groups, and adequately protects against axillary recurrence unless the axilla is extensively involved.

References

Adami HO, Graffman S, Johansson H, Rimsan A (1978) Survival and recurrence five years after selective treatment for breast cancer. Br J Cancer 38: 624–630

Almarick R, Santamaria F, Robert F et al (1982) Radiation therapy with or without primary limited surgery for operable breast cancer: a 20-year experience at the Marseilles Cancer Institute. Cancer 49: 30–34

Cancer Research Campaign Work Party (1980) Cancer Research Campaign (King's/Cambridge) trial for early breast cancer. Lancet ii: 55–60

Carter CL, Allen C, Henson DE (1989) Relation of tumor size, lymph node status, and survival in 24740 breast cancer cases. Cancer 63: 181–187

Clarke D, Martinez A, Cox R et al (1982) Breast edema following staging axillary node dissection in patients with breast carcinoma by radical radiotherapy. Cancer 49: 2295

Clarke DH, Le MG, Sarrazin D et al (1985) Analysis of local-regional relapses in patients with early breast cancers treated by excision and radiotherapy: experience of the Institute Gustave-Roussy. Int J Radiat Oncol Biol Phys 11: 137–145

Cody HS, Egeli RA, Urban JA (1984) Rotter's node metastases: therapeutic and prognostic considerations in early breast carcinoma. Ann Surg 199: 266–270

Danforth DN, Findlay PA, McDonald HD et al (1986) Complete axillary lymph node dissection for Stage I–II carcinoma of the breast. J Clin Oncol 4: 655–662

Davies GC, Millis RR, Hayward JL (1980) Assessment of axillary lymph node status. Ann Surg 192: 148–151

Dewar JA, Sarrazin D, Benhamou E et al (1987) Management of the axilla in conservatively treated breast cancer: 592 patients treated at the Institute Gustave-Roussy. Int J Radiat Oncol Biol Phys 13: 475–481

Fisher B, Redmond C, Fisher ER et al (1985) Ten-year results of a randomized trial comparing radical mastectomy and total mastectomy with or without radiation. N Engl J Med 312: 674–681

Fisher ER, Swamidoss S, Lee CH et al (1978) Detection and significance of occult axillary node metastases in patients with invasive breast cancer. Cancer 42: 2025–2031

Forrest APM, Roberts MM, Cant E, Shivas AA (1976) Simple mastectomy and pectoral node biopsy. Br J Surg 63: 569–575

Fowble B, Gray R, Gilchrist K et al (1988) Identification of a subgroup of patients with breast cancer and histologically positive axillary nodes receiving adjuvant chemotherapy who may benefit from postoperative radiotherapy. J Clin Oncol 6: 1107–1117

Graversen HP, Blichert-Toff M, Andersen JA et al (1988) Breast cancer: risk of axillary recurrence in node-negative patients following partial dissection of the axilla. Eur J Surg Oncol 14: 407–412

Griem KL, Henderson IC, Gelman R et al (1987) The 5-year results of a randomized trial of adjuvant radiation therapy after chemotherapy in breast cancer patients treated with mastectomy. J Clin Oncol 5: 1546–1555

Haffty BG, Fischer D, Rose M et al (1991) Prognostic factors for local recurrence in the conservatively treated breast cancer patient: a cautious interpretation of the data. J Clin Oncol 9: 997–1003

Hayward J (1984) The principles of breast cancer surgery. Breast Cancer Res Treat 4: 61–68

Hayward J, Caleffi M (1987) The significance of local control

in the primary treatment of breast cancer. Arch Surg 122: 1244–1247
Kinne DW, Petrek JA, Osborne MP et al (1989) Breast carcinoma in situ. Arch Surg 124: 33–36
Kissin MW, Price AB, Thompson EM et al (1982) The inadequacy of axillary sampling in breast cancer. Lancet 1: 1210–1211
Kissin MW, Querci della Rovere G, Easton D, Westburg G (1986) Lymphoedema and breast cancer. Br J Surg 73: 580–584
Kitchen PRB, McLennan R, Mursell A (1980) Node-positive breast cancer: a comparison of clinical and pathological findings and assessment of axillary clearance. Aust NIJ Surg 50: 580–583
Lagios MD, Westdahl PR, Margolin FR, Rose MR (1982) Duct carcinoma in situ: relationship of extent of noninvasive disease to the frequency of occult invasion, multicentricity, lymph node metastases, and short-term treatment failures. Cancer 50: 1209–1314
Larson D, Weinstein M, Goldberg I et al (1988) Edema of the arm as a function of the extent of axillary surgery in patients with Stage I–II carcinoma of the breast treated with primary radiotherapy. Int J Radiat Oncol Biol 12: 1575–1582
McCready DR, Hortobagyi GN, Kau SW et al (1989) The prognostic significance of lymph node metastases after preoperative chemotherapy for locally advanced breast cancer. Arch Surg 124: 21–25
National Cancer Institute (1988) Clinical alert. May 16
Osborne MP, Orniston N, Harmer CL et al (1984) Breast conservation in the treatment of early breast cancer: a 20-year follow-up. Cancer 53: 349–355
Osteen RT, Smith B (1990) Results of conservative surgery and radiation therapy for breast cancer. Surg Clin N Am 70: 1005–1021
Parl FF, Schmidt BP, Dupont WD, Wagner RK (1984) Prognostic significance of estrogen receptor status in breast cancer in relation to tumor stage, axillary node metastases and histopathologic grading. Cancer 54: 2237–2242
Recht A, Pierce SM, Abner A et al (1991) Regional nodal failure after conservative surgery and radiotherapy for early-stage breast carcinomas. J Clin Oncol 9: 988–996
Rose CM, Botnick LE, Weinstein M et al (1983) Axillary sampling in the definitive treatment of breast cancer by radiation therapy and lumpectomy. Radiat Oncol Biol Phys 9: 339–344
Rose MA, Henderson IC, Gelman R et al (1989) Premenopausal breast cancer patients treated with conservative surgery, radiotherapy, and adjuvant chemotherapy have a low risk of local failure. Int J Radiat Oncol Biol Phys 17: 711–717
Rose MA, Olivotto I, Koufman C et al (1989) Conservative surgery and radiation therapy for early breast cancer: long-term cosmetic results. Arch Surg 124: 153–157
Rosen PP (1980) Axillary lymph node metastases in patients with occult noninvasive breast carcinoma. Cancer 46: 1298–1306
Rosen PP, Saigo PE, Braun DW et al (1981) Axillary micro- and macrometastases in breast cancer: prognostic significance of tumor size. Ann Surg 194: 585–591.
Rosen PP, Lesser ML, Kinne DW, Beattie EJ (1983) Discontinuous or "skip" metastases in breast carcinomas: analysis of 1228 axillary dissections. Ann Surg 197: 276–287
Rosner D, Lane WW (1991) Should all patients with node-negative breast cancer receive adjuvant therapy? Identifying additional subsets of low-risk patients who are highly curable by surgery alone. Cancer 68: 1482–1494
Sarrazin D, Le M, Arriagada R et al (1989) Ten year results of a randomized trial comparing a conservative treatment to mastectomy in early breast cancer. Radiother Oncol 14: 177
Senofsky GM, Moffat FL, Davis K et al (1991) Total axillary lymphadenectomy in the management of breast cancer. Arch Surg 126: 1336–1342
Silverstein MJ, Rosser RJ, Gierson ED (1987) Axillary lymph node dissection for intraductal breast carcinoma – is it indicated? Cancer 59: 1819–1824
Silverstein MJ, Waisman JR, Gamagami P et al (1990) Intraductal carcinoma of the breast (208 cases): clinical factors influencing treatment choice. Cancer 66: 102–108
Temple WJ, Jenkins M, Alexander F et al (1989) Natural history of in situ breast cancer in a defined population. Ann Surg 210: 653–657
Veronesi U, Saccozzi R, Del Vecchio M et al (1981) Comparing radical mastectomy with quadrantectomy, axillary dissection and radiotherapy in patients with small cancers of the breast. N Engl J Med 305: 6–11
Winchester DP (1991) Adjuvant therapy for node-negative breast cancer: the use of prognostic factors in selecting patients. Cancer 67: 1741–1743
Wolmark N, Fisher B (1982) Surgery in the primary treatment of breast cancer. Breast Cancer Res Treat 1: 339–348

5 How Much of the Effect of Chemotherapy Is Due to Hormonal Manipulation?

NIGEL P. M. SACKS, ROGER P. A'HERN, and MICHAEL BAUM

CONTENTS

5.1 Introduction . . . 35
5.2 Evidence for Hormonal Manipulation . . . 36
5.3 Evidence Against Hormonal Manipulation . . . 38
5.4 Discussion . . . 39
5.5 Conclusions . . . 42
References . . . 42

5.1 Introduction

Despite the widely held belief that there is a lack of progress in the management of patients with breast cancer, remarkable advances in fact have been made. It has now been conclusively shown that a treatment intervention given after surgery for operable or early breast cancer can improve long-term survival as well as perturb the natural history of breast cancer. Administering adjuvant systemic therapy to patients presenting with seemingly localized early breast cancer (currently comprising approximately 70% of cases) was initiated by the realization that subclinical metastatic disease is usually present at the time of first diagnosis.

The recently updated worldwide overview of over 75000 women with early breast cancer randomized in systemic adjuvant therapy trials (EARLY BREAST CANCER TRIALISTS' COLLABORATIVE GROUP 1992) confirms that hormone manipulation or prolonged (greater than 1 month) cytotoxic polychemotherapy (more than one drug) can reduce the annual odds of death by approximately 30% and that this benefit may possibly be increased by combining the two modalities. Thus, highly significant reductions in the annual rate of both recurrence and death can be achieved by tamoxifen, by ovarian ablation (in patients aged under 50 years), and by polychemotherapy. The benefits of chemotherapy were seen in all patients aged under 70 years regardless of their menopausal status, with nearly twice the benefit seen in women under 50 years; it was not possible to estimate the effect in patients aged over 70 years because statistical power was inadequate. In patients under 50 years, the benefits in terms of recurrence and death were similar with either prolonged polychemotherapy or ovarian ablation. The odds reductions observed were also consistent with the hypothesis that ovarian ablation has effects which are independent of the chemotherapy effect and also that chemotherapy has effects which are independent of the ovarian ablation effect. These results are of vital clinical importance as they bring to a head the issue of how much the effect of chemotherapy is due to an indirect effect on ovarian function – are these treatments equivalent or do they both have a role? While systemic cytotoxic chemotherapy with an alkylating agent such as cyclophosphamide has many hormonal effects in patients with breast cancer (ROSE and DAVIS 1980), the major effect is to induce a chemical ovarian ablation in a proportion of premenopausal patients. As adjuvant cyclophosphamide, methotrexate, and 5-fluorouracil (CMF) therapy has no significant effect on pituitary or adrenal function (DNISTRIAN et al. 1983), we will concentrate on the effects of systemic cytotoxic chemotherapy on ovarian endocrine function.

These observations have stimulated several investigators to study whether this induction of ovarian failure is the most important component of the chemotherapy effect in premenopausal patients and whether the incidence of chemotherapy-induced amenorrhoea (CIA) can be correlated with the rate of recurrence and overall mortality. In this chapter, we present data both supporting and refuting the assertion that the effect of chemotherapy is due to a "chemical castration" – the permanent cessation of ovarian function immediately following administration of chemotherapy (time to onset varies from

NIGEL P. M. SACKS, M. D., Associate Professor, Department of Surgery, The Royal Marsden Hospital, Fulham Road London, SW 3 6JJ, UK; ROGER P. A'HERN, M.Sc., Statistician in Computing, The Royal Marsden Hospital, Fulham Road London, SW3 6JJ, UK; MICHAEL BAUM, M.D., Professor; Department of Surgery, The Royal Marsden Hospital, Fulham Road, London, SW3 6JJ, UK study to study). We then draw conclusions made from the available published data.

5.2 Evidence for Hormonal Manipulation

Several investigators have examined the endocrine effect of adjuvant cytotoxic polychemotherapy, which prolongs the 10-year relapse-free survival (RFS) and overall survival in premenopausal breast cancer patients: CMF given for six 28-day cycles is the most common combination. ROSE and DAVIS (1980) studied both the ovarian and adrenal function in premenopausal patients before and at intervals during adjuvant therapy with CMF, CMF plus prednisone (CMFP), and CMFP plus tamoxifen (CMFPT). Amenorrhoea developed within 10 months of starting therapy in 13 of 15 patients (average age 42 $\pm$ 6 years) treated with CMF, in 8 of 10 patients (average age 41 $\pm$ 7 years) receiving CMFP, and in all 13 (average age 38 $\pm$ 6 years) CMFPT-treated patients. The amenorrhoeic patients receiving CMF showed a reduction in plasma levels of total oestrogens (oestrone plus oestradiol) and an increase in plasma levels luteinizing and follicle-stimulating hormones (LH and FSH), indicating that these cytotoxic drugs directly suppressed ovarian function. Plasma androstenedione levels, which in premenopausal women are derived equally from the ovaries and the adrenals, were also reduced, while the plasma dehydroepiandrosterone sulphate level, a steroid of predominantly adrenal origin, was unaffected. The addition of prednisone to CMF further decreased the secretion of androstenedione, which by peripheral aromatization is an important precursor of oestrogens; presumably this decrease resulted from adrenal suppression. The authors also found that the addition of tamoxifen to CMFP caused an initial increase in total oestrogens without any significant change in plasma LH or FSH. SAMMAN et al. (1978) confirmed this study and were also the first to show that premenopausal patients rendered amenorrhoeic (mean age 44.9 $\pm$ 5.8 years) were significantly older than those who were not affected in this way (mean age 33.5 $\pm$ 4.4 years; $p < 0.001$). Their patients who developed amenorrhoea also had elevated LH and FSH levels (before and after LH-releasing hormone, LH-RH, stimulation) and had significantly lower plasma oestradiol levels when compared with those who had not become amenorrhoeic.

The Guy's/Manchester group also studied the effect of adjuvant CMF on ovarian function as part of a prospective randomized trial in 74 axillary node-positive premenopausal women (defined as last menstrual period within 1 year of entry into trial) with operable breast cancer (RICHARDS et al. 1990; PADMANABHAN et al. 1986). The hormonal changes they found were similar to the above studies confirming ovarian suppression by CMF in most cases. After a median follow-up of 47 months, 50%, 70%, and 80% of the 35 patients receiving CMF became permanently amenorrhoeic within 3, 6, and 12 months, respectively. In contrast, only five of the no treatment (control) group of 39 patients became permanently amenorrhoeic within 12 months of starting the trial ($p < 0.001$). The eight treated patients who did not develop amenorrhoea were significantly younger (median age 35 years; range 25–38 years) than those who did develop it (median age 46; range 35–55 years; $p < 0.01$). The LUDWIG BREAST CANCER STUDY GROUP (1985b) found in their Trial I that 89% of 134 CMFP-treated patients who were menstruating within 6 months of study entry had amenorrhoea for at least one 3-month interval during therapy. Menses resumed in only 19% (21/111) of the women who experienced amenorrhoea and whose menstrual history was reported beyond 18 months of study entry. The Eastern Cooperative Oncology Group (ECOG) adjuvant chemotherapy trial showed that amenorrhoea occurred in only 21% of patients aged under 40 years given a CMF-containing regimen compared with 49% of patients more than 40 years ($p < 0.05$) given the same drugs (TORMEY et al. 1990).

It can be concluded from the above that adjuvant CMF chemotherapy causes amenorrhoea due to ovarian suppression in a large proportion of premenopausal patients and is more common in premenopausal women aged 40 years or more. However, comparison of data is difficult because a number of questions are left open in each study. First, the definition of premenopausal status varies from the occurrence of menses within 6 weeks prior to commencing adjuvant chemotherapy (BIANCO et al. 1991) to the presence of menstrual activity during the previous 12 months (RICHARDS et al. 1990; TORMEY et al. 1990). Second, the definition of CIA varies; although most studies use cessation of menses for at least 3 months from the commencement of chemotherapy as the criterion to define CIA, the ECOG study required 12 months without any menstrual activity. Finally, there is a close direct relationship between the induction of amenorrhoea and increasing age of the premenopausal patient with an inverse relationship between the time of onset of CIA and patient age.

The important question raised by several of the above studies is whether the occurrence of amenorrhoea in premenopausal patients given chemotherapy is associated with a longer RFS or overall survival than that seen in patients who do not become amenorrhoeic? The Ludwig group (GOLDHIRSCH et al. 1990; INTERNATIONAL BREAST CANCER STUDY GROUP 1990) also found a slightly higher RFS at 4 years for patients who experienced amenorrhoea (53%) compared with that for patients who continued to menstruate (44%; $p = 0.91$). In the 19% (21/111) of those whose menses resumed after cessation of chemotherapy, the RFS was 48%, slightly lower than that for patients who maintained loss of menses (57%, $p = 0.26$). Furthermore, in the ECOG study it was observed that patients developing amenorrhoea had a significantly better survival ($p = 0.001$) than those who did not develop amenorrhoea, with the greatest effect in the patients with oestrogen receptor (ER)-negative tumours. In the recently updated Guy's/Manchester trial (RICHARDS et al. 1990), none of the 77% (69/90) of premenopausal patients (menstrual data available in 90 of the total 97 patients) who developed amenorrhoea resumed menses within 12 months. Thirty-seven per cent (11/30) of patients aged 40 years or less and 97% (58/60) of those aged 41 years or more developed amenorrhoea. Patients with CMF-induced amenorrhoea had a significantly better RFS (74% at 5 years) than either the control group (35% at 5 years; $p > 0.001$) or those patients who received CMF, but continued to menstruate (46% at 5 years; $p = 0.005$). However, within the subgroup of CMF-treated patients aged 40 years or less, no difference in RFS was noted between those who developed amenorrhoea (46% at 5 years) and those who continued to menstruate (51% at 5 years; $p = 0.9$). In contrast to the survival benefit from CMF seen in their premenopausal women aged 41–54 years ($n = 64$), the Guy's/Manchester trial did not show any improvement in RFS in postmenopausal women. They also found a significantly better RFS for premenopausal CMF-treated patients aged 41–54 years than for postmenopausal CMF-treated patients of the same age ($p = 0.002$).

The prognostic role of CMF-induced amenorrhoea was recently studied in further detail by BIANCO et al. (1991) in 221 premenopausal node-positive breast cancer patients given six or nine courses of adjuvant regimens containing CMF. They used strict definitions of premenopausal status: the occurrence of last normal menses within 6 weeks of initiation of chemotherapy and CMF-induced amenorrhoea, and the cessation of menses for at least 3 months not later than 3 months from the end of chemotherapy. Amenorrhoea occurred in 75% (166/221) of patients and they also found a strong correlation between the development of amenorrhoea and increasing patient age. There was an inverse linear correlation between the patient's age and the time to development of amenorrhoea ($r = -0.42$, $p < 0.001$). At median follow-up of 69 months, the RFS of amenorrhoeic patients was significantly better than those who maintained normal menses (Mantel-Byar χ-square = 10.95, $p < 0.001$, relative hazard = 0.50). Multivariate evaluation of the prognostic role of CMF-induced amenorrhoea confirmed that its occurrence was independently associated with a better prognosis (relative hazard = 0.43; 95% CI 0.24–0.77) and that there was no significant interaction between menstrual status and other conventional prognostic factors. They found no difference in RFS in those developing temporary as opposed to permanent amenorrhoea (Mantel-Byar χ-square = 0.77; $0.30 < p < 0.40$).

In the Ludwig Group's Trial I (LUDWIG BREAST CANCER STUDY GROUP 1985b), 85% (340/399) of premenopausal patients (menses within 6 months of starting chemotherapy) given CMF developed amenorrhoea for at least 3 months during treatment; these patients had a longer 4-year RFS than the 59 premenopausal patients who did not develop amenorrhoea ($p = 0.006$). This association was primarily observed in patients under 35 years of age and was not statistically significant in analysis stratified by age. Menstrual function was re-established in 20% of those who developed amenorrhoea during treatment (55% of patients under 40 years old and 11% of patients over 40 years old) and the RFS was similar in those who did and did not resume menses (75% vs 78%, 4-year RFS). The Danish Breast Cancer Cooperative Group recently reported a large prospective randomized trial ($n = 1032$) which demonstrated that cyclophosphamide alone improved RFS only in those patients who experienced drug-induced amenorrhoea, whereas CMF was equally effective in improving RFS in those who experienced amenorrhoea and those who did not (BRINCKER et al. 1987).

The recent publication of the worldwide overview results by the EARLY BREAST CANCER TRIALISTS' COLLABORATIVE GROUP (1992) provides irrefutable evidence that adjuvant systemic therapy given after surgery for seemingly localized breast cancer can alter the natural history of the disease. Highly significant reductions in the annual rate both of recurrence and death are produced by ovarian ablation below age 50 years (26% ± 6% for recurrence and 25% ± 7% for mortality) and by prolonged polychemotherapy (37% ± 5% for recurrence and 27% ± 6% for mortality; $2p < 0.00001$). The effect of polychemotherapy in relation to age was examined in the overview and, for both RFS and overall survival, there is a strong statistically significant indication of a greater effect among younger women than older women. It was found, however, that while the effect of polychemotherapy on mortality is still statistically significant among women aged over 50 years (13% ± 4%; $1p < 0.002$) it is only half as great as that seen among women under 50 years (24% ± 5%; $1p < 0.00001$). In view of the small numbers it was not possible to determine whether among women of similar age, menopausal status is correlated with the response to chemotherapy. Therefore, it is reasonable to use the cut-off age of 50 years as a surrogate end point for the menopause. Among the 1746 women aged under 50 years treated by ovarian ablation, there was a highly significant improvement in recurrence-free survival (26% ± 6%; $2p < 0.0001$) and in overall survival (25% ± 7%; $2p < 0.001$). These effects of ovarian ablation seemed to be somewhat smaller in the presence of added chemotherapy. For the 1326 women aged over 50 years undergoing ovarian ablation, the overview results were not significant for recurrence or for mortality with no obvious heterogeneity between the different trial results in either end point.

5.3 Evidence Against Hormonal Manipulation

The results from some of the above studies show some association between the cessation of menses in response to chemotherapy and patient outcome. However, the results from several other studies are contradictory. The Ludwig Trial II (International Breast Cancer Study Group 1990) of CMFP for node-positive patients suggests that the effects of amenorrhoea are partly confounded by the ER content of the tumour. The trial showed that CIA was associated with a longer RFS only in patients aged under 35 years and in those with ER-positive primary tumours. In a Milan trial (Bonadonna et al. 1985), CMF failed to produce a therapeutic benefit in postmenopausal women, and the 10-year RFS of 37.2% and 31.6% in the patients aged under 40 years who did and did not have CIA were not any different. In addition, the Milan group found that oophorectomy at first relapse was associated with a response rate of 24.5% (13/53) in those who had received prior adjuvant CMF, compared with a 41.7% (5/12) response rate in controls who had not received CMF. Furthermore, women who had drug-induced amenorrhoea exhibited a higher response rate (30%) than those who did not have this side effect (20%). Bonadonna and his colleagues concluded that these results further contribute to dispelling the theory that amenorrhoea is equivalent to permanent ovarian failure, although this opinion is in stark contrast to the previously discussed findings of several endocrine laboratory studies of ovarian function during adjuvant chemotherapy.

As discussed previously, the Guy's/Manchester group (Richards et al. 1990) found that patients with CMF-induced amenorrhoea had a significantly better 5-year RFS (74%) than those who continued to menstruate (46%; $p = 0.005$). However, as drug-induced amenorrhoea was so strongly related to age (37% in patients under 40 years compared with 97% in patients over 40 years) they looked in more detail at the influence of amenorrhoea in CMF-treated patients and controls aged under 40 years. The CMF-treated patients aged under 40 years had a significantly improved 5-year RFS, but there was no difference between those who developed amenorrhoea and those who continued to menstruate (46% vs 51%; $p = 0.9$). The CMF-treated patients aged under 40 years had a worse survival than those aged over 40 years (46% vs 74%; $p = 0.001$). At least part of the reason for this may be that the older patients reached natural menopause sooner. The National Surgical Adjuvant Breast and Bowel Project (NSABP) group (Fisher et al. 1979, 1986) also reported a lack of association between RFS with depressed ovarian function induced by melphalan. Using an indirect comparison, the improved survival obtained with melphalan was higher in younger patients, who had a lower incidence of CIA, than in older women. However, no detailed analysis was carried out to evaluate the exact relationship between the occurrence of CIA and the effect of therapy. In a prospective randomized trial, the Danish Breast Cancer Cooperative Group (Brincker et al. 1987) found that adjuvant cyclophosphamide alone and the combination CMF improved, to a similar degree, RFS significantly ($p = 0.0001$), but CMF had a greater overall survival advantage than cyclophosphamide alone. The RFS of both control patients and those treated with CMF did not differ significantly, regardless of the presence or absence of amenorrhoea. However, in patients treated with cyclophosphamide alone, the group with amenorrhoea had a significantly better RFS than the group without amenorrhoea ($p = 0.02$) and, in this same subgroup, ER-positive patients had significantly better RFS than the ER-negative group ($p = 0.015$).

In the cohort of patients with node-positive disease from the Ludwig V trial (GOLDHIRSCH et al. 1990), a single cycle of preoperative CMF was associated with a 4-year RFS of 38% compared with 66% ($p < 0.0001$) for patients who received CMF for 6 months. This difference was claimed to be due to the chemotherapy effect; the difference in 4-year RFS of 68% compared with 61% ($p = 0.05$) in those who did and did not become amenorrhoeic was claimed to be due to the endocrine effect of chemotherapy-induced suppressed ovarian function. However, on close inspection of the data, only 31% of the node-positive CMF developed amenorrhoea compared with the incidence of 68% found in those receiving 6 or 9 months of adjuvant CMF. While 30% of those patients aged under 40 years given prolonged CMF developed amenorrhoea, 56% (19/34) of these resumed menses within 15 months of the onset of amenorrhoea.

An informal literature overview of the comparative RFS in those women developing CIA and those who did not is presented in Table 5.1. The hazard ratios and their standard errors were estimated from the published percentage of RFS at 4 or 5 years and the overall p value for the comparison of the curves. In the case of the Ludwig I trial, the actual hazard ratio was available in the published paper (LUDWIG BREAST CANCER STUDY GROUP 1985a). This overview shows a very convincing effect on improving RFS for the group experiencing amenorrhoea.

5.4 Discussion

The only data that will yield a definitive answer to how much of the effect of chemotherapy is due to ovarian suppression will come from randomized trials with four arms: an untreated arm (A), a chemotherapy-alone arm (C), an ovarian ablation-alone arm (B), and a combined chemotherapy and ovarian ablation arm (D). This is a 2×2 factorial design, as shown diagrammatically below:

	nil	ovarian ablation
nil	A	B
chemotherapy	C	D

The difference between the effect of chemotherapy assessed by comparing arms C and A and the effect of chemotherapy obtained by comparing arms D and B would indicate how much of the effect of chemotherapy was due to ovarian suppression. If chemotherapy acted only by ovarian suppression, then D and B would be identical, i.e. there would be no benefit of adding chemotherapy to ovarian ablation. If the difference between C and A were identical to the treatment effect between D and B, then the two effects would be independent – none of the effect of chemotherapy would be due to ovarian suppression. Obviously, the evidence suggests that neither of these two extremes is true.

Can anything be inferred from the data available in the overview? If the only mechanism explaining the effect of adjuvant cytotoxic chemotherapy is that it causes drug-induced amenorrhoea, then this would imply two features that could be expected to appear in the overview. First, the treatment effect seen in pre- and postmenopausal women would differ, and there would be no treatment effect in postmenopausal women. This is not found to be the case. For RFS there is a trend towards greater effects of polychemotherapy at younger than at older ages ($2p = 0.006$), but even among women aged 60–69 years, polychemotherapy still produces a 20% ($\pm 5\%$) delay in the detection of relapse ($1p < 0.0001$). Second, since chemotherapy does not result in complete ovarian suppression in all patients, it would be expected that the size of the effect of chemotherapy would be less than the size of the effect of ovarian ablation. This is not supported by indirect comparisons that can be made from the overview results: ovarian ablation shows odds reductions of 30% ($\pm 9\%$) and 28% ($\pm 9\%$) for recurrence and mortality, respectively; the corresponding figures for chemotherapy are 37% ($\pm 5\%$) and 27% ($\pm 6\%$), respectively.

Both these pieces of evidence suggest that chemotherapy does not act by ovarian suppression alone. Is it possible to estimate plausible ranges for the relative effects of chemotherapy and ovarian

Table 5.1. Overview of comparative relapse-free survival in those women who developed chemotherapy-induced amenorrhoea and those who did not

Reference		Percentage relapse free for 5 or 4 years		p Value
		Amenorrhoea	Nonamenorrhoea	
Goldhirsch et al (1990)		70	63	0.05
Ludwig Breast Cancer Study Group (1985a)		53	44	0.91
Bianco et al (1991)		57	32	0.001
Brincker et al (1987)	C	75	62	0.02
	CMF	67	68	0.92
Richards et al (1990)		74	46	0.005
Ludwig Breast Cancer Study Group (1985b)				
Beex et al (1988)		76	45	0.03
				Overall

Estimated hazard ratio (95% CI)
(Amenorrhoea : nonamenorrhoea)

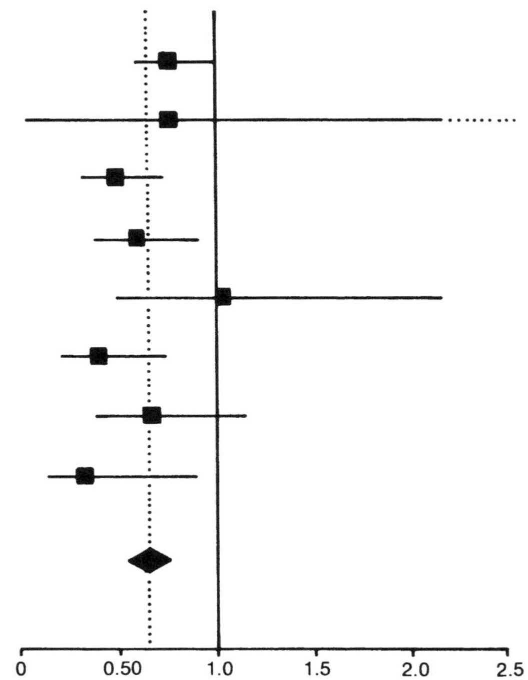

The overall hazard ratio was 0.64 (95% CI, 0.56–0.76; $2p < 0.001$). The heterogeneity χ-square = 9.1 (not significant)

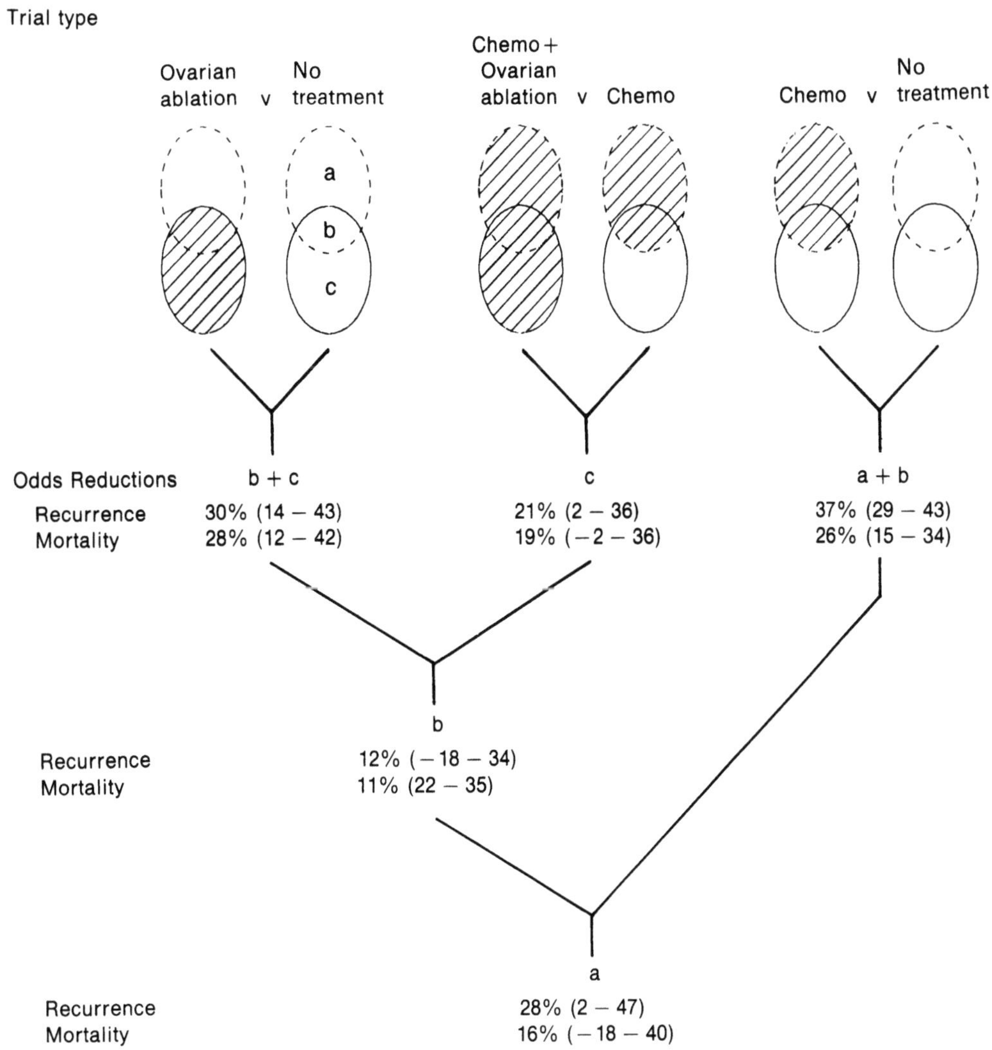

Fig. 5.1. Indirect estimates of the size of the independent chemotherapy effect (*a*), independent ovarian effect (*c*), and their shared effect (*b*). *Numbers in parentheses* indicate the 95% confidence interval. (From EARLY BREAST CANCER TRIALISTS' COLLABORATIVE GROUP 1992)

ablation? We have done this in Fig. 5.1, estimating the sizes of the independent chemotherapy effect, the independent ovarian ablation effect, and the shared effect from indirect comparisons performed in the overview. The estimated sizes of these effects are odds reductions of 28% (95% CI, 2–47), 21% (95% CI, 2–36), and 12% (95% CI, – 18–34), respectively, in terms of recurrence. The corresponding figures for mortality are 16% (95% CI, – 18–40), 19% (95% CI, – 2–36), and 11% (95% CI, – 22–35). This suggests that for both these endpoints the shared effect is less than the independent effects of each treatment, although the wide confidence intervals and method of calculation need to be taken into account in interpreting these figures.

In the trials presented in the worldwide overview there was no randomized trial directly comparing adjuvant chemotherapy with and without oophorectomy. While age is obviously closely related to menopausal status, the cut-off used in the overview, above or below age 50, is a valid surrogate cut-off for subdividing pre- and postmenopausal women. In the overview of over 11 000 women given cytotoxic polychemotherapy, only 225 women under age 50 were *known* to be postmenopausal, while among women over 50 years only 911 were *known* to be premenopausal. These numbers of patients with atypical menopausal status were far too small to determine whether, among women of similar age groups, menopausal status is correlated with response to chemotherapy. For overall survival the trend towards greater effect among younger women is even less significant ($2p = 0.01$) than for recurrence. The absolute effect of polychemotherapy on mortality among women aged over 50 years was a 12% ± 4% reduction in the annual odds of death ($1p < 0.002$) compared with that of 25% ± 5% seen in women aged under 50 years ($1p < 0.00001$).

5.5 Conclusions

What definite conclusion about the mechanism of the effect of adjuvant chemotherapy can be drawn from the published data presented above? There are several irrefutable statements that can be made: Prolonged adjuvant cytotoxic chemotherapy produces a highly significant reduction in the risk of recurrence and death from breast cancer irrespective of age (up to 70 years); the magnitude of this effect is greater in women under 50 years than in those aged 50 years or over; oophorectomy in women aged under 50 years is associated with similar improvements in RFS and overall survival to that seen with adjuvant chemotherapy; the incidence of drug-induced amenorrhoea is higher in older women (40–49 years) than in younger women (under 40 years), although survival rates in these age groups are similar, and the majority of studies show a correlation between the induction of amenorrhoea by chemotherapy and improved survival.

Ovarian ablation, therefore, comprises a major component of the benefit obtained with the use of cytotoxic chemotherapy. However, several details, such as determining the extent played by the mechanism of chemotherapy in premenopausal women, still need clarification. The results of current trials addressing the place of adjuvant ovarian ablation (usually with an LH-RH analogue) in addition to prolonged polychemotherapy are awaited with great interest.

References

Beex LVAM, McKenzie MA, Raemaekers JMM et al (1988) Adjuvant chemotherapy in premenopausal patients with primary breast cancer: relation to drug-induced amenorrhoea, age, and the PR status of the tumor. Eur J Cancer Clin Oncol 24: 719–721

Bianco AR, Del Mastro L, Gallow E et al (1991) Prognostic role of amenorrhoea induced by adjuvant chemotherapy in premenopausal patients with early breast cancer. Br J Cancer 63: 799–803

Bonadonna G, Valagussa P, Rossi A et al (1985) Ten year experience with CMF-based adjuvant chemotherapy in resectable breast cancer. Breast Cancer Res Treat 5: 95–115

Brincker H, Rose C, Rank F et al (1987) Evidence of a castration-mediated effect of adjuvant cytotoxic chemotherapy in premenopausal breast cancer. J Clin Oncol 5: 1771–1778

Dnistrian AM, Schwartz MK, Fracchia AA et al (1983) Endocrine consequences of adjuvant therapy in premenopausal and postmenopausal breast cancer patients. Cancer 51: 803–807

Early Breast Cancer Trialists' Collaborative Group (1992) Systemic treatment of early breast cancer by hormonal, cytotoxic, or immune therapy – 133 randomized trials involving 31000 recurrences and 24000 deaths among 75000 women. Lancet 339: 1–15, 71–85

Fisher B, Sherman B, Rocketter H et al (1979) L-Phenylalanine mustard (L-PAM) in the management of premenopausal patients with primary breast cancer. Lack of association of disease-free survival with depression of ovarian function. Cancer 44: 487–491

Fisher B, Fisher ER, Redmond C (1986) Ten year results from the NSABP clinical trial evaluation the use of L-phenylalanine mustard (L-PAM) in the management of primary breast cancer. J Clin Oncol 4: 929–941

Goldhirsch A, Gelber RD, Castiglione M (1990) The magnitude of endocrine effects of adjuvant chemotherapy for premenopausal breast cancer patients. Ann Oncol 1: 183–188

International Breast Cancer Study Group (1990) Late effects of adjuvant oophorectomy and chemotherapy upon premenopausal breast cancer patients. Ann Oncol 1: 30–35

Ludwig Breast Cancer Study Group (1985a) Chemotherapy with or without oophorectomy in high-risk premenopausal patients with operable breast cancer. J Clin Oncol 3: 1059–1067

Ludwig Breast Cancer Study Group (1985b) A randomized trial of adjuvant combination chemotherapy with or without prednisone in premenopausal breast cancer patients metastases in one to three axillary lymph nodes. Cancer Res 45: 4454–4459

Padmanabhan N, Howel A, Rubens RD (1986) Mechanism of action of adjuvant chemotherapy in early breast cancer. Lancet 11: 411–414

Richards MA, O'Reilly SM, Howell A, Rubens RD (1990) Adjuvant CMF in node positive breast cancer: Guy's/Manchester trial at 8 years. J Clin Oncol 8: 2032–2039

Rose D, Davis TE (1980) Effects of adjuvant chemo-hormonal therapy on the ovarian and adrenal function of breast cancer patients. Cancer Res 40: 4043–4047

Samman NA, DeAsis DN, Buzdar AV, Blumenschein GR (1978) Pituitary – ovarian function in breast cancer patients on adjuvant chemotherapy. Cancer 41: 2084–2087

Tormey DC, Gray R, Gilchrist K et al (1990) Adjuvant chemohormonal therapy with cyclophosphamide, methotrexate, 5-fluorouracil, and prednisone (CMFP) or CMFP plus tamoxifen compared with CMF for premenopausal breast cancer patients. An Eastern Cooperative Oncology Group Trial. Cancer 65: 200–206

6 Chemotherapy for Node-Negative Breast Cancer

RICHARD J. EPSTEIN and I. CRAIG HENDERSON

CONTENTS

6.1	Introduction	43
6.2	Definition of Lymph Node-Negativity	43
6.2.1	Positive Lymph Nodes	43
6.2.2	Negative Lymph Nodes	44
6.3	Mechanisms of Adjuvant Chemotherapeutic Action	44
6.3.1	General Aspects of Cytotoxic Drug Action	44
6.3.2	Adjuvant Chemotherapeutic Action	44
6.3.3	Models Predicting Efficacy of Adjuvant Node-Negative Chemotherapy	45
6.3.3.1	Enhanced Curability	45
6.3.3.2	Diminishing Returns	45
6.3.3.3	Similar Proportions	45
6.4	Patient Benefit from Adjuvant Chemotherapy	46
6.4.1	Clinical Studies	46
6.4.2	Optimal Scheduling of Adjuvant Chemotherapy	46
6.4.3	Cost-Effectiveness	48
6.5	Toxicity of Adjuvant Chemotherapy	48
6.5.1	Short-Term Toxicity	48
6.5.2	Long-Term Toxicity	49
6.6	Prognostic Factors in Node-Negative Disease	49
6.6.1	Prognostic Algorithms	49
6.6.1.1	Flow Cytometry	49
6.6.1.2	Cathepsin D	50
6.6.2	Disease Aggression and Therapeutic Benefit	50
6.6.2.1	Hormone Receptor Status	50
6.6.2.2	Expression of c-*erb*B-2	51
6.7	New Horizons in Adjuvant Node-Negative Chemotherapy	51
6.7.1	Node Dissection	51
6.7.2	Clinical Protocols	52
6.8	Conclusion	52
	References	53

RICHARD J. EPSTEIN, M. D., Instructor in Medicine, Harvard Medical School, Attending Physician, Breast Evaluation Clinic, Dana-Farber Cancer Institute, 44 Binney Street, Boston, MA 02115, USA; I. CRAIG HENDERSON, M. D., Professor of Medicine, Chief, Medical Oncology, Director, Clinical Oncology Program, UCSF Cancer Center, Mount Zion USF Medical Center, 505 Parnassus Avenue, San Francisco, CA 94143, USA

6.1 Introduction

The role of adjuvant cytotoxic therapy in lymph node-negative disease remains an ongoing debate in breast cancer management. The data base for this discussion has been greatly strengthened in recent years by the publication of several large overviews of adjuvant systemic breast cancer therapy, the most recent of which analyzes results from randomized studies of 75000 women (EARLY BREAST CANCER TRIALISTS' COLLABORATIVE GROUP 1992). In this chapter we present some of the issues related to these new data in an effort to help individual physicians assess for themselves the current status of adjuvant chemotherapy for node-negative premenopausal breast cancer patients.

6.2 Definition of Lymph Node-Negativity

6.2.1 Positive Lymph Nodes

To appreciate what is meant by the term 'node-negative,' it is useful first to consider what is understood by the designation of node-positive breast cancer. According to conventional tumor biology, spread of primary neoplasia to neighboring lymph nodes constitutes metastatic disease; the presence of these regional metastases correlates positively with subsequent development of distant disease (KOSCIELNY et al. 1989). Survival improvements related to surgical resection of the axilla have proven difficult to detect (FISHER et al. 1985a), although it remains possible that a small proportion of patients gain survival benefit from this procedure. Nonetheless, these and other empiric observations (FISHER et al. 1980, 1991; CUZICK et al. 1987) are consistent with the broad notion that breast cancer is a systemic disease, the outcome of which is largely unaffected by local measures (FISHER et al. 1980; KOSCIELNY et al. 1989).

At first glance, this paradigm seems inconsistent with a number of clinical observations. Chief among these is the finding that up to 30% of newly diagnosed breast cancer patients with established axillary lymph node involvement (i.e., systemic involvement) will enjoy long-term survival and perhaps cure (EARLY BREAST CANCER TRIALISTS' COLLABORATIVE GROUP 1992). This paradox is reinforced by the results of the National Surgical Adjuvant Breast and Bowel Project (NSABP) B-04 study which demonstrated that only 18% of clinically node-negative patients treated with mastectomy alone required treatment for axillary recurrence after 10 years of follow-up, even though 40% of a matched randomized cohort were found to have lymph node involvement at initial axillary dissection (FISHER et al. 1985a). Hence, there appear to be distinct biologic subsets concealed beneath the blanket designation of 'node-positive disease' (ADAIR et al. 1974).

6.2.2 *Negative Lymph Nodes*

The presence or absence of macroscopic tumor spread to the resected axillary lymph glands is the single strongest predictor of breast cancer outcome (SHEK and GODOLPHIN 1988). Despite the relatively strong predictive power of this feature, however, approximately 30% of node-negative patients remain destined to die from their disease (HAAGENSEN 1977). How can a patient have negative lymph nodes yet still succumb to metastatic disease? At least three possibilities exist:

1. Tumor cell metastases may selectively bypass (i.e., fail to seed) the axillary lymphatics in some patients (CARTER et al. 1989), reflecting either anatomic considerations (KOSCIELNY et al. 1989) or the existence of specific cell-surface 'homing receptors' mediating tumor organotropism (BENCHIMOI et al. 1989; GÜNTHERT et al. 1991);
2. True-positive lymph nodes may not be dissected out during a limited operation (DANFORTH et al. 1986); or
3. Routine histochemistry may be insufficiently sensitive to detect occult lymph node micrometastases.

It is interesting to note that this last hypothesis gained little support from early studies. HUVOS et al. (1971) reported a 94% 8-year survival for patients with axillary micrometastases (defined as nodal deposits less than 2 mm in diameter) compared with 82% for 'true' node-negative and 62% for conventional (macrometastatic) node-positive patients. Similarly, FISHER et al. (1978) found no significant survival difference between patients with 'true' node-negative disease and those with axillary micrometastases. In contrast, a more recent study has suggested that occult nodal metastases are strongly predictive of reduced disease-free and overall survival ($p = 0.003$ and 0.002, respectively, after 5 years of follow-up) (INTERNATIONAL LUDWIG BREAST CANCER STUDY GROUP 1990). The true prognostic significance of axillary node micrometastases therefore appears unresolved at the present time.

Like 'node-positive,' the term 'node-negative' is best regarded as a relative rather than an absolute concept: some node-positive tumors behave like typical node-negatives, while a similar proportion of node-negative tumors behave like typical node-positives. This raises the possibility that the early phases of tumor cell dissemination and metastatic growth may prove to be less critical in dictating disease outcome than is presently assumed – a point particularly relevant to the understanding of adjuvant chemotherapeutic action.

6.3 Mechanisms of Adjuvant Chemotherapeutic Action

6.3.1 *General Aspects of Cytotoxic Drug Action*

Precisely how cytotoxic chemotherapy works in established disease is not known (EPSTEIN 1990). Drug-induced deoxyribonucleic acid (DNA) damage is the most readily measurable association of cytotoxicity in experimental systems, but the genetic material is by no means an exclusive drug target (TRITTON and YEE 1982; PIEPER et al. 1989). The biochemical basis for combination drug synergy (GOLDIN 1984; LOTAN and NICOLSON 1988) is little better understood today than a decade ago. Selective targeting of drug toxicity to tumor cells continues to elude clinical investigators, while the varying chemosensitivity of different tumor types remains largely unexplained (WELCH 1987). These uncertainties invite caution in ascribing explanations for the efficacy of cytotoxic therapy in the setting of measurable neoplastic disease.

6.3.2 *Adjuvant Chemotherapeutic Action*

How chemotherapy exerts its effect in the adjuvant setting is even less clear. From a hypothetical standpoint, such therapy may exert its action via any of several mechanisms:

- Direct tumor cytoreduction (CHAN and SCHECHTER 1989);
- Induction of tumor cell 'differentiation' (TEILLAUD et al. 1989; BRAMBILLA 1991);
- Abrogation of hormone-dependent tumor growth via hormonal suppression (DNISTRIAN et al. 1983; BRINCKER et al. 1987); or
- Destruction of mitogen-secreting mesenchymal cells within the tumor microenvironment (CULLEN et al. 1991; ARTEAGA et al. 1989).

Of these candidate mechanisms, the one which has been most keenly debated is the endocrine alternative; this issue is reviewed in detail in Chap. 5 in this volume and elsewhere (EPSTEIN 1988). The relative contributions of the remaining mechanisms remain unknown. Perhaps the most intriguing of these is the last-mentioned one, since numerous lines of evidence implicate paracrine regulatory pathways in the control of human breast tumor cell growth (RO et al. 1989a; PERES et al. 1987; BASSET et al. 1990). Such a mechanism might be expected to contribute to prolongation of disease-free interval in the adjuvant setting, and/or palliative tumor 'responses' without improved survival in the metastatic setting. While there have been some negative studies consistent with the latter expectation (POWLES et al. 1980), others have suggested that chemoresponsiveness of advanced disease is associated with significant survival prolongation (A'HERN et al. 1988; FALKSON et al. 1991). Survival improvement in disseminated disease may thus contribute to the observation that survival differences in adjuvant studies are only about half as large as the disease-free survival differences (EARLY BREAST CANCER TRIALISTS' COLLABORATIVE GROUP 1992), since control groups may derive survival benefit from treatment after relapse.

6.3.3 *Models Predicting Efficacy of Adjuvant Node-Negative Chemotherapy*

6.3.3.1 Enhanced Curability

The average node-negative patient appears to have a smaller tumor burden than the average node-positive patient (CARTER et al. 1989; KOSCIELNY et al. 1984). This observation is consistent with the hypothesis that node-negative patients fated to suffer recurrence are intrinsically more curable by adjuvant therapy than are their node-positive counterparts (COOPER 1991). Preclinical studies support this line of reasoning. Less advanced lesions tend to be better vascularized, with consequent enhancements of oxygenation, cytotoxic drug delivery, and chemosensitivity (RICE et al. 1986). Gompertzian models of cancer cell kinetics also predict that higher growth fractions will accompany smaller tumor volumes (MENDELSOHN 1960). Such enhancements of growth fraction are associated with marked tumor cell chemosensitization in vitro (WEICHSELBAUM et al. 1978; EPSTEIN et al. 1989). A weakness of this argument is that its central premise of smaller total body tumor burden in the critical subset of 'false-negative' node-negative patients is empirically unsupported. Furthermore, early tumor detection improves cancer-specific mortality by only 25% following local therapy for breast cancer (EDDY 1989) and has not been proven to enhance therapeutic outcome in some other malignancies (CHILVERS et al. 1989).

6.3.3.2 Diminishing Returns

The most pessimistic view of node-negative chemotherapy holds that recurrent disease in node-negative patients is typically less aggressive than that seen in a matched recurrent node-positive cohort. Such reductions in tumor aggression might reasonably be expected to be associated with a more benevolent natural history (hence a smaller capacity for therapeutic benefit) as well as with lower tumor growth fractions (with consequent reductions in chemosensitivity, as discussed above); both of these factors might be anticipated to reduce, or even abnegate, the extent of therapeutic benefit. Hence, this view is diametrically opposed to the biologic differences forecast by the 'enhanced curability' model; its weakness is that it elects to deny the in vivo possibility that less advanced (smaller volume) tumors may actually exhibit greater chemosensitivity than their node-positive (larger volume) counterparts, perhaps even to the extent of overshadowing the projected therapeutic disadvantage of having a smaller contingent at risk.

6.3.3.3 Similar Proportions

A third line of reasoning is that node-negative tumors destined to recur are best regarded as 'occult' node-positive tumors which have been misdiagnosed, and that recurrent node-negative and

Table 6.1. Comparison of therapeutic efficacy in node-positive and node-negative breast cancer patient subsets treated with adjuvant cytotoxic therapy

Number of positive nodes[a]	Number of patients[a]	Reduction in annual odds			
		Recurrence[a]		Death[a]	
		%	SD	%	SD
0	2833	29	6	16	8
1-3	2244	29	6	18	7
4 +	1424	24	4	13	8

[a] Test for trend $p > 0.1$

node-positive disease are thus biologically and therapeutically similar entities. Hence, if adjuvant chemotherapy prevents a quarter of the 70% of node-positive patients from recurring – thus conferring an absolute benefit on 17.5% of all patients treated – then this line of reasoning predicts that chemotherapy for node-negative disease will benefit a quarter of 30%, or 7.5%. In contrast to the other models presented, this model derives strong support from data provided by overviews of randomized clinical studies (Table 6.1). Indeed, the Early Breast Cancer Trialists' Collaborative Group concluded, with respect to both disease-free and overall survival, that 'nodal status has little effect on the proportional risk reductions produced by tamoxifen and by polychemotherapy, both of which are highly significant even for node-negative patients ($p < 0.0001$)' (Early Breast Cancer Trialists' Collaborative Group 1992). Hence, adjuvant chemotherapy appears to have similar relative efficacy in node-negative and node-positive patients.

6.4 Patient Benefit from Adjuvant Chemotherapy

6.4.1 Clinical Studies

Early studies of adjuvant chemotherapy for stage I breast cancer yielded mixed results (Nissen-Meyer et al. 1978; Seminglazov et al. 1985), but interpretation of these results is confounded by use of single agents, suboptimal treatment duration, or both. One subsequent study reported a dramatic treatment-related survival benefit in a small group of node-negative patients who experienced disease-free survival at 6 years of 88% compared with 46% in the control arm (Bonadonna et al. 1987). However, the unexpectedly poor outcome of the control group in this study has cast doubt upon the generalizability of these results. More recently, several studies of node-negative chemotherapy have been published in which the results are impressively concordant. Four large studies were published in 1989 (Fisher et al. 1989; Mansour et al. 1989; Ludwig Breast Cancer Study Group 1989; Morrison et al. 1989); of these, three reported significant prolongation of disease-free survival (with the weakest results yielding $p < 0.004$), but not overall survival (Fisher et al. 1989; Mansour et al. 1989; Ludwig Breast Cancer Study Group 1989). These similarities are particularly striking given that patient selection criteria and protocol designs were quite different in these studies. With respect to the latter point, the most impressive enhancement of disease-free survival occurred in the study with the greatest toxicity (Mansour et al. 1989). In contrast, the negative trial failed to detect any improvement in disease-free survival 7 years following adjuvant therapy of node-negative disease (Morrison et al. 1989). This apparent inconsistency may be explained by the substitution of chlorambucil for cyclophosphamide in this study (although randomized data do not as yet support this explanation; Senn et al. 1989), or else by the finding that node-negative patients with worse prognostic features tend to be included in some studies of adjuvant chemotherapy (Henderson et al. 1990). More likely than either of these explanations, however, is the fact that the absolute benefit of adjuvant chemotherapy in node-negative disease is quite small (Early Breast Cancer Trialists' Collaborative Group 1992) and could thus go undetected due to the play of chance in a single study. Pooled results from a recent overview of randomized outcome data are shown in Fig. 6.1, confirming a small but significant benefit of therapeutic intervention in this context.

6.4.2 Optimal Scheduling of Adjuvant Chemotherapy

Palliation of metastatic breast cancer may be prejudiced by administration of low-dose as opposed to full-dose cytotoxic therapy (Bonadonna and Valagussa 1981; Tannock et al. 1988). Extrapolation from these and similar data might logically suggest that high-dose treatment will produce analogous therapeutic improvements over results achievable using standard regimens (De Vita 1986; Hryniuk 1988). Although some preliminary studies

Recurrence (all ages) in polychemotherapy trials

Annual rates in		years 0–4	years 5–9 (or 5+)	years 10+
N neg	Cytotoxic	6 06 % SD 0 37	4 08 % SD 0 51	
	Control	8 50 % SD 0 44	3 99 % SD 0 52	
N pos	Cytotoxic	12 70 % SD 0 32	6 98 % SD 0 44	5 57 % SD 0 94
	Control	17 82 % SD 0 41	8 37 % SD 0 54	4 98 % SD 1 11

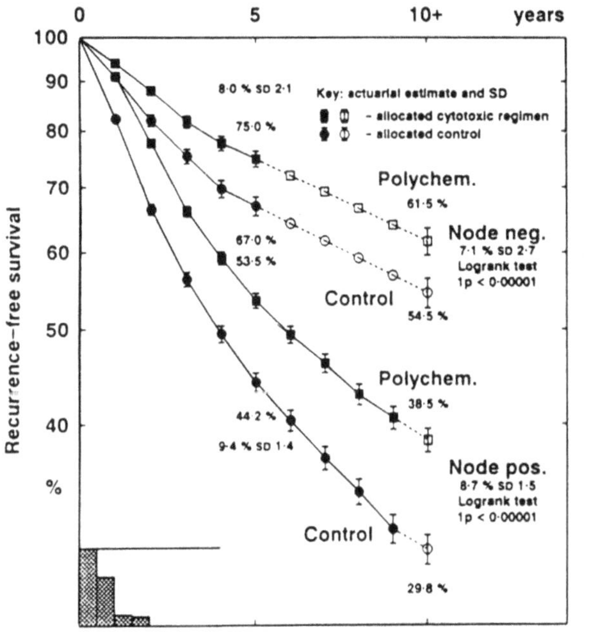

Mortality (all ages) in polychemotherapy trials

Annual rates in		years 0–4	years 5–9 (or 5+)	years 10+
N neg	Cytotoxic	3 23 % SD 0 26	4.59 % SD 0 49	
	Control	3 99 % SD 0 29	4 85 % SD 0 52	
N pos	Cytotoxic	7 47 % SD 0 23	7 47 % SD 0 40	4 94 % SD 0 79
	Control	8 73 % SD 0 26	9 90 % SD 0 49	7 65 % SD 1 14

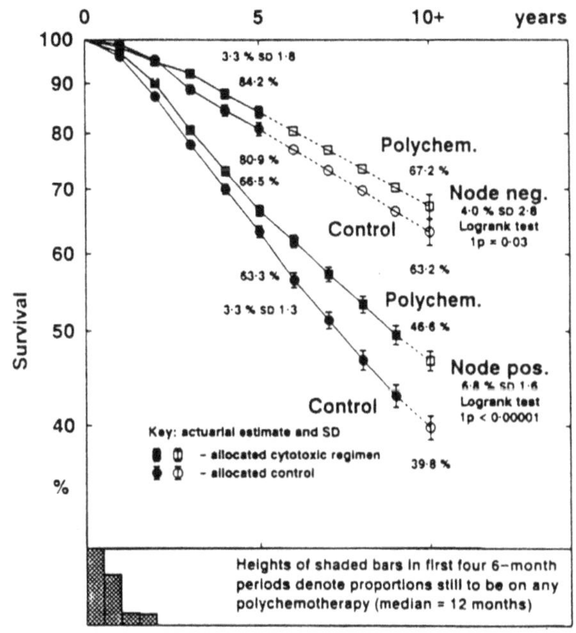

Fig. 6.1. Overview of disease-free and overall survival outcomes in node-positive and node-negative breast cancer patients managed with or without adjuvant chemotherapy (From Early Breast Cancer Trialists' Collaborative Group 1992, with permission).

of adjuvant dose-intensive chemotherapy failed to detect a significant survival benefit when compared with standard-dose therapy (Richards et al. 1990; Ang et al. 1989), larger studies are needed to resolve this issue. It has been pointed out that dose-intensity per se may prove to be less critical than the relative intensities of drugs administered in combination (Gelman 1990), and a benefit for high-dose therapy may yet emerge in some therapeutic scenarios, including the adjuvant setting. Routine use of this approach for node-negative patients does not appear justified by published data at the present time, however. Whether inclusion of doxorubicin (Adriamycin) in cytotoxic regimens significantly improves the outcome of adjuvant chemotherapy in node-negative patients also remains uncertain. What is clear from overview analysis is that many varieties of polychemotherapy confer greater benefit than single-agent therapy; in contrast, prolonged course of adjuvant chemotherapy following mastectomy, venous thromboembolic events occurred chemotherapy of standard (6-month) duration (Early Breast Cancer Trialists' Collaborative Group 1992). This negative result may be pertinent to optimization of patient quality-of-life, since durations of adjuvant therapy exceeding 6 months have been associated with substantial increases in psychiatric morbidity when compared with shorter durations (Hughson et al. 1986).

How is adjuvant chemotherapy best combined with other therapeutic modalities in the node-negative setting? Combination chemohormonal therapy has not yet been proven to produce a substantial survival advantage for patients with advanced breast cancer (Australian and New Zealand Breast Cancer Trials Group 1986), and in vitro data raise the possibility that such combinations may be therapeutically counterproductive if administered simultaneously (Hug et al. 1985; Osborne et al. 1989). In the adjuvant setting, however, overview analysis has suggested a substantial reduction in the odds of death associated with the sequential combination of chemotherapy and either oophorectomy or tamoxifen in premenopausal women with stage II disease (Early Breast Cancer Trialists' Collaborative Group 1992). The implications of these data for routine management of node-negative disease are not yet clear. Optimal scheduling of adjuvant chemotherapy with respect to radiation therapy similarly remains an open debate. A recent retrospective analysis indicated that node-positive patients in whom adjuvant radiation was delayed until completion of chemotherapy sustained a higher incidence of local recurrence than did patients treated with initial radiation (RECHT et al. 1991). Again, it remains premature to extrapolate these nonrandomized results to the routine management of node-negative patients.

6.4.3 Cost-Effectiveness

A major advance in cancer therapy over the last decade has been the finding that treatment of node-positive premenopausal breast cancer patients with adjuvant chemotherapy confers a 20% to 25% relative mortality reduction in patients followed for 10 years (EARLY BREAST CANCER TRIALISTS' COLLABORATIVE GROUP 1992). At an all-inclusive cost of less than $5000 for an average 6-month course, such treatment may now constitute one of the most cost-effective interventions in contemporary medical practice (EPSTEIN 1992). As alluded to above, the 1992 Early Breast Cancer Trialists' Collaborative Group overview indicated that chemotherapy of premenopausal patients with node-negative disease is associated with moderate absolute improvement of 10-year disease-free survival (7.1% $\pm$ 2.7%) and small increments in overall survival (4.0% $\pm$ 2.8%) (EARLY BREAST CANCER TRIALISTS' COLLABORATIVE GROUP 1992) (Fig. 6.1). Do these improvements in disease-free survival constitute a valid end point for toxic and expensive therapy? Patients may perceive this to be the case and choose such therapy notwithstanding the expectation that overall survival is only marginally affected. The theoretical cost of such therapy has been estimated by one group to be approximately $50 000 per quality-adjusted life year (QALY) assuming improved disease-free but not overall survival (HILLNER and SMITH 1991). Reliable calculations of cost-effectiveness in this context, however, will require many years of follow-up (and, in particular, disease-related deaths) to provide more precise quantitative evaluation of long-term benefits and toxicities.

6.5 Toxicity of Adjuvant Chemotherapy

The importance of confirming a net quality-of-life benefit conferred by palliative chemotherapy has been widely acknowledged in recent years (RUBENS 1990). As daunting as the task of converting subjective patient data into objective clinical research is, performing such audits in the adjuvant node-negative context poses even more complex methodologic difficulties. Since these patients by definition have no symptoms to palliate, and since most have good prognoses even without systemic therapy, accurate quantitation of both short- and long-term toxicities is all the more critical to an evaluation of net therapeutic benefit. For the purposes of this discussion it will be assumed that such toxicity is identical in node-positive and node-negative subjects.

6.5.1 Short-Term Toxicity

Adjuvant chemotherapeutic toxicities are often unanticipated by patients. One distressing and unexpected side effect occurring in up to 45% of patients is weight gain (LOVE et al. 1989; HUNTINGTON 1985; HEASMAN et al. 1985). Fatigue, which was judged in one series to be the worst-tolerated side effect of adjuvant breast cancer chemotherapy (KNOBF 1986), affected 59% of patients in this study yet was anticipated by only 8% (LOVE et al. 1989). Similarly, hair loss was anticipated by 44% of patients, but was experienced by 89% (LOVE et al. 1989). This same study confirmed that nausea, vomiting, and hair loss occur significantly more often with doxorubicin-based regimens than with cyclophosphamide, methotrexate, and 5-fluorouracil (CMF)-based ones ($p < 0.01$). Recent pediatric studies of patients treated with anthracycline have also generated concern regarding delayed expression of myocardial toxicity 10–20 years after doxorubicin use, a complication previously assumed to be evident during or soon after therapy (LIPSHULTZ et al. 1991; YEUNG et al. 1991). On the positive side, one study reported a nonsignificant trend towards lower patient anxiety in a cohort undergoing chemotherapy than in randomized controls with no treatment (CASSILETH et al. 1986). One serious complication of adjuvant chemotherapy which has only recently been recognized is arterial thrombosis (HEALEY et al. 1987; DONALDSON et al. 1990), a potentially devastating event which may be related to cytotoxic-induced alterations in blood coagulability (ROGERS et al. 1988; BALDWIN and COSGRIFF 1985). This development has been reported in as many as 1%–2% of patients undergoing adjuvant therapy (WALL et al. 1989). In another study of 433 patients treated with a 2-year course of adjuvant chemotherapy following mastectomy, venous thromboembolic events occurred in 5% (WEISS et al. 1981). These considerations emphasize that the decision to prescribe adjuvant chemotherapy is not a casual one, particularly in node-negative patients with additional good prognostic features.

6.5.2 *Long-Term Toxicity*

Unlike adjuvant tamoxifen (McDONALD and STEWART 1991), adjuvant chemotherapy remains unable to boast beneficial nononcologic side effects – with the occasional exception, perhaps, of minor effects such as improved psoriasis. A particular concern has been the development of second malignancies (especially leukemias) in response to mutagenesis induced by cytotoxicity, a phenomenon well-recognized following use of alkylating agents for other malignancies (KALDOR 1990). The literature concerning this complication in the adjuvant setting is conflicting, with different studies reporting markedly increased (FISHER et al. 1985b; ANDERSSON et al. 1990), unchanged (VALAGUSSA et al. 1987), or dramatically reduced (HORTOBAGYI et al. 1986; ARRIAGADA and RUTQVIST 1991) incidences of second malignancy. Of these studies, the association of leukemia with adjuvant L-phenylalanine mustard (L-PAM, melphalan) is perhaps the most striking (FISHER et al. 1985b). The Danish study reported a 7% incidence of leukemic transformation within the first 37 months following initiation of chemotherapy (5 of 71 patients), representing a 339-fold increased relative risk of leukemia (ANDERSSON et al. 1990). In the Italian study, no cases of acute leukemia were seen in a cohort of 666 patients treated with CMF and followed for more than 10 years; the cumulative frequency of solid tumor development was the same in patients treated with CMF as in controls treated with surgery alone (4.2% versus 4.0%) (VALAGUSSA et al. 1987). Recently, however, a French study has reported a 10-year 5%–6% incidence of new primary malignancies in 509 patients treated with adjuvant radiotherapy and 1986 patients treated with surgery alone, compared with only a 1% incidence in 604 patients randomized to receive adjuvant chemotherapy (ARRIAGADA and RUTQVIST 1991); as in the Italian report, no leukemias occurred in any treatment subset. These latter results echo the findings of an earlier publication which reported a 1.3% incidence of second malignancy in patients treated with adjuvant cyclophosphamide, Adriamycin, and 5-fluorouracil (CAF) compared with 4.8% in historical controls (HORTOBAGYI et al. 1986). Hence, the literature concerning second malignancies following adjuvant chemotherapy remains little more conclusive than 5 years ago (HENDERSON and GELMAN 1987).

A controversy brewing over the widespread use of adjuvant node-negative chemotherapy in American women relates to the induction of premature menopause in many of these patients. Chemotherapy induces amenorrhea in 80% of premenopausal patients; for patients younger than 40 years, this development is irreversible in 50%, whereas for patients aged over 40 years rendered amenorrheic, fewer than 10% will menstruate again (HORTOBAGYI et al. 1986). The possibility of this complication in node-negative breast cancer patients who have not completed childbearing mandates serious discussion.

6.6 Prognostic Factors in Node-Negative Disease

There are two general strategies for improving the therapeutic index of a given intervention: improve efficacy and reduce toxicity. In the case of node-negative breast cancer, most efforts have been focused on reducing toxicity; as will be discussed, however, this strategy cannot necessarily be pursued in isolation from the first. The most straightforward approach to reducing chemotherapeutic toxicity for node-negative patients is to identify the patient subset which is most likely (or least likely) to benefit from treatment.

6.6.1 *Prognostic Algorithms*

Much enthusiasm exists for developing a breast tumor 'prognostic index' based on available biologic parameters (McGUIRE et al. 1990; LEVINE et al. 1991; TODD et al. 1987; HOLLAND and VERBEEK 1990). Indeed, the American Joint Committee on Cancer (AJCC) is reportedly already in the process of developing an electronic pocket-sized staging apparatus (WINCHESTER 1991). While long-term prospective randomized studies remain the empirical gold standard of clinical research, no such data have yet been published. Numerous retrospective studies have been published, however, which provide hypotheses for prospective testing.

6.6.1.1 Flow Cytometry

Relatively few studies have assessed the value of flow cytometry in node-negative disease. Although studies of tumor DNA ploidy in this patient subpopulation have produced inconsistent results (Fallenius et al. 1988; Muss et al. 1989), the largest flow cytometric study of node-negative patients demonstrated both ploidy and S-phase fraction to be important predictors of disease-free and overall survival in this cohort (Clark et al. 1989). This retrospective analysis of 345 frozen tumor specimens documented a probability of 5-year disease-free survival of 88% in patients with diploid tumors and 74% in patients with aneuploid tumors. S-phase fraction was not significantly associated with disease-free survival in patients with aneuploid tumors, but a highly significant association was documented in those with diploid tumors (Clark et al. 1989).

6.6.1.2 Cathepsin D

Cathepsin D is an estrogen-dependent intracellular protease which is commonly overexpressed in human breast cancer cells (Capony et al. 1989). In vitro data have confirmed that overexpression plays a pathogenic role in modulating the malignant phenotype of affected cells (Garcia et al. 1990), while in vivo expression has been retrospectively correlated with tumor metastatic propensity (Thorpe et al. 1989). Some of the inconsistencies in the literature on cathepsin D appear to reflect differences in monoclonal antibody-based detection assays. One study, for example, reported a correlation between this marker and adverse prognosis in node-negative but not node-positive patients (Tandon et al. 1990), while another reported a similar correlation in node-positive but not node-negative patients (Namer et al. 1989). Still other studies have reported significant associations of cathepsin D expression with improved prognosis in both node-positive (Henry et al. 1990) and node-negative disease (Granata et al. 1991); in the latter study, co-expression of estrogen receptors (ER) and cathepsin D correlated with significant improvements in both disease-free ($p = 0.02$) and overall survival ($p = 0.01$). Provided that assay techniques can be standardized, however, measurement of cathepsin D remains a promising marker for future studies in node-negative disease.

The status of other prognostic factors is discussed below and elsewhere in this review, but some readers may find a more comprehensive discussion helpful (McGuire et al. 1990; Henderson 1991). Although beyond the scope of this review, many other markers have shown promise as prognostic indicators: these include epidermal growth factor receptors, heat-shock proteins, haptoglobin-related proteins, laminin receptors, factor VIII immunocytochemistry, and tumor glycosylation (Brooks and Leathem 1991). However, the extent to which such molecular markers predict chemotherapeutic benefit – as opposed to disease aggression per se – remains an issue infrequently addressed.

6.6.2 Disease Aggression and Therapeutic Benefit

Whether adjuvant chemotherapy offers maximal benefit to those node-negative patients in greatest jeopardy of recurrence remains conjectural. Retrospective analyses such as those described above may provide strong circumstantial evidence implicating a particular clinical feature with disease aggression and, in so doing, help define high-risk patient subsets within the node-negative population; if this approach is able to be implemented with sufficient precision, therapeutic toxicity may be reduced. This is not synonymous with identifying a patient subset which will benefit from therapy, however, since it is possible that those very factors conferring the aggressive-disease phenotype may also confer chemotherapeutic resistance. This issue has been addressed in the metastatic setting, where it has been found that rapidly proliferating tumors with high S-phase fractions (Remvikos et al. 1989), tritiated thymidine uptake (Sulkes et al. 1979), or thymidine kinase levels (Zhang et al. 1984) tend to have higher response rates, albeit often associated with shorter response durations (Remvikos et al. 1989). While no such studies are yet available in the adjuvant setting, such caveats may be worth keeping in mind.

6.6.2.1 Hormone Receptor Status

Many reports have implicated ER negativity as a marker of tumor aggression (Blamey et al. 1980; Knight et al. 1977). Receptor-positive patients tend to outlive their receptor-negative counterparts (Huseby et al. 1988), perhaps in part due to superior hormone-responsiveness following development of distant disease (Blanco et al. 1984; Goldhirsch et al. 1988). A number of small studies have suggested that disease-free survival following initial diagnosis may be unaffected by hormone receptor status (Huseby et al. 1988; Caldarola et al. 1986;

References

A'Hern RP, Ebbs SR, Baum MB (1988) Does chemotherapy improve survival in advanced breast cancer? A statistical overview. Br J Cancer 57: 615–618

Adair F, Berg J, Joubert L, Robbins GF (1974) Long-term follow-up of breast cancer patients: the 30-year report. Cancer 33: 1145–1150

Alanko A, Heinonen E, Scheinin TM et al (1984) Oestrogen and progesterone receptors and disease-free interval in primary breast cancer. Br J Cancer 50: 667–672

Ali IU, Campbell G, Lidereau R, Callahan R (1988) Amplification of c-*erb*B-2 and aggressive human breast tumors? Science 240: 1795–1796

Andersson M, Philip P, Pedersen-Bjergaard J (1990) High risk of therapy-related leukemia and preleukemia after therapy with prednimustine, methotrexate, 5-fluorouracil, mitoxantrone, and tamoxifen for advanced breast cancer. Cancer 65: 2460–2464

Ang P, Buzdar AU, Smith TL et al (1989) Analysis of dose intensity in doxorubicin-containing adjuvant chemotherapy in stage II and III breast carcinoma. J Clin Oncol 7: 1677–1684

Arriagada R, Rutqvist LE (1991) Adjuvant chemotherapy in early breast cancer and incidence of new primary malignancies. Lancet 338: 535

Arteaga CL, Kitten LJ, Coronado EB et al (1989) Blockade of the type I somatomedin receptor inhibits growth of human breast cancer cells in athymic mice. J Clin Invest 84: 1418–1423

Australian and New Zealand Breast Cancer Trials Group (1986) A randomized trial in postmenopausal patients with advanced breast cancer comparing endocrine and cytotoxic therapy given sequentially or in combination. J Clin Oncol 4: 186–193

Baldwin P, Cosgriff T (1985) Anti-thrombin III levels during adjuvant CMF therapy. Proc Am Soc Clin Oncol 4: 63

Basset P, Bellocq JP, Wolf C et al (1990) A novel metalloproteinase gene specifically expressed in stromal cells of breast carcinomas. Nature 348: 699–704

Belanger D, Moore M, Tannock I (1991) How American oncologists treat breast cancer: an assessment of the influence of clinical trials. J Clin Oncol 9: 7–16

Benchimoi S, Fuks A, Jothy S et al (1989) Carcinoembryonic antigen, a human tumor marker, functions as an intercellular adhesion molecule. Cell 57: 327–334

Benner SE, Clark GM, McGuire WL (1988) Steroid receptors, cellular kinetics, and lymph node status as prognostic factors in breast cancer. Am J Med Sci 296: 59–66

Blamey RW, Bishop HM, Blake JRS (1980) Relationship between primary breast tumor receptor status and patient survival. Cancer 46: 2765–2769

Blanco G, Alavaikko M, Ojala A et al (1984) Estrogen and progesterone receptors in breast cancer: relationships to tumor histopathology and survival of patients. Anticancer Res 4: 383–390

Bonadonna G, Valagussa P (1981) Dose response effect of adjuvant chemotherapy in breast cancer. N Engl J Med 304: 10–15

Bonadonna G, Valagussa P, Zambetti M et al (1987) Milan adjuvant trials for stage I–II breast cancer. In: Salmon SE (ed) Adjuvant therapy of cancer V. Grune and Stratton, New York

Borg A, Linell F, Idvall I et al (1989) HER-2/*neu* amplification and comedo type breast carcinoma. Lancet i: 1268–1269

Borg A, Tandon AK, Sigurdsson H et al (1990) HER-2/*neu* amplification predicts poor survival in node-positive breast cancer. Cancer Res 50: 4332–4337

Brambilla E, Moro S, Gazzeri S et al (1991) Cytotoxic chemotherapy induces cell differentiation in small-cell lung carcinoma. J Clin Oncol 9: 50–61

Brincker H, Rose C, Rank F et al (1987) Evidence of a castration-mediated effect of adjuvant cytotoxic chemotherapy in premenopausal breast cancer. J Clin Oncol 5: 1771–1778

Brooks SA, Leathem AJC (1991) Prediction of lymph node involvement in breast cancer by detection of altered glycosylation in the primary tumor. Lancet 338: 71–74

Caldarola L, Volterrani P, Caldarola B et al (1986) The influence of hormone receptors and hormonal adjuvant therapy on disease-free survival in breast cancer: a multifactorial analysis. Eur J Cancer Clin Oncol 22: 151–155

Capony F, Rougeot P, Montcourrier V et al (1989) Increased secretion, altered processing, and glycosylation of procathepsin D in human mammary cancer cells. Cancer Res 49: 3904–3909

Carter CL, Allen C, Henson DE (1989) Relation of tumor size, lymph node status, and survival in 24740 breast cancer cases. Cancer 63: 181–187

Cassileth BR, Knuiman MW, Abeloff MD et al (1986) Anxiety levels in patients randomized to adjuvant therapy versus observation for early breast cancer. J Clin Oncol 4: 972–974

Chan C, Schechter G (1989) In vitro evidence for dose-dependent cytotoxicity as the predominant effect of low dose ara-C on human leukemic and normal marrow cells. Cancer Chemother Pharmacol 23: 87–94

Chilvers CED, Saunders M, Bliss JM et al (1989) Influence of delay in diagnosis on prognosis in testicular teratoma. Br J Cancer 59: 126–128

Clark GM, Dressler LG, Owens MA et al (1989) Prediction of relapse or survival in patients with node-negative breast cancer by DNA flow cytometry. N Engl J Med 320: 627–633

Cohen JA, Weiner DB, More KF et al (1989) Expression pattern of the *neu* (NGL) gene-encoded growth factor receptor protein (p185^{neu}) in normal and transformed epithelial tissues of the digestive tract. Oncogene 4: 81–88

Cooper MR (1991) The role of chemotherapy for node-negative breast cancer. Cancer 67: 1744–1747

Cullen KJ, Smith HS, Hill S, Rosen N, Lippman ME (1991) Growth factor messenger RNA expression by human breast fibroblasts from benign and malignant lesions. Cancer Res 51: 4978–4985

Cuzick J, Stewart H, Peto R et al (1987) Overview of randomized trials comparing radical mastectomy without radiotherapy against simple mastectomy with radiotherapy in breast cancer. Cancer Treat Rep 71: 7–14

D'Emilia J, Bulovas K, D'Ercole K et al (1989) Expression of the c-*erb*B-2 gene product (p185) at different stages of neoplastic progression in the colon. Oncogene 4: 1233–1239

Danforth DN, Findlay PA, McDonald HD (1986) Complete axillary lymph node dissection for stage I–II carcinoma of the breast. J Clin Oncol 4: 655–662

Davis BW, Gelber R, Goldhirsch A et al (1985) Prognostic significance of peritumoral invasion in clinical trials of adjuvant therapy for breast cancer with axillary lymph node metastases. Hum Pathol 16: 1212–1218

De Vita VT (1986) Dose-response is alive and well. J Clin Oncol 4: 1157–1159
De Vita VT (1989) Breast cancer therapy: exercising all our options. N Engl J Med 320: 527–529
Dnistrian AM, Schwarz MK, Fracchia AA et al (1983) Endocrine consequences of CMF adjuvant therapy in premenopausal and postmenopausal breast cancer patients. Cancer 51: 803–807
Donaldson MC, Bettinger LA, Epstein R (1990) Acute arm ischemia associated with cervical ribs and adjuvant chemotherapy for breast cancer. J Vasc Med Biol 2: 86–89
Early Breast Cancer Trialists' Collaborative Group (1992) Systemic treatment of early breast cancer by hormonal, cytotoxic, or immune therapy. Lancet 339: 1–15, 71–85
Eddy DM (1989) Screening for breast cancer. Ann Intern Med 111: 389–399
Epstein RJ (1988) The clinical biology of hormone-responsive breast cancer. Cancer Treat Rev 15: 33–51
Epstein RJ (1990) Drug-induced DNA damage and tumor chemosensitivity. J Clin Oncol 8: 2062–2084
Epstein RJ (1992) Does the breast cancer dollar make sense? Eur J Cancer 28: 486–491
Epstein R, Watson J, Smith P, Bleehen N (1989) Oestrogen enhances topisomerase II synthesis in an activated G1-phase subset of human breast cancer cells. Int J Cancer 44: 501–505
Falkson G, Tormey DC, Cary P et al (1991) Long-term survival of patients treated with combination chemotherapy for metastatic breast cancer. Eur J Cancer 27: 973–977
Fallenius AG, Franzen SA, Auer GU (1988) Predictive value of nuclear DNA content in breast cancer in relation to clinical morphologic factors: a retrospective study of 227 consecutive cases. Cancer 62: 521–530
Fentiman IS, Mansel RE (1991) The axilla: not a no-go zone. Lancet 337: 221–223
Fisher B, Redmond CK, Fisher ER (1980) The contribution of NSABP trials of primary breast cancer therapy to an understanding of tumor biology: an overview of findings. Cancer 46: 1009–1025
Fisher B, Redmond C, Fisher ER et al (1985a) Ten-year results of a randomized clinical trial comparing radical mastectomy and total mastectomy with or without radiation. N Engl J Med 312: 674–681
Fisher B, Rockette H, Fisher ER et al (1985b) Leukemia in breast cancer patients following adjuvant chemotherapy or postoperative radiation: the NSABP experience. J Clin Oncol 3: 1640–1658
Fisher B, Redmond C, Fisher ER et al (1988) Relative worth of estrogen or progesterone receptor and pathologic characteristics of differentiation as indicators of prognosis in node negative breast cancer patients: findings from National Surgical Adjuvant Breast and Bowel Project Protocol B-06. J Clin Oncol 6: 1076–1087
Fisher B, Redmond C, Dimitrov NV et al (1989) A randomized clinical trial evaluating sequential methotrexate and fluorouracil in the treatment of patients with node-negative breast cancer who have estrogen-receptor negative tumors. N Engl J Med 320: 473–478
Fisher B, Anderson S, Fisher ER et al (1991) Significance of ipsilateral breast tumour recurrence after lumpectomy. Lancet 338: 327–331
Fisher ER, Sass R, Fisher B et al (1984) Pathologic findings from the NSABP for breast cancers (protocol no. 4). X. Discriminants of tenth year failure. Cancer 53: 712–723
Fisher ER, Swamidoss S, Lee CH (1978) Detection and significance of occult axillary lymph node metastases in patients with invasive breast cancer. Cancer 42: 2025–2031
Garcia M, Derocq D, Pujol P, Rochefort H (1990) Overexpression of transfected cathepsin D in transformed cells increases their malignant phenotype and metastatic potency. Oncogene 5: 1809–1814
Gelman RS (1990) Keeping an open mind about the doses of chemotherapy. JNCI 82: 6–7
Goldhirsch A, Gelber R, Castiglione M (1988) Relapse of breast cancer after adjuvant treatment in premenopausal and perimenopausal women: patterns and prognosis. J Clin Oncol 6: 89–97
Goldhirsch A, Gelber RD, Castiglione M (1990) The magnitude of endocrine effects of adjuvant chemotherapy for premenopausal breast cancer patients. Ann Oncol 1: 183–188
Goldin A (1984) Dosing and sequencing for antineoplastic synergism in combination chemotherapy. Cancer 54: 1155–1159
Granata G, Coradini D, Cappelletti V, DiFronzo G (1991) Prognostic relevance of cathepsin D versus oestrogen receptors in node-negative breast cancers. Eur J Cancer 27: 970–972
Günthert U, Hofmann M, Rudy W et al (1991) A new variant of glycoprotein CD44 confers metastatic potential to rat carcinoma cells. Cell 65: 13–24
Gusterson BA, Machin LG, Gullick WJ et al (1988) Immunohistochemical distribution of c-*erb*B-2 in infiltrating and in situ breast cancer. Int J Cancer 42: 842–845
Haagensen CD (1977) Treatment of curable carcinoma of the breast. Int J Radiat Biol Phys 2: 975–980
Haynes RB (1990) Loose connections between peer-reviewed clinical journals and clinical practice. Ann Intern Med 113: 724–728
Healey B, Tormey DC, Gray R et al (1987) Arterial and venous thrombotic events in ECOG adjuvant breast cancer trials. Proc Am Soc Clin Oncol 6: 54
Heasman KZ, Sutherland HJ, Campbell JA et al (1985) Weight gain during adjuvant chemotherapy for breast cancer. Breast Cancer Res Treat 5: 195–200
Hellman S, Hellman DS (1991) Of mice but not men: problems of the randomized clinical trial. N Engl J Med 324: 1585–1589
Henderson IC (1991) Prognostic factors. In: Harris JR, Hellman S, Henderson IC, Kinne DW (eds) Breast diseases. Lippincott, Philadelphia
lowing adjuvant chemotherapy? Too soon to tell. J Clin Oncol 5: 1135–1137
Henderson IC, Hayes DF, Parker LM et al (1990) Adjuvant systemic therapy for node-negative patients. Cancer 65: 2132–2147
Henry JA, McCarthy AL, Angus B et al (1990) Prognostic significance of the estrogen-related protein, cathepsin D, in breast cancer: an immunohistochemical study. Cancer 65: 265–271
Hillner BE, Smith TJ (1991) Efficacy and cost effectiveness of adjuvant chemotherapy in women with node-negative breast cancer: a decision-analysis model. N Engl J Med 324: 160–168
Holland R, Verbeek ALM (1990) Prognostic assessment in node-negative breast cancer patients. J Clin Oncol 8: 1451–1453
Hortobagyi GN, Buzdar AU, Marcus CE, Smith TL (1986) Immediate and long-term toxicity of adjuvant chemotherapy regimens containing doxorubicin in trials at MD Anderson Hospital and Tumor Institute. NCI Monogr 1: 105–109
Howell A, Barnes DM, Harland RNL et al (1984) Steroid hormone receptors and survival after first relapse in breast cancer. Lancet i: 588–591

Hryniuk WM (1988) More is better. J Clin Oncol 6: 1365–1367
Hug V, Hortobagyi GN, Drewinko B, Finders M (1985) Tamoxifen citrate counteracts the antitumor effects of cytotoxic drugs in vitro. J Clin Oncol 3: 1672–1677
Hughson AVM, Cooper AF, McArdle CS, Smith DC (1986) Psychological impact of adjuvant chemotherapy in the first two years after mastectomy. Br Med J 293: 1268–1272
Huntington MO (1985) Weight gain in patients receiving adjuvant chemotherapy for carcinoma of the breast. Cancer 56: 472–474
Huseby R, Ownby H, Frederick J et al (1988) Node-negative breast cancer treated by modified radical mastectomy without adjuvant therapies: variables associated with disease recurrence and survivorship. J Clin Oncol 6: 83–88
Huvos AG, Hutter RVP, Berg JW (1971) Significance of axillary macrometastases and micrometastases in mammary cancer. Ann Surg 173: 44–46
Iglehart JD, Kraus MH, Langton BC et al (1990) Increased *erb*B-2 gene copies and expression in multiple stages of breast cancer. Cancer Res 50: 6701–6707
International (Ludwig) Breast Cancer Study Group (1990) Prognostic importance of occult axillary lymph node micrometastases from breast cancers. Lancet 335: 1565–1568
Kaldor J (1990) Second cancer following chemotherapy and radiotherapy: an epidemiological perspective. Acta Oncol 29: 647–655
Knight WA, Livingston RB, Gregory EJ, McGuire WL (1977) Estrogen receptor as an independent prognostic factor for early recurrence in breast cancer. Cancer Res 37: 4669–4671
Knobf MT (1986) Physical and psychologic distress associated with adjuvant chemotherapy in women with breast cancer. J Clin Oncol 4: 678–684
Korn EL, Baumrind S (1991) Randomised clinical trials with clinician-preferred treatment. Lancet 337: 149–152
Koscielny S, Tubiana M, Le MG et al (1984) Breast cancer: relationship between the size of the primary tumour and the probability of metastatic dissemination. Br J Cancer 49: 709–715
Koscielny S, Le MG, Tubiana M (1989) The natural history of human breast cancer: the relationship between involvement of axillary lymph nodes and the initiation of distant metastases. Br J Cancer 59: 775–782
Kury F, Sliutz G, Schemper M et al (1990) HER-2 oncogene amplification and overall survival of breast carcinoma patients. Eur J Cancer 26: 946–949
Lee AKC, DeLellis RA, Silverman ML et al (1990) Prognostic significance of peritumoral lymphatic and blood vessel invasion in node-negative carcinoma of the breast. J Clin Oncol 8: 1457–1465
Levine MN, Browman GP, Gent M et al (1991) When is a prognostic factor useful? A guide for the perplexed. J Clin Oncol 9: 348–356
Lipshultz SE, Colan SD, Gelber RD et al (1991) Late cardiac effects of doxorubicin therapy for acute lymphoblastic leukemia in childhood. N Engl J Med 324: 808–815
Lotan R, Nicolson G (1988) Can anticancer therapy be improved by sequential use of cytotoxic and cytostatic (differentiating or immunomodulating) agents to suppress tumor cell phenotypic diversification? Biochem Pharmacol 37: 149–154
Love RR, Leventhal H, Easterling DV, Nerenz DR (1989) Side effects and emotional distress during cancer chemotherapy. Cancer 63: 604–612
Ludwig Breast Cancer Study Group (1989) Prolonged disease-free survival after one course of perioperative adjuvant chemotherapy for node-negative breast cancer. N Engl J Med 320: 491–496
Mansour EG, Gray R, Shatila AH et al (1989) Efficacy of adjuvant chemotherapy in high-risk node-negative breast cancer. N Engl J Med 320: 485–490
McDonald CC, Stewart HJ (1991) Fatal myocardial infarction in the Scottish adjuvant tamoxifen trial. Br Med J 303: 435–437
McGuire WL, Tandon AK, Allred DC et al (1990) How to use prognostic factors in axillary node-negative breast cancer patients. JNCI 82: 1006–1015
Mendelsohn ML (1960) The growth fraction: a new concept applied to tumors. Science 132: 1496
Morrison JM, Howell A, Kelly KA et al (1989) West Midlands Oncology Association trials of adjuvant chemotherapy in operable breast cancer: results after a median follow-up of 7 years. I. Patients without involved axillary lymph nodes. Br J Cancer 60: 919–924
Muss HB, Kute TE, Case LD et al (1989) The relation of flow cytometry to clinical and biologic characteristics in women with node negative primary breast cancer. Cancer 64: 1894–1900
Namer M, Etienne MC, Fontana X et al (1989) Prognostic value of total cathepsin D in breast cancer. Breast Cancer Res Treat 14: 135–139
National Cancer Institute (1988) Treatment alert issued for node-negative breast cancer. J Natl Cancer Inst 80(8): 550–551
Nissen-Meyer R, Kjellgren K, Malmio K et al (1978) Surgical adjuvant chemotherapy: results with one short course with cyclophosphamide after mastectomy for breast cancer. Cancer 41: 2088–2098
O'Reilly SM, Barnes DM, Camplejohn RS et al (1991) The relationship between c-*erb*B-2 expression, S-phase fraction and prognosis in breast cancer. Br J Cancer 63: 444–446
Osborne CK, Kitten E, Arteaga CL (1989) Antagonism of chemotherapy-induced cytotoxicity for human breast cancer cells by antiestrogens. J Clin Oncol 7: 710–717
Padmanabhan N, Howell A, Rubens RD (1986) Mechanism of action of adjuvant chemotherapy in early breast cancer. Lancet ii: 411–414
Paik S, Hazan R, Fisher ER et al (1990) Pathological findings from the National Surgical Adjuvant Breast and Bowel Project: prognostic significance of *erb*B-2 protein overexpression in primary breast cancer. J Clin Oncol 8: 103–109
Paterson MC, Dietrich KD, Danyluk J et al (1991) Correlation between c-*erb*B-2 amplification and risk of recurrent disease in node-negative breast cancer. Cancer Res 51: 556–567
Peres R, Betsholtz C, Westermark B, Heldin C (1987) Frequent expression of growth factors for mesenchymal cells in human mammary carcinoma cell lines. Cancer Res 47: 3425–3429
Perren TJ (1991) c-*erb*B2 oncogene as a prognostic marker in breast cancer. Br J Cancer 63: 328–332
Pieper R, Futscher B, Erickson L (1989) Transcription-terminating lesions induced by bifunctional alkylating agents in vitro. Carcinogenesis 10: 1307–1314
Powles TJ, Coombes RC, Smith IE et al (1980) Failure of chemotherapy to prolong survival in a group of patients with metastatic breast cancer. Lancet i: 580–582
Recht A, Come SE, Gelman RS et al (1991) Integration of conservative surgery, radiotherapy, and chemotherapy for the treatment of early-stage node-positive breast cancer: sequencing, timing, and outcome. J Clin Oncol 9: 1662–1667
Remvikos Y, Beuzeboc A, Zajdela N et al (1989) Correlation

of pre-treatment proliferative activity of breast cancer with the response to cytotoxic chemotherapy. JNCI 81: 1383–1387

Rice GC, Hoy CA, Schimke RT (1986) Transient hypoxia enhances the frequency of dihydrofolate reductase gene amplification in Chinese hamster ovary cells. Proc Natl Acad Sci USA 83: 5978–5982

Richards MA, O'Reilly SM, Howell A et al (1990) Adjuvant cyclophosphamide, methotrexate, and fluorouracil in patients with axillary node-positive breast cancer: an update of the Guy's/Manchester trial. J Clin Oncol 8: 2032–2039

Ro J, Bresser J, Ro J et al (1989a) SIS/PDGF-B expression in benign and malignant human breast lesions. Oncogene 4: 351–354

Ro J, El Naggar A, Ro JY (1989b) c-*erb*B-2 amplification in node-negative human breast cancer. Cancer Res 49: 6941–6945

Rogers JS, Murgo AJ, Fontana JA, Raich PC (1988) Chemotherapy for breast cancer decreases plasma protein C and protein S. J Clin Oncol 6: 276–281

Rosen PP, Groshen S, Kinne DW (1991) Prognosis in T2 N0 M0 stage I breast carcinoma: a 20-year follow-up. J Clin Oncol 9: 1650–1661

Rosen PP, Groshen S, Saigo PE et al (1989) A long-term follow-up study of survival in stage I (T1 N0 M0) and stage II (T1 N1 M0) breast carcinoma. J Clin Oncol 7: 355–366

Rubens RD (1990) Auditing palliative cancer chemotherapy. Eur J Cancer 26: 1023–1025

Seminglazov VF, Bavli J, Moiseyenko VM et al (1985) Clinical trials on adjuvant chemotherapy for breast cancer. Cancer 57: 1957–1960

Senn HJ, Goldhirsch A, Jungi WF et al (1989) LMF vs CMF as adjuvant chemotherapy in operable breast cancer. Proc ECCO 5: 1989

Shek LLM, Godolphin W (1988) Model for breast cancer survival: relative prognostic roles of axillary nodal status, TNM stage, estrogen receptor concentration, and tumor necrosis. Cancer Res 48: 5565–5569

Slamon DJ, Clark GM, Wong SG et al (1987) Human breast cancer: correlation of relapse and survival with amplification of the HER-2/*neu* oncogene. Science 235: 177–182

Sulkes A, Livingston RB, Murphy WK (1979) Tritiated thymidine labeling index and response in human breast cancer. JNCI 62: 513–515

Tandon AK, Clark GM, Chamness GC et al (1990) Cathepsin D and prognosis in breast cancer. N Engl J Med 322: 297–302

Tannock IF, Boyd NF, DeBoer G et al (1988) A randomized trial of two dose levels of cyclophosphamide, methotrexate, and fluorouracil chemotherapy for patients with metastatic breast cancer. J Clin Oncol 6: 1377–1387

Teillaud J, Fourcade A, Huppert J et al (1989) Effect of doxorubicin on mouse hybridoma B cells: stimulation of immunoglobulin synthesis and secretion. Cancer Res 49: 5123–5129

Thorpe SM, Rochefort H, Garcia M et al (1989) Association between high concentrations of Mr 52000 cathepsin D and poor prognosis in primary human breast cancer. Cancer Res 49: 6008–6014

Todd JH, Dowle C, Williams MR et al (1987) Confirmation of a prognostic index in primary breast cancer. Br J Cancer 56: 4849–492

Tritton T, Yee G (1982) The anticancer agent Adriamycin can be actively cytotoxic without entering cells. Science 217: 248–250

Valagussa P, Tancini G, Bonadonna G (1987) Second malignancies after CMF for resectable breast cancer. J Clin Oncol 5: 1138–1142

Wall JG, Weiss RB, Norton L et al (1989) Arterial thrombosis associated with adjuvant chemotherapy for breast carcinoma: a cancer and leukemia group B study. Am J Med 87: 501–508

Weichselbaum RR, Hellman S, Piro AS et al (1978) Proliferation kinetics of a human breast cancer cell line in vitro following treatment with 17-β-estradiol and 1-β-D-arabinofuranosylcytosine. Cancer Res 38: 2339–2346

Weiss RB, Tormey DC, Holland JF, Weinberg VE (1981) Venous thrombosis during multimodal treatment of primary breast cancer. Cancer Treat Rep 65: 677–679

Welch D (1987) Biologic considerations for drug targeting in cancer patients. Cancer Treat Rev 14: 351–358

Winchester DP (1991) Adjuvant therapy for node-negative breast cancer: the use of prognostic factors in selecting patients. Cancer 647: 1741–1743

Yeung ST, Yoong C, Spink J et al (1991) Functional myocardial impairment in children treated with anthracyclines for cancer. Lancet 337: 816–818

Zhang HJ, Kennedy BJ, Kiang DT (1984) Thymidine kinase as a predictor of response to chemotherapy in advanced breast cancer. Breast Cancer Res Treat 4: 221–225

7 Treatment of the Peripheral Lymphatics: Rationale, Indications, and Techniques

Eric A. Strom, Marsha D. McNeese, and Gilbert H. Fletcher

CONTENTS

7.1	Introduction	57
7.2	Anatomy of the Lymphatics of the Breast	57
7.3	Probability of Regional Lymphatic Involvement and Recurrence: Surgical Series	58
7.3.1	Representative Studies: Haagensen and Milan Trials	59
7.3.2	Discussion	61
7.4	Postoperative Irradiation of the Lymphatics	61
7.4.1	Results of Nonrandomized Trials	61
7.4.2	Results of Randomized Trials	62
7.4.2.1	National Surgical Adjuvant Breast and Bowel Project	62
7.4.2.2	Stockholm	63
7.4.2.3	Institute Gustave-Roussy: Treatment of the Internal Mammary Chain	64
7.5	Impact of Systemic Therapy on Locoregional Control	64
7.5.1	Eastern Cooperative Oncology Group	65
7.6	Combined Irradiation and Systemic Therapy	65
7.6.1	Helsinki	65
7.6.2	Danish Breast Cancer Cooperative Trials	65
7.7	Meta-analyses of Postoperative Irradiation	67
7.8	Indications and Techniques of Irradiation	68
7.8.1	Treatment Technique of Regional Lymphatics	69
7.8.1.1	Internal Mammary Chain	69
7.8.1.2	Supraclavicular Fossa and Axillary Apex	69
7.8.1.3	Midaxilla	69
7.8.1.4	Lymphatics During Breast-Preserving Therapy	70
7.9	Conclusions	70
	References	71

7.1 Introduction

The rationale for delivery of irradiation after surgical removal of macroscopic tumor is to sterilize occult deposits of tumor in regional tissue. The areas at risk may include residual breast tissue, surrounding skin and connective tissue, and the regional lymphatics. Regional lymph node irradiation is frequently performed in patients with breast cancer who present with advanced stage disease, but the efficacy of such radiation in patients with limited stage breast cancer continues to remain controversial despite decades of study. Results of clinical trials and sequelae of regional lymphatic radiation vary because of patient selection factors, treatment practice patterns, and design flaws in some clinical trials.

In this chapter we assess the effect of regional lymphatic treatment by addressing two specific issues:

1. Does treatment of the lymphatics improve local control?
2. Does treatment of the lymphatics improve survival?

While some would argue that improving survival is the only end point by which treatment efficacy should be measured, the effect of improved locoregional control on the quality of life should also be considered.

7.2 Anatomy of the Lymphatics of the Breast

The skin and glandular tissue of the breast drain to two primary lymph node basins: the axillary and the internal mammary chains (IMC). Additionally, lymph nodes can be identified within the substance of the breast (intramammary nodes), below the pectoralis major (subpectoral, interpectoral, or Rotter's nodes), and in the supraclavicular fossa.

The axilla is bordered medially by the serratus anterior muscle, anteriorly by the pectoralis major and minor muscles, and posteriorly by the converging muscles and fascia of the subscapular region. The apex of the axilla lies below the midclavicle. Within this space, lymph nodes lie in proximity to

Eric A. Strom, M. D., Assistant Professor of Radiotherapy; Marsha D. McNeese, M. D., Associate Professor of Radiotherapy, Gilbert H. Fletcher, M. D., Professor; Department of Radiotherapy, Division of Radiotherapy, The University of Texas, M. D. Anderson Cancer Center, 1515 Holcombe Boulevard, Houston, TX 77030, USA

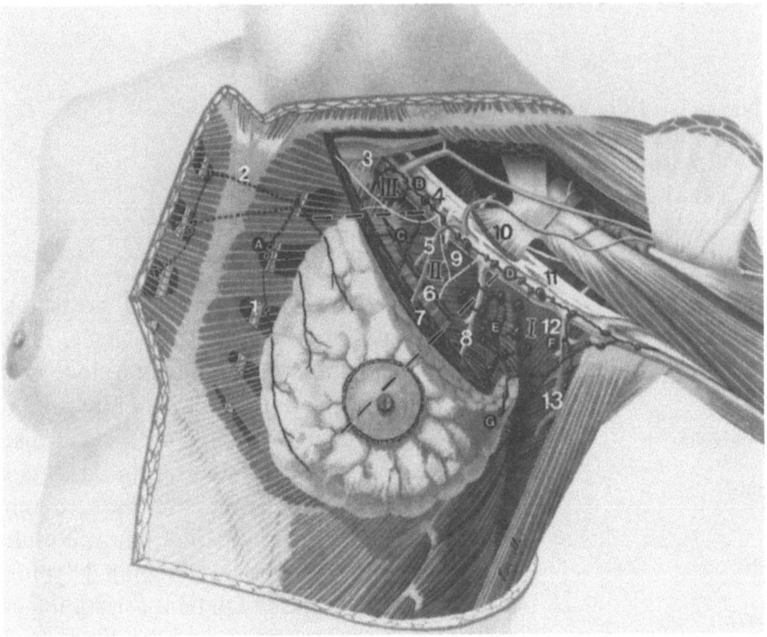

Fig. 7.1. Anatomy of the breast and lymphatics. *1*, Internal mammary artery and vein; *2*, substernal cross drainage to contralateral internal mammary lymphatic chain; *3*, subclavius muscle and Halsted's ligament; *4*, lateral pectoral nerve (from lateral cord); *5*, pectoral branch from thoracoacromial vein; *6*, pectoralis minor muscle; *7*, pectoralis major muscle; *8*, lateral thoracic vein; *9*, medial pectoral nerve (from medial cord); *10*, pectoralis minor muscle; *11*, median nerve; *12*, subscapular vein; *13*, thoracodorsal vein; *A*, Internal mammary lymph nodes; *B*, apical lymph nodes; *C*, interpectoral (Rotter's) lymph nodes; *D*, axillary vein lymph nodes; *E*, central lymph nodes; *F*, scapular lymph nodes; *G*, external mammary lymph nodes: *I*, level I lymph nodes, lateral to lateral border of pectoralis minor muscle; *II*, level II lymph nodes, behind pectoralis minor muscle; *III*, level III lymph nodes, medial to medial border of pectoralis minor muscle. (From OSBORNE 1987)

the vascular structures. The axillary nodes are conveniently divided into three anatomic groups: The proximal group (level I) is located inferior (lateral) to the pectoralis minor muscle, the middle group (level II) directly beneath the pectoralis minor muscle and the distal (high) group (level III) superior to the pectoralis minor muscle along the axillary vein (Fig. 7.1).

The internal mammary nodes lie in the intercostal spaces and drain the central and inner portions of the breast. These nodes and lymphatic structures are found on either side of the internal mammary vessels, usually within 3 cm of the lateral margin of the sternum (Fig. 7.2). While nodes can usually be identified in the first three intercostal spaces, they are also identified in the fourth and fifth interspaces in 47% and 12%, respectively, of patients undergoing extended radical mastectomy (URBAN and MARJANI 1971).

The major route of spread to the supraclavicular nodes is through the axillary chain. While patients may rarely present with supraclavicular adenopathy without axillary involvement, supraclavicular node involvement generally indicates advanced regional disease and is associated with a grave prognosis. Since 1988, the AJC Staging System has categorized ipsilateral supraclavicular disease as M1 (metastatic).

7.3 Probability of Regional Lymphatic Involvement and Recurrence: Surgical Series

There is a direct relationship between the size and location of the primary breast neoplasm and the probability of nodal metastasis. Larger primary tumors have a higher probability of axillary involvement than small ones (NEMOTO et al. 1980; SCHOTTENFELD et al. 1976) (Table 7.1). Similarly, outer quadrant lesions are more likely to have associated axillary nodal metastases than inner quadrant lesions of the same size. The clinical and pathologic status of the axillary nodes is an important indicator of the risk of subsequent local recurrence and distant metastasis (FISHER et al. 1983).

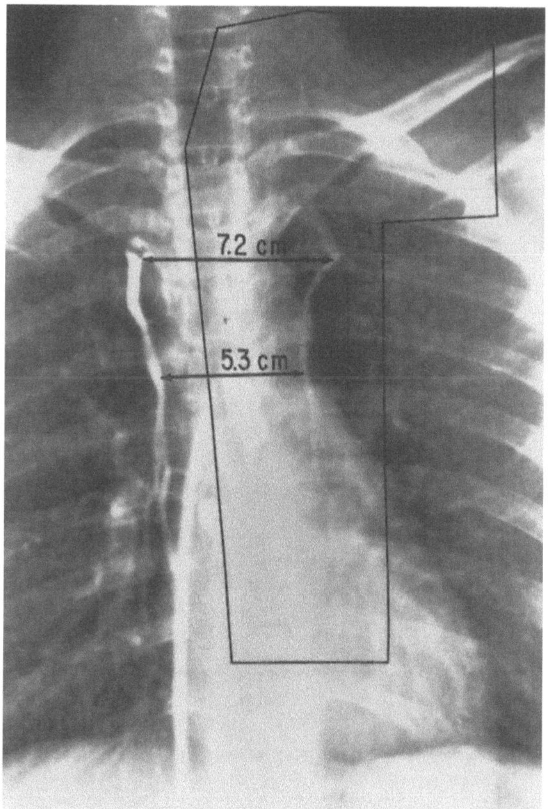

Fig. 7.2. Venogram of the internal mammary vessels showing anatomic target volume. (From FLETCHER and MONTAGUE 1978)

The probability of internal mammary node involvement is related both to location of the primary lesion and to the presence or absence of axillary node involvement. In series published by HANDLEY (1975), URBAN and MARJANI (1971), BUCALOSSI et al. (1971), and LI and SHEN (1984), sequential patients underwent extended radical mastectomy with dissection of the internal mammary node groups. The probability of pathologic involvement of the internal mammary nodes in these patients is shown in Table 7.2.

Recognizing that the supraclavicular nodes were a potential site of residual tumor, Halsted, early in his career, attempted to remove these nodes as a part of his radical mastectomy. Because of the excessive morbidity of routine dissection of the supraclavicular fossa, he shortly abandoned this procedure. Additionally, it was recognized by HAAGENSEN and STOUT (1943), as early as the 1940s, that clinically evident supraclavicular nodal disease conferred a poor prognosis and thus became one of the criteria of clinical inoperability. As a result, there are few or no data relating clinical parameters with the probability of pathologic involvement of the supraclavicular nodes.

There is, however, inferential data to suggest that the risk of subclinical disease in the supraclavicular fossa is substantial. In patients with axillary nodal involvement 19%–33% have disease in the axillary apex (ROSEN et al. 1983; VERONESI et al. 1987; PIGOTT et al. 1984; DANFORTH et al. 1986). Similarly, up to 25% of patients with positive axillary nodes treated with mastectomy alone eventually manifest disease in supraclavicular nodes (PATERSON and RUSSELL 1959; ROBBINS et al. 1966).

The probability of locoregional recurrence after standard mastectomy is a function of the size of the primary tumor, size and number of axillary lymph nodes involved, presence of skin or chest wall involvement, and the type of surgical procedure performed. The results of mastectomy alone for patients with operable breast cancer are seen in Table 7.3. After mastectomy, most patients with stage I and stage II disease have a less than 10% risk of locoregional tumor recurrence. However, patients with positive axillary nodes, especially those with four or more nodes involved, are at higher than standard risk for locoregional recurrence and distant metastasis (DONEGAN et al. 1966; HAAGENSEN 1986; ROSENMAN et al. 1986; HOPTON et al. 1989; DECK and KERN 1976; DAO and NEMOTO 1963; LEE 1984; FISHER et al. 1970).

7.3.1 Representative Studies: Haagensen and Milan Trials

C. D. Haagensen, during half a century of performing the classic radical mastectomy at the Columbia University College of Physicians and Surgeons, noted a clear relationship between the number of axillary nodes found to contain metastasis and the frequency of chest wall recurrence. He consistently performed the radical mastectomy as described by Halsted, removing all the skin over the breast and both pectoral muscles and performing a complete axillary dissection, including skeletonizing of the axillary vein. In his review of 562 patients with Colombia stage A and B (operable) breast cancer, only 4% of patients with one to three positive axillary lymph nodes subsequently developed a chest wall recurrence. In contrast, patients with four or more positive nodes had a 22% probability of local recurrence, and patients with eight or more positive nodes, a 42%

Table 7.1. National Survey by the American College of Surgeons on the probability of nodal metastasis by size of primary in 12881 patients (adapted from NEMOTO et al. 1980)

Size of primary tumor (cm)	Number of patients with positive nodes (n)	Number of patients with negative nodes (n)	Probability of nodal metastasis (%)
0.1–0.5	42	105	29
0.6–1.0	237	723	25
1.1–2.0	1380	2664	34
2.1–3.0	1413	2033	41
3.1–4.0	960	957	50
4.1–5.0	641	494	56
5.1 +	795	437	65

Table 7.2. Probability of internal mammary node metastasis

Reference	Axillary nodal status	IMC nodes histologically positive (%)			Total patients (*n*)
		Outer quadrants	Inner or central primary	Any quadrant	
URBAN and MARJANI (1971)	N –	13	16		384
	N +	42	53		341
BUCALOSSI et al. (1971)	N – and N +	14	27		1213
	N0			17	660
	N1			29	553
HANDLEY (1975)	N –	4	10		465
	N +	21	48		535
LI and SHEN (1984)	N –	2	9		607
	N +	25	35		635

IMC, internal mammary chain; N –, node-negative; N +, node-positive; N0, no regional lymph node metastasis; N1, metastasis to movable ipsilateral axillary nodes

Table 7.3. Probability of local recurrence after mastectomy[a]

Reference	Total number of patients (*n*)	Recurrence (%)			
		Node-negative patients	Node-positive patients	Patients with 1–3 positive lymph nodes	Patients with 4 + positive lymph nodes
DECK and KERN (1976)	1027	4	11		
HAAGENSEN (1986)	935	3		4	22
HOPTON et al. (1989)	829	13	29		
VALAGUSSA et al. (1978)	716	8	27		
DONEGAN et al. (1966)	703	6	26	12	38
ROSENMAN et al. (1986)	404	4		17	22
LEE (1984)	320	6		11	31
FISHER et al. (1970)	269	8	24	24	31

[a] The locoregional recurrence rates were analysed in patients who underwent surgery only.

local recurrence rate after radical mastectomy (HAAGENSEN 1986).

The Instituto Nazionale Tumori reported on the patterns of relapse and survival following mastectomy without any further therapy on 716 patients consecutively treated from 1964 to 1968 (VALAGUSSA 1978). These patients had clinically staged primary tumors, and the axilla was pathologically evaluated in all cases. Of the 335 patients with histologically negative axillary nodes, only 8% developed a locoregional recurrence at 10 years, whereas 26.9% of patients with histologically proven nodal metastasis developed locoregional disease. Since over 90% of node-negative patients never manifested locoregional recurrence, this study suggests that those patients who have negative axillary nodes would not benefit from locoregional irradiation.

7.3.2 *Discussion*

These studies, plus the contributions of other authors, have clearly established the consistent relationship between the intensity of axillary nodal infestation with tumor and the likelihood of locoregional recurrence. The early pioneers of breast cancer therapy accepted the view that neoplastic cells spread in an orderly fashion, first to regional nodes and only later from these nodal deposits to visceral sites. In view of the identification of certain high-risk groups, it was reasonable to recommend adjuvant irradiation, not only to prevent locoregional recurrences, but also to prevent dissemination of disease. The changing perception of the biology of breast cancer spread has caused some clinicians to underestimate the value of locoregional therapy. Many clinicians hypothesize that breast cancer is systemic from inception, and that nodal disease is merely an indicator of this process. This bias can result in overlooking clinical data that support the use of regional irradiation in certain high-risk populations.

7.4 Postoperative Irradiation of the Lymphatics

Randomized trials to assess the usefulness of postoperative irradiation have been performed for the last half of this century. While many of these trials were well-designed for their day, we now understand that many had serious design flaws for various reasons. Often some of the region at risk was not treated, suboptimal doses of radiation were delivered (often with orthovoltage), and many of these trials included large numbers of patients who were node-negative and thus at low risk for locoregional disease. Such patients would not be expected to show a benefit from postmastectomy irradiation and, therefore, any treatment efficacy for high-risk patients would potentially be obscured. Finally, many trials were multi-institutional and had considerable variation in treatment techniques, making comparison of patient populations more difficult. These issues have therefore resulted in the continuing discussion regarding the efficacy of locoregional irradiation in breast cancer.

7.4.1 *Results of Nonrandomized Trials*

At the University of Texas M. D. Anderson Cancer Center, postoperative irradiation has been given routinely to high-risk patients since 1959 (MONTAGUE and FLETCHER 1980; 1985). With the development of the electron beam in 1963, comprehensive treatment of the volume at risk became technically easy (FLETCHER et al. 1968; FLETCHER 1972; TAPLEY et al. 1982). Although the indications for postoperative treatment evolved over the years, patients generally received treatment if they had any of the following:

1. Positive axillary nodes;
2. Primaries larger than 5 cm; or
3. Medial primary tumors (MONTAGUE 1972; FLETCHER 1980).

Between 1963 and 1977, 941 patients with carcinoma of the breast received peripheral lymphatic irradiation alone or with chest wall irradiation after a radical or modified radical mastectomy. None of the patients received adjuvant chemotherapy (FLETCHER et al. 1989). The incidence of histologically involved axillary nodes was 70%. The lymphatics of the apex of the axilla, the supraclavicular area, and the IMC were irradiated in patients with histologically positive axillary nodes and in patients with central or inner quadrant primaries, regardless of the axillary status. Chest wall irradiation was added to the peripheral lymphatic irradiation primarily when there was a heavy involvement of the axillary nodes or a large primary tumor. At 10 and 20 years, the respective disease-free survival rates are 55% and 50% for all patients, 44% and 40% for all patients with positive nodes, 56% and 48% for the patients with one to three positive

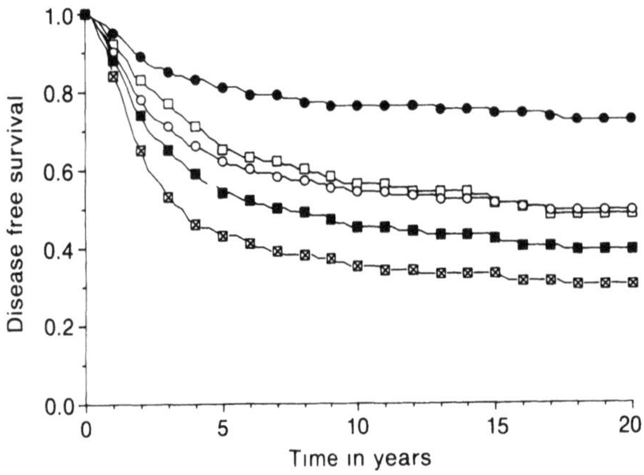

Fig. 7.3. Disease-specific survival in M.D. Anderson series of patients treated with mastectomy and postoperative irradiation. (From Fletcher et al. 1989). ○ Overall group Axillary histology 941 pts.; ● negative nodes 262 pts.; ■ positive nodes 679 pts.; □ 1–3 pos nodes 332 pts.; ⊠ ≥ 4 pos nodes 347 pts.

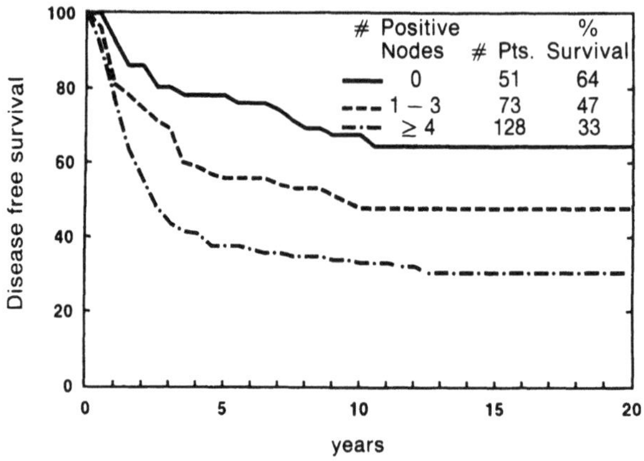

Fig. 7.4. Actuarial disease-free survival of stage III patients with breast cancer treated with mastectomy and irradiation only at M.D. Anderson. (From Strom et al. 1991)

nodes, and 33% and 30% for the patients with four or more positive nodes. Comparison of the mortality curves between the general population and the breast cancer patients seems to indicate a cured fraction, since the curves become parallel at 17 years (Fig. 7.3).

A significant fraction of patients with locoregionally advanced (stage III) carcinoma of the breast were also treated with mastectomy and radiation alone (Strom et al. 1991). Between 1955 and 1984, 376 patients were treated in this manner. In 124 patients, the surgical management was confined to removal of the breast alone. In 252 patients, dissection of the axilla was performed either by extended total, modified radical, or classic radical mastectomy. The follow-up period ranged between 8 and 34 years (median 17 years). At 10 years, the actuarial disease-specific, relapse-free survival (DSRFS) rate for the entire group was 40%, and the actuarial locoregional control rate was 82%. For the 202 patients with stage IIIA disease, the DSRFS was 48% and the locoregional control rate was 88%. For those 174 patients with stage IIIB disease, the figures were 30% and 74%, respectively. In the 252 patients in whom the axilla was assessed, the number of positive nodes was a powerful predictor of both locoregional control and survival. The DSRFS rates at 10 years for patients with zero, one to three, and four or more positive nodes were 63%, 48%, and 30%, respectively (Fig. 7.4). The actuarial locoregional control rates at 10 years exceeded 95% for patients with up to three positive nodes, versus 75% for those with four or more nodes. Although some clinicians would argue that all patients with locally advanced carcinoma of the breast have occult systemic metastasis, these results clearly demonstrate that this is not true and that local treatment alone cures a significant proportion of these patients.

7.4.2 Results of Randomized Trials

7.4.2.1 National Surgical Adjuvant Breast and Bowel Project

The National Surgical Adjuvant Breast and Bowel Project (NSABP) has designed many multi-institutional trials in breast cancer. Two of these trials, B-02 (Fisher et al. 1970) and B-04 (Fisher et al. 1980; 1985) are pertinent to assess the role of radiotherapy for this disease.

From 1961 to 1965, the NSABP enrolled 1882 patients into protocol B-02. After conventional radical mastectomy, patients were randomly assigned to receive postoperative radiotherapy versus observation. A second randomization for node-positive patients compared treatment with triethylthiophosphamide (TSPA) to placebo. An additional 142 patients in control groups from other NSABP studies were added for the analysis. Radiotherapy was to be directed to the axillary apex, internal mammary, and supraclavicular regions only (the chest wall was not treated) to a dose of 3500 Roentgens (R) in 3 weeks or 4500 R in 5 weeks. About one-quarter were treated with orthovoltage irradiation, the remainder with ^{60}Co photons. Because 569 patients were declared ineligible after randomization and 210 patients had incomplete data available, 41% of the patients enrolled were subsequently withdrawn from analysis. At 5 years, no significant advantage in relapse-free survival was observed in those patients who received postoperative irradiation. Irradiated patients had fewer regional recurrences, but proportionally more distant metastases as site of first failure, although the final proportion of patients developing metastatic disease was the same in both groups. Since the chest wall was not irradiated, there were similar rates of local failure in both groups.

In 1971, the NSABP began protocol B-04, a prospective randomized trial including 1665 women to compare alternative local and regional treatments of breast cancer, all of which employed breast removal. The patients were treated by radical mastectomy alone, total ("simple") mastectomy without axillary dissection but with regional irradiation, or total mastectomy without irradiation. Axillary dissection was performed in this subgroup only if nodes subsequently became positive. This trial was designed to examine the use of radiotherapy after total mastectomy without axillary dissection. Postoperative radiotherapy was used to treat disease, both occult and clinically evident, in the axilla, as well as subclinical disease in the chest wall and supraclavicular and internal mammary nodes.

Of the patients treated with modified radical mastectomy, 38.6% had tumor in the axillary nodes. Presumably a similar percentage of patients in the other treatment arms had axillary involvement. Locoregional failure was low in all groups, but lowest in the irradiated group. There were no significant differences in disease-free survival, distant disease-free survival, or overall survival at 10 years among the three treatment groups in patients with clinically negative axilla.

Patients with clinically negative nodes who were treated by total mastectomy alone who later required an axillary dissection because of recurrence were *not* deemed to have had a treatment failure at that time unless the nodes could not be completely removed. Additionally, the NSABP only reported first site of failure, rather than cumulative rates. Therefore, the true rate of axillary node recurrence after total mastectomy remains somewhat obscure.

Although these trials are frequently discounted because of problems already discussed, perhaps two useful conclusions can be made from these and similar trials. First, radiotherapy confers no additional benefit to patients at low risk of residual subclinical disease. Furthermore, treatment of only part of the volume at risk may result in higher than expected local failure rates as compared to similarly staged patients receiving comprehensive irradiation.

7.4.2.2 Stockholm

Some of the largest and best designed trials to assess the role of postoperative radiotherapy after mastectomy have been the Stockholm trials. The results of these prospective, randomized clinical trials were originally analyzed by Wallgren et al. (1986) and updated by Rutqvist et al. (1989). The first trial was started in 1971 and included 960 pre- and postmenopausal patients with operable disease. This three-arm study compared results of preoperative and postoperative radiotherapy, including chest wall and regional lymphatic irradiation, to 45 Gy in 5 weeks versus surgery alone. All patients underwent a modified radical mastectomy. Major protocol variations occurred in less than 4% of patients.

At a mean follow-up of 13.5 years, there was a sustained improvement of the recurrence-free survival with either preoperative or postoperative radiotherapy when compared to surgery alone ($p < 0.001$). There was no difference between the radiotherapy arms. Among node-positive cases, radiation reduced the frequency of both locoregional recurrence ($p < 0.001$) and distant metastasis ($p < 0.001$) (Fig. 7.5). Among node-negative patients the cumulative incidence of locoregional failure at 10 years was 23% in the surgical group versus 5% in the irradiated group. The corresponding figures for the node-positive patients were 55% and 21%. In the node-positive patients, the cumulative incidence of distant metastasis at 10 years was 48% in the irradiated group versus 65% in the surgical control group. These observations strongly suggest that distant dissemination in node-positive patients can originate from residual foci of tumor on the chest wall and in the regional lymph nodes. No adverse effect from radiation on long-term survival was observed in this study.

The second study, started in 1976, compared postmastectomy radiation with adjuvant chemotherapy (cyclophosphamide, methotrexate, 5-fluorouracil, CMF) in pre- and postmenopausal high-risk patients. At a mean follow-up of 6.5 years there was no significant difference in recurrence-free survival between the two treatments. However, postmenopausal patients fared significantly better with radiotherapy ($p < 0.01$), with radiation more

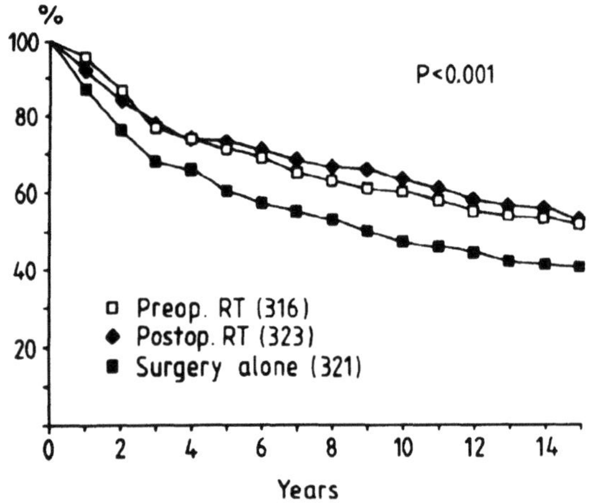

Fig. 7.5. Disease-specific survival for patients in Stockholm randomized trial. (From RUTQVIST et al. 1989)

effective than adjuvant chemotherapy in reducing both distant metastases ($p < 0.01$) and locoregional recurrences ($p < 0.001$).

7.4.2.3 Institute Gustave-Roussy: Treatment of the Internal Mammary Chain

Based on the realization that 40%–60% of axillary node-positive patients with medial tumors would have pathologic evidence of tumor in the IMC, the Institute Gustave-Roussy initiated a series of trials to assess the value of various forms of treatment (ARRIAGADA et al. 1988; LE et al. 1990). Between 1958 and 1978, patients undergoing mastectomy for operable breast cancer and histologically positive axillary nodes were treated in one of four methods: IMC dissection, IMC irradiation, both, or neither. A total of 1195 patients was included in the analysis, with all women under 70 years of age, tumors less than 7 cm in size, and histologically positive nodes. Patients with T4 lesions were excluded. From 1958 to 1963 and from 1968 to 1972, IMC dissection and postoperative radiotherapy were undertaken for all patients with histologic evidence of axillary node metastasis, regardless of tumor site. Additionally, some patients with medial quadrant lesions and negative axillae underwent both IMC dissection and radiotherapy. From 1963 to 1968, IMC dissection without postoperative irradiation was performed according to randomization in a multicenter trial. From 1972 to 1978, node-positive patients were randomized between peripheral lymphatic irradiation versus no further treatment (Table 7.4).

The 10-year risk of death from all causes was decreased ($p = 0.06$) for all patients who received IMC treatment of any kind versus those who did not, but statistically significant benefit was seen only in the subgroup of patients with medial quadrant lesions whose survival ($p = 0.01$) and risk of metastasis ($p = 0.05$) were significantly improved (Fig. 7.6). Postoperative locoregional irradiation decreased the risk of locoregional recurrences ($p = 0.001$). This effect was independent of location of the primary tumor or surgical management of the lymph nodes. Of the 270 patients living 15 years or more after the treatment, no detrimental effect of radiotherapy on survival was seen.

7.5 Impact of Systemic Therapy on Locoregional Control

There are sufficient data from the above trials to show that well-performed, consistently designed radiotherapy decreases the rate of locoregional disease recurrence. Additionally, those large trials that examined comprehensive irradiation to the entire volume at risk showed a small, but statistically significant, improvement in disease-specific and

Table 7.4. Patient characteristics in the Institut Gustave-Roussy study of internal mammary node treatment (from ARRIAGADA et al. 1988)

	Without IMCD, without RT	With IMCD, without RT	Without IMCD, with RT	With IMCD, with RT
Number of patients	135	102	523	435
Mean age (years)	53	52	52	50
Primary size (mm)	34	39	33	37
Medial tumors (%)	44	51	38	64
4 + Positive axillary nodes (%)	27	40	41	53

IMCD, internal mammary chain dissection; RT, radiation therapy

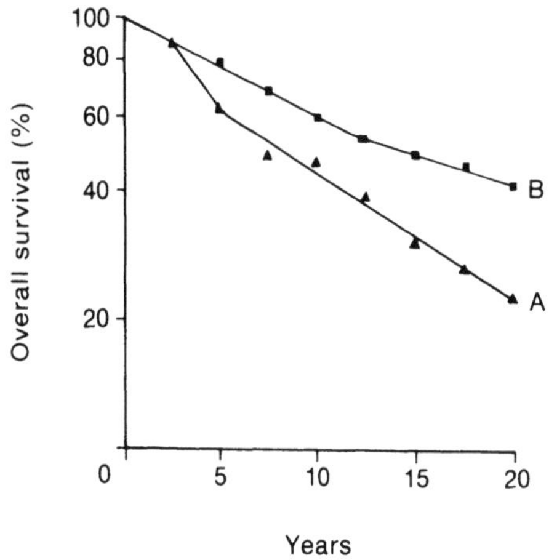

Fig. 7.6. Survival of patients in Institut Gustave-Roussy study of internal mammary node treatment. Patients with medial tumors. *A*, No treatment of internal mammary chain; *B*, treatment of internal mammary chain ($p = 0.01$). (From Arriagada et al. 1988)

overall survival, predominantly in patients with positive axillary nodes.

The effect of adjuvant chemotherapy on locoregional control has not been fully established. Well-performed studies seem to demonstrate conflicting results. If the mechanism of action of systemic therapy is by reduction of systemic micrometastases, then it may also have beneficial locoregional effects as well. Some even postulate that this presumed effect eliminates the need for locoregional irradiation. In the Milan trial, which compared the results of adjuvant treatment with or without CMF, the relapse-free survival was improved from 31% in the control group to 43% in the treated group (Bonadonna 1986). The local failure rates, however, of the treated group (11.6%) versus the control group (14.5%) were not significantly different. Other trials have also demonstrated minimal effect on locoregional disease even when different chemotherapeutic regimens are used, including those containing doxorubicin (Adriamycin) (Table 7.5).

7.5.1 Eastern Cooperative Oncology Group

Fowble et al. (1988), in a report on 627 patients entered into the Eastern Cooperative Oncology Group (ECOG) adjuvant chemotherapy trials from 1978 to 1982, demonstrated in a multivariate analysis that some subgroups of patients with breast cancer and histologically positive axillary nodes were particularly likely to benefit from postoperative radiotherapy even though they received systemic chemotherapy. The chance of patients with four to seven axillary nodes or tumor size greater than 5 cm developing an isolated locoregional recurrence was almost equal to the risk of distant metastases. It is suggested that these patients, who are at an intermediate risk of distant metastasis, may be most likely to benefit from irradiation (Table 7.6).

7.6 Combined Irradiation and Systemic Therapy

7.6.1 Helsinki

A randomized trial from Helsinki has been useful in demonstrating the efficacy of combining each therapeutic modality (Grohn et al. 1984; Klefstrom et al. 1987). In this trial, 120 patients with stage IIIA breast cancer were randomized to one of three arms after modified radical mastectomy: either locoregional irradiation alone, systemic therapy (vincristine, doxorubicin, and cyclophosphamide) for six cycles, or both chemotherapy and irradiation. At both 36 and 60 months, radiotherapy preferentially reduced local failure relative to the chemotherapy arm, whereas systemic therapy reduced the number of distant failures. Forty percent of patients treated with chemotherapy alone developed locoregional recurrence, suggesting that locoregional recurrence is not markedly reduced by adjuvant chemotherapy. The best disease-free survival and local control rates were obtained in the combined modality arm (Fig. 7.7).

7.6.2 Danish Breast Cancer Cooperative Trials

The largest of the combined modality trials that assess the contribution of locoregional irradiation are the Danish Breast Cancer Cooperative Group Trials (Overgaard et al. 1988; 1990). Pre- and postmenopausal patients with T3, T4 tumors and/or positive axillary nodes were eligible for participation in the study. The initial treatment for all patients was mastectomy with axillary dissection, with removal of all gross tumor. A total of 1473 pre- and perimenopausal patients were randomized to receive either CMF chemotherapy alone or CMF plus comprehensive irradiation, and 1120 postmenopausal patients were randomized to receive tamoxifen alone versus tamoxifen plus irradiation.

Table 7.5. Incidence of locoregional recurrence in node-positive patients receiving postmastectomy adjuvant chemotherapy (adapted from FOWBLE 1991)

Reference	Chemotherapy	Locoregional recurrence (%)				Follow-up (years)
		All patients	Patients with 1–3 positive lymph nodes	Patients with 4 or more positive lymph nodes	Patients with T_3 tumors	
BONADONNA et al. (1986)	CMF	9	5	14[a] 21[b]	–	8
STEFANIK et al. (1985)	CMF	19	9	36	27	5
TORMEY et al. (1983)	CMF	–	–	18	–	2.8[d]
	CMFVP	–	–	10	–	
FOWBLE et al. (1988)	CMF (PT)	11	7	15	19	3
RAO et al. (1985)	CMF or L-PAMFT	18	6	24	31	5.2[d]
LEE (1984)	CMF, L-PAMFT	20	9	27	–	4.4[d]
GOLDHIRSCH and GELBER (1986)[c]	CMFP	11	8	15	–	4[d]
GRIEM et al. (1987)	CMF/MF	14	5	–	–	4.4[d]
	CA			20	–	
SYKES et al. (1989)	AC	–	10	10	28	2.9

C, cyclophosphamide; M, methotrexate; F,5-fluorouracil; V, vincristine; P, prednisone; A, doxorubicin (Adriamycin); T, tamoxifen; L-PAM, L-phenylalanine mustard
[a] Four to ten positive nodes
[b] More than ten positive nodes
[c] Premenopausal patients only
[d] Median

Table 7.6. ECOG study on Locoregional recurrence (adapted from FOWBLE et al. 1988)

Probability of isolated locoregional recurrence after chemotherapy alone

Number of positive lymph nodes (*n*)	Number of patients (*n*)	Isolated local recurrence (%)	Distant metastasis (%)	Recurrence isolated local recurrence (%)
1 to 3	310	7	17	29
4 to 7	181	15	21	42
> 7	136	15	47	24

Isolated recurrence by site

Chest wall (%)	Axilla (%)	Supraclavicular nodes (%)	Infraclavicular nodes (%)	Multiple nodal sites (%)	Chest wall and nodes (%)
53	11	23	1	7	4

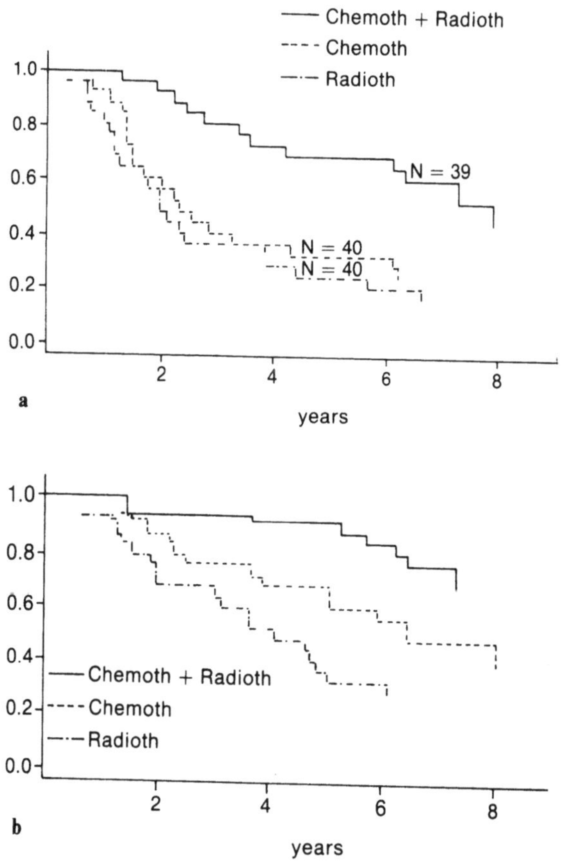

Fig. 7.7a, b. Helsinki randomized trial. **a** Disease-free survival. **b** Overall survival. (From KLEFSTROM et al. 1987)

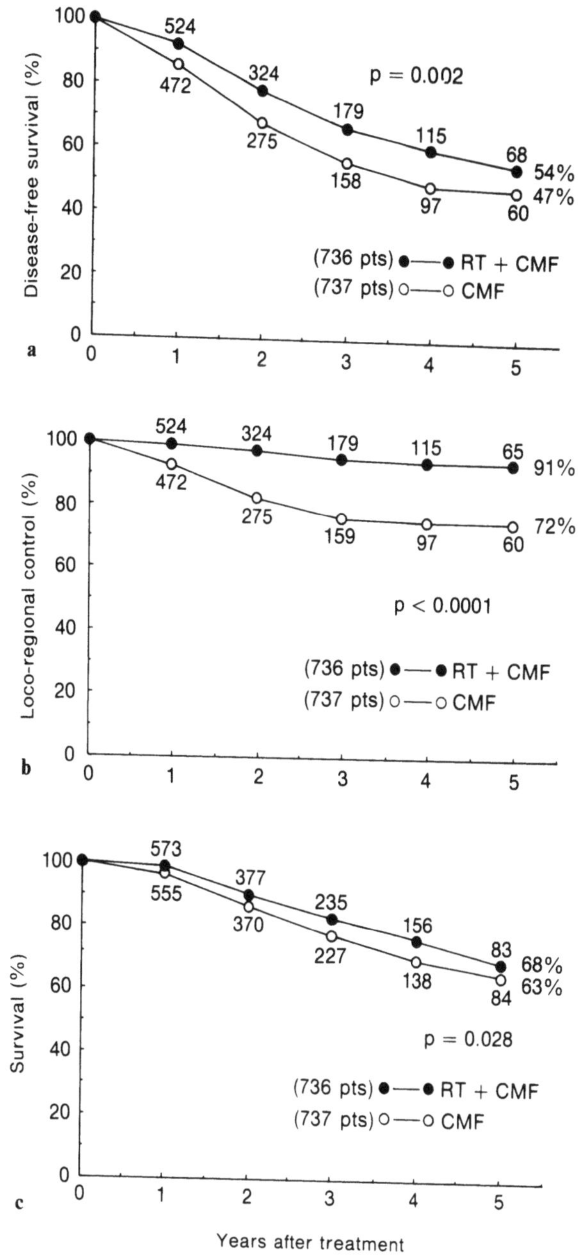

Fig. 7.8a–c. Danish Breast Cancer Cooperative Group Trial. Premenopausal patients. **a** Disease-free survival; **b** locoregional control; **c** overall survival. (From OVERGAARD et al. 1990)

At 5 years, the actuarial locoregional recurrence rate was significantly lower in the irradiated patients, regardless of the type of systemic therapy used. Furthermore, disease-free survival was significantly improved in both pre- and postmenopausal irradiated patients compared with those who had only systemic treatment. At the time of analysis, premenopausal patients treated in the combined modality arm had a significantly superior overall survival than those receiving chemotherapy alone (Figs. 7.8, 7.9).

7.7 Meta-analyses of Postoperative Irradiation

In attempt to evaluate the results of the early randomized trials of postmastectomy irradiation, CUZICK et al. (1987) combined the survival rates of 7941 patients entered into ten randomized trials. An overview of the mortality results of these trials in which radiotherapy was a randomized option after simple or radical mastectomy was analyzed. No difference was found in survival in the first 10 years of follow-up, but an excess of deaths was observed among patients given radiotherapy ($p < 0.001$) at 15 years. This has led some clinicians to attempt to decrease the use of radiotherapy, believing that these trials clearly demonstrate excess long-term mortality.

On closer review, a number of problems are identified. First, most of the patients included in these trials were node-negative. Adjuvant radiation can only benefit those patients who have disease in

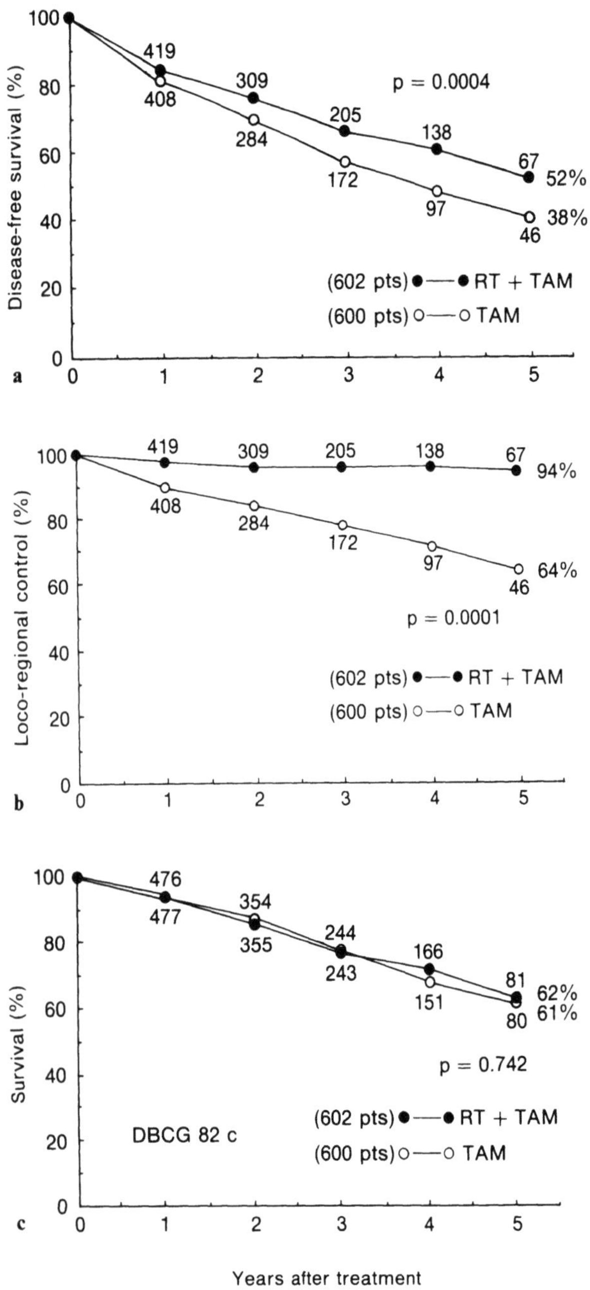

Fig. 7.9a–c. Danish Breast Cancer Cooperative Group Trial. Postmenopausal patients. **a** Disease-free survival; **b** locoregional control; **c** overall survival. (From OVERGAARD et al. 1990)

the areas treated and can only improve survival if there is occult locoregional disease but no occult distant metastasis. To quote FLETCHER (1976): "Patients who do not have disease in nodal areas do not require treatment to these areas and those who have occult distant metastases will not be cured by the extra treatment." Therefore, it is understandable that no benefit is seen when patients with a low risk of locoregional disease are irradiated.

Furthermore, many of the patients were treated using radiation techniques and principles that are now clearly outmoded and potentially dangerous. Orthovoltage was used in many of the trials, and some did not irradiate the entire region at risk (e.g., lymphatic irradiation alone). Doses and treatment schedules did not always deliver a dose sufficient to sterilize subclinical tumor. Most important, many patients had excessive normal tissue, particularly cardiac tissue, irradiated.

7.8 Indications and Techniques of Irradiation

The use of postoperative irradiation of the peripheral lymphatics has evolved in the past two decades. It is now clear that regional nodal recurrence rates and chest wall recurrence rates parallel one another. Patients with small primary tumors and negative axillary nodes have a very small risk of locoregional failure. Those with locally advanced tumors or multiple axillary node metastases are at high risk for both peripheral lymphatic recurrence and chest wall recurrence. It is therefore uncommon to irradiate the lymphatics alone. Instead, most patients who are to be irradiated should receive comprehensive locoregional treatment.

Treatment of the IMC is important for patients with inner and centrally located primary tumors and positive axillary nodes. The possibility of loss of survival benefit due to late cardiac damage suggests that the parasternal nodes are optimally treated with electron beam irradiation or by inclusion in tangential chest wall fields.

Less information exists about irradiation of the peripheral lymphatics for patients undergoing breast-preserving therapy. It is reasonable to infer that the presence of high-risk factors as identified above would still apply. Additional considerations must be taken into account for these patients: excessive lung or heart irradiation should be avoided, as should undertreatment of the primary tumor site due to field junctions.

Based on these concepts, current treatment recommendations are as follows: Postmastectomy irradiation to the chest wall and lymphatics of the chest is recommended for patients at high risk of locoregional recurrence, that is, patients with the following:

(1) more than four of the axillary nodes histologically positive and/or extranodal extension into axillary connective tissue;
(2) a primary tumor of at least 5 cm or accompanied by erythema, ridging, peau d'orange, skin or chest wall invasion; or
(3) presence of axillary nodes that are greater than 2.5 cm, fixed or matted (i.e., N2 presentation). In this patient population, irradiation clearly improves rates of local control, and probably also has a positive impact on survival.

The indications for postoperative irradiation can be summarized as follows:

1. Patients with stage III breast carcinoma (T3–4, or N2–3); include patients with ipsilateral supraclavicular nodes.
2. Patients with stage II breast carcinoma with any of the following:
   - Four or more lymph nodes containing tumor or extranodal tumor
   - Vascular, perineural, lymphatic invasion
   - Skin or muscle invasion
   - Tumor at margin of resection

The following detailed description of the technical aspects of treatment of the regional lymphatics has recently been published elsewhere (McNeese et al. 1992).

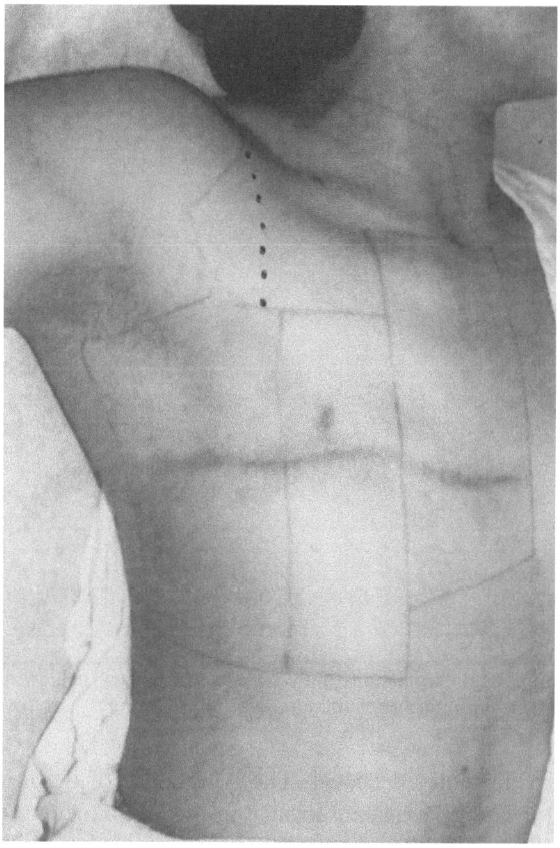

Fig. 7.10. Field arrangements to treat peripheral lymphatics and chest wall with electrons

7.8.1 Treatment Technique of Regional Lymphatics

7.8.1.1 Internal Mammary Chain

Treatment of the ipsilateral IMC is indicated for patients with medially or centrally located tumors when the axillary nodes have been demonstrated to contain tumor. After mastectomy, the electron beam is used as it makes it possible to avoid underlying cardiac and mediastinal tissue. Skin tolerance may necessitate a few treatments with photons, but the dose to cardiac structures should be kept as low as possible. To provide more than 98% local control, 50 Gy to 25 fractions is sufficient.

7.8.1.2 Supraclavicular Fossa and Axillary Apex

Since skip metastasis is extremely uncommon, treatment of the axillary apex and supraclavicular fossa is rarely indicated when there is minimal or no involvement of the dissected axilla. The supraclavicular fossa is irradiated in all patients with locally advanced disease, when four or more axillary nodes contain tumor, or when the midaxilla is to be treated. When small nodes are removed from the axilla without extranodal extension seen in the axillary fat, there is no need to irradiate the midaxilla with photons. Electron beam irradiation (usually 9 or 10 MeV) is ideal for treating the anterior structures of the apical nodes and supraclavicular area. Subclinical disease is controlled more than 98% of the time when 50 Gy is delivered (Fig. 7.10).

7.8.1.3 Midaxilla

Postoperative irradiation of the midaxilla is indicated if there are large (> 2.5 cm), fixed, or matted nodes, or if there is evidence of gross extranodal disease. The midaxilla is also routinely treated when delivering preoperative irradiation, or if the

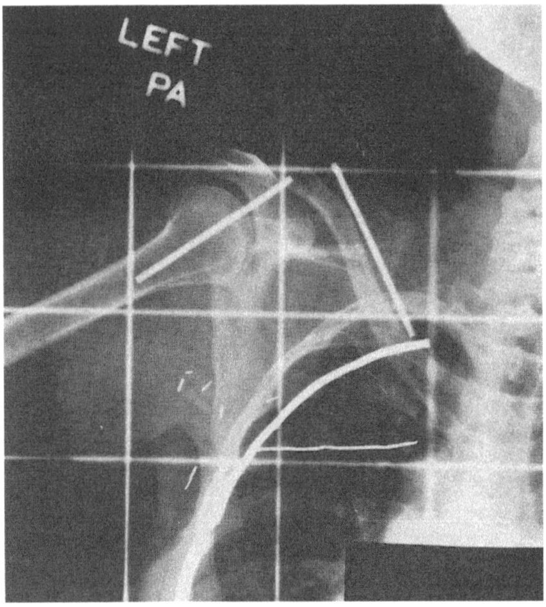

Fig. 7.11. Simulation film of posterior axillary field with clips outlining lymphatic anatomy

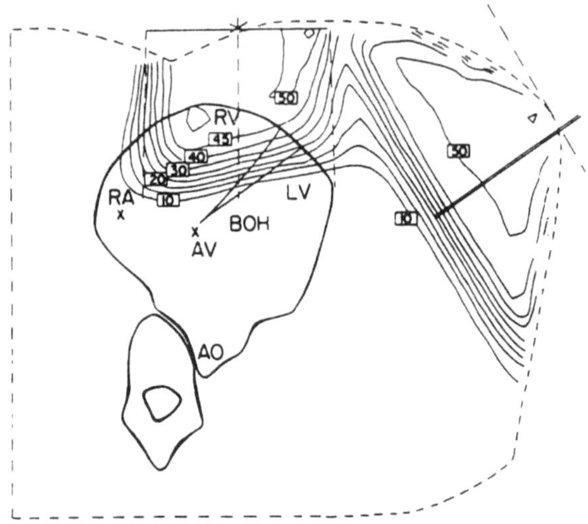

Fig. 7.12. Dosimetry using 12 MeV electrons to treat the internal mammary chain. The breast is treated with 7 MV tangents. *RV*, right ventricle; *LV*, left ventricle; *RA*, right atrium; *AV*, atrioventricular node; *AO*, aorta; *BOH*, bundle of His. (From JANJAN et al. 1989)

axilla is not dissected. The lymphatics of the low (or lateral) axilla are located in the midplane of the thorax. As the lymphatics are followed proximally in continuity with the subclavicular vessels, they are found closer to the anterior surface of the thorax. Therefore, they are treated with parallel-opposed photon beams, loaded primarily from the anterior. The anterior field encompasses the low to midaxilla, the axillary apex, the supraclavicular fossa, and the low jugular nodes, using a 15° lateral tilt to minimize treatment of the spinal cord and esophagus. The field receives 50 Gy as specified at D_{max}. The posterior photon field covers only the low and midaxilla (Fig. 7.11) and supplements the midaxilla to a dose of 40–50 Gy.

7.8.1.4 Lymphatics During Breast-Preserving Therapy

Since most patients treated by breast conservation have early stage disease, they tend to have a lower risk for regional nodal disease than patients with more advanced disease. After segmental resection in patients with medial tumors and positive axillary nodes, it is desirable to include the internal mammary nodes in the treatment volume, either by including these nodes in the tangential fields used to treat the breast, or by using a separate electron beam field (Fig. 7.12). Geometric disadvantages occur frequently. When the IMC is treated with the electron beam there is a risk of undertreatment to some of the medial area of the breast and/or overlap in medial portions of the breast. Large amounts of lung and, on the left, cardiac tissue, can be seen when the entire volume is treated with tangents alone. Care must be exercised to balance the potential benefit of IMC irradiation with these potential disadvantages (JANJAN 1989). As a rule, the primary tumor bed should not be split by the junction of electron and photon fields due to the possibility of not treating the primary tumor bed adequately. The inclusion of left ventricle should be avoided as much as possible, particularly in this era, when a majority of patients also receive doxorubicin or other cardiotoxic chemotherapy.

7.9 Conclusions

From the above studies a number of conclusions may be reached. First, postoperative radiotherapy consistently decreases locoregional failure rates in high-risk patients. This effect is most pronounced in patients with four or more lymph nodes involved with tumor and patients with locoregionally advanced disease. Second, postoperative radiotherapy improves disease-specific and overall survival in this patient population. This is best demonstrated in large studies where standard doses are delivered with consistent techniques to the entire volume at risk – the chest wall and draining lymphatics. Those studies that suggest an overall survival detriment were based on poorly performed trials (based on current standards) and used questionable statistical methods. Third, treatment of the IMC is important, particularly for patients with inner quadrant and central lesions and evidence of axillary metastasis. Care should be taken not to place field junctions over a primary tumor bed or to include a significant amount of ventricle in patients with left-sided lesions. Finally, the benefit of comprehensive irradiation persists even when systemic chemotherapy is used.

Acknowledgements. This investigation was supported in part by grants CA06294 and CA16627 by the National Cancer Institute, Department of Health and Human Services.

References

Arriagada R, Le MG, Mouriesse H et al (1988) Long-term effect of internal mammary chain treatment. Results of a multivariate analysis of 1195 patients with operable breast cancer and positive axillary nodes. Radiother Oncol 11(3): 213–222

Bonadonna G, Valagussa P, Tancini G et al (1986) Current status of Milan adjuvant chemotherapy trials for node-positive and node-negative breast cancer. NCI Monogr 1986(1): 45–49

Bucalossi P, Veronesi U, Zingo L, Cantu C (1971) Enlarged mastectomy for breast cancer. Review of 1213 cases. Am J Roentgenol Radium Ther Nucl Med 111(1): 119–122

Cuzick J, Stewart H, Peto R et al (1987) Overview of randomized trials of postoperative adjuvant radiotherapy in breast cancer. Cancer Treat Rep 71(1): 15–29

Danforth DJ, Findlay PA, McDonald HD et al (1986) Complete axillary lymph node dissection for stage I–II carcinoma of the breast. J Clin Oncol 4(5): 655–662

Dao TL, Nemoto T (1963) The clinical significance of skin recurrence after radical mastectomy in women with cancer of the breast. Surg Obstet Gynecol 117: 447

Deck KB, Kern WH (1976) Local recurrence of breast cancer. Arch Surg 111(4): 323–325

Donegan WL, Perez MC, Watson FR (1966) A biostatistical study of locally recurrent breast carcinoma. Surg Gynecol Obstet 122(3): 529–540

Fisher B, Slack NH, Cavanaugh PJ et al (1970) Postoperative radiotherapy in the treatment of breast cancer: results of the NSABP clinical trial. Ann Surg 172(4): 711–732

Fisher B, Montague E, Redmond C et al (1980) Findings from the NSABP Protocol No. B-04: comparison of radical mastectomy with alternative treatments for primary breast cancer. I. Radiation compliance and its relation to treatment outcome. Cancer 46(1): 1 13

Fisher B, Bauer M, Wickerham DL et al (1983) Relation of number of positive axillary nodes to the prognosis of patients with primary breast cancer. an NSABP update. Cancer 52(9): 1551–1557

Fisher B, Bauer M, Margolese R et al (1985) Ten-year results of a randomized clinical trial comparing radical mastectomy and total mastectomy with or without radiation. N Engl J Med 312(11): 674–681

Fletcher GH (1972) Local results of irradiation in the primary management of localized breast cancer. Cancer 29(3): 545–551

Fletcher GH (1976) Reflections on breast cancer. Int J Radiat Oncol Biol Phys 1(7–8): 769–779

Fletcher GH (1980) Textbook of Radiotherapy. Lea and Febiger, Philadelphia, p 959

Fletcher GH, Montague ED, White EC (1968) Evaluation of irradiation of the peripheral lymphatics in conjunction with radical mastectomy for cancer of the breast. Cancer 21(5): 791–797

Fletcher GH, Montague ED (1978) Does adequate irradiation of the internal mammary chain and supraclavicular nodes improve survival rates? Int J Radiat Oncol Biol Phys 4: 481–492

Fletcher GH, McNeese MD, Oswald MJ (1989) Long-range results for breast cancer patients treated by radical mastectomy and postoperative radiation without adjuvant chemotherapy: an update. Int J Radiat Oncol Biol Phys 17(1): 11–14

Fowble B (1991) The role of postmastectomy adjuvant radiotherapy for operable breast cancer. In: Fowble B, Goodman RL, Glick JH, Rosato EF (eds) Breast cancer treatment: a comprehensive guide to management. Mosby Year Book, St. Louis, pp 289–309

Fowble B, Gray R, Gilchrist K et al (1988) Identification of a subgroup of patients with breast cancer and histologically positive axillary nodes receiving adjuvant chemotherapy who may benefit from postoperative radiotherapy. J Clin Oncol 6(7): 1107–1117

Goldhirsch A, Gelber R (1986) Adjuvant treatment for early breast cancer: the Ludwig breast cancer studies. NCI Monogr 1986(1): 55–70

Griem KL, Henderson IC, Gelman R et al (1987) The 5-year results of a randomized trial of adjuvant radiation therapy after chemotherapy in breast cancer patients treated with mastectomy. J Clin Oncol 5(10): 1546–1555

Grohn P, Heinonen E, Klefstrom P, Tarkkanen J (1984) Adjuvant postoperative radiotherapy, chemotherapy, and immunotherapy in stage III breast cancer. Cancer 54(4): 670–674

Haagensen CD (1986) Results with Halsted's radical mastectomy. In: Haagensen CD (ed) Disease of the breast, 3rd edn. Saunders, Philadelphia, pp 903–932

Haagensen CD, Stout AP (1943) Carcinoma of the breast: criteria of operability. Annals of Surgery 118: 859–870, 1032–1051

Handley RS (1975) Carcinoma of the breast. Ann R Coll Surg Engl 57(2): 59–66

Hopton DS, Thorogood J, Clayden AD, MacKinnon D (1989) Histological grading of breast cancer: significance of grade on recurrence and mortality. Eur J Surg Oncol 15(1): 25–31

Janjan NA, Gillin MT, Prows J et al. (1989) Dose to the cardiac vascular and conduction systems in primary breast irradiation. Med Dosim 14: 81–87

Klefstrom P, Grohn P, Heinonen E et al (1987) Adjuvant postoperative radiotherapy, chemotherapy, and immunotherapy in stage III breast cancer. II. 5-year results and influence of levamisole. Cancer 60(5): 936–942

Lee YN (1984) Breast carcinoma: patterns of recurrence and metastasis after mastectomy. Am J Clin Oncol 7: 443

Le MG, Arriagada R, de Vathaire F et al (1990) Can internal mammary chain treatment decrease the risk of death for patients with medical breast cancer and positive axillary lymph nodes? Cancer 66(11): 2313–2318

Li KY, Shen ZZ (1984) An analysis of 1,242 cases of extended radical mastectomy. Breast 10: 10–19

McNeese MD, Fletcher GH, Levitt SH (1992) Breast cancer. In: Levitt SH, Tapley ND (eds) Levitt and Tapley's technological basis of radiation therapy: practical clinical applications, 2nd edn. Lea and Febiger, Philadelphia, pp 232–247

Montague ED (1972) Adaptation of irradiation techniques to various types of surgical procedures for breast cancer. Cancer 29(3): 557–560

Montague ED, Fletcher GH (1980) The curative value of irradiation in the treatment of nondisseminated breast cancer. Cancer 46(4): 995–998

Montague ED, Fletcher GH (1985) Local regional effectiveness of surgery and radiation therapy in the treatment of breast cancer. Cancer 55(9): 2266–2272

Nemoto T, Vana J, Bedwani RN et al (1980) Management and survival of female breast cancer: results of a national survey by the American College of Surgeons. Cancer 45(12): 2917–2924

Osborne MP (1987) Breast development and anatomy. In: Harris JR, Hellman S, Henderson KC, Kinne DW (eds) Breast disease. Lippincott, Philadelphia, pp 1–14

Overgaard M, Christensen JJ, Johansen H et al (1988) Postmastectomy irradiation in high-risk breast cancer patients. Present status of the Danish Breast Cancer Cooperative Group trials. Acta Oncol 27(6A): 707–714

Overgaard M, Christensen JJ, Johansen H et al (1990) Evaluation of radiotherapy in high-risk breast cancer patients: report from the Danish Breast Cancer Cooperative Group (DBCG 82) Trial. Int J Radiat Oncol Biol Phys 19(5): 1121–1124

Paterson R, Russell MH (1959) Clinical trials in malignant disease. Part III. Breast cancer: evaluation of postoperative radiotherapy. J Fac Radiol (London) 10: 175–180

Pigott J, Nichols R, Maddox WA, Balch CM (1984) Metastases to the upper levels of the axillary nodes in carcinoma of the breast and its implications for nodal sampling procedures. Surg Gynecol Obstet 158(3): 255–259

Rao AF, Murthy AK, Hendrickson FR et al (1985) Analysis of risk factors for locoregional failure in Stage II breast carcinoma treated with mastectomy and adjunctive chemotherapy. Int J Radiat Oncol Biol Phys II [Suppl. I]: 151

Robbins GF, Lucas JC, Fracchia AA (1966) An evaluation of postoperative prophylactic radiation therapy in breast cancer. Surg Gynecol Obstet 122: 979–982

Rosen PP, Lesser ML, Kinne DW, Beattie EJ (1983) Discontinuous or "skip" metastases in breast carcinoma. Analysis of 1228 axillary dissections. Ann Surg 197(3): 276–283

Rosenman J, Bernard S, Kober C et al (1986) Local recurrences in patients with breast cancer at the North Carolina Memorial Hospital (1970–1982). Cancer 57(7): 1421–1425

Rutqvist LE, Cedermark B, Glas U et al (1989) Radiotherapy, chemotherapy, and tamoxifen as adjuncts to surgery in early breast cancer: a summary of three randomized trials. Int J Radiat Oncol Biol Phys 16(3): 629–639

Schottenfeld D, Nash AG, Robbins GF, Beattie EJ (1976) Ten-year results of the treatment of primary operable breast carcinoma: A summary of 304 patients evaluated by the TNM system. Cancer 38(2): 1001–1007

Stefanik D, Goldberg R, Byrne P et al (1985) Local-regional failure in patients treated with adjuvant chemotherapy for breast cancer. J Clin Oncol 3: 660–665

Strom EA, McNeese MD, Fletcher GH et al (1991) Results of mastectomy and postoperative irradiation in the management of locoregionally advanced carcinoma of the breast. Int J Radiat Oncol Biol Phys 21(2): 319–323

Sykes HF, Sim DA, Wong CJ et al (1989) Local-regional recurrence in breast cancer after mastectomy and adriamycin-based adjuvant chemotherapy: evaluation of the role of postoperative radiotherapy. Int J Radiat Oncol Biol Phys 16(3): 641–647

Tapley ND, Spanos WJ, Fletcher GH et al (1982) Results in patients with breast cancer treated by radical mastectomy and postoperative irradiation with no adjuvant chemotherapy. Cancer 49(6): 1316–1319

Tormey DC, Weinberg VE, Holland JF et al (1983) A randomized trial of five and three drug chemotherapy and chemoimmunotherapy in women with operable node-positive breast cancer. J Clin Oncol 1(2): 138–145

Urban JA, Marjani MA (1971) Significance of internal mammary lymph node metastases in breast cancer. Am J Roentgenol Radium Ther Nucl Med 111(1): 130–136

Valagussa P, Bonadonna G, Veronesi U (1978) Patterns of relapse and survival following radical mastectomy. Analysis of 716 consecutive patients. Cancer 41(3): 1170–1178

Veronesi U, Rilke F, Luini A et al (1987) Distribution of axillary node metastases by level of invasion: an analysis of 539 cases. Cancer 59(4): 682–687

Wallgren A, Arner O, Bergstrom J et al (1986) Radiation therapy in operable breast cancer: results from the Stockholm trial on adjuvant radiotherapy. Int J Radiat Oncol Biol Phys 12(4): 533–537 [Erratum published in Int J Radiat Oncol Biol Phys 1987 13(1): 149]

8 What Is the Value of Clinical Trials?

SEYMOUR H. LEVITT and LARS-ERIK RUTQVIST

CONTENTS

8.1 Introduction 73
8.2 "Is It Too Much to Expect that Cancer Trials Should Be Well-Designed, Appropriately Conducted, and Honestly Presented" (Tobias and Tattersall 1985)? 74
8.2.1 Randomized Clinical Trials 74
8.2.2 Meta-Analysis 75
8.3 Adjuvant Therapies in Treating Breast Cancer: Assessing Specific Trials 76
8.3.1 Radiation Therapy 76
8.3.2 Chemotherapy 77
8.4 Discussion 78
8.5 Conclusion 79
References 79

8.1 Introduction

Few subjects in the treatment of disease arouse so much emotion and concern as does that of cancer, and particularly breast cancer. And similar to all emotionally laden issues, there is difficulty letting go of long-held views of treatment that have provided some degree of help and subsequent security for both physicians who administer treatment and for patients who receive it. It is expected, therefore, that controversy develops when new therapies are proposed or introduced that challenge these existing views. Yet challenging established views, many of which are vigorously defended with only nonrandomized experience, is critical to improving treatment results for early breast cancer.

SEYMOUR H. LEVITT, M. D., Head and Professor, Department of Therapeutic Radiology – Radiation Oncology, University of Minnesota, Box 494, UMHC, Harvard Street at East River Road, Minneapolis, MN 55455, USA; LARS-ERIK RUTQVIST, M. D., Director, Oncologic Center, Radiumhemmet, Karolinska Hospital, 104-01 Stockholm, Sweden

Treating early breast cancer with adjuvant therapies is one such challenge to long-held treatment views favoring radical or modified radical mastectomy. The controversy incited over this challenge hinges on the small impact adjuvant chemotherapy and radiation therapy have had on overall survival in early breast cancer patients. (There is no controversy over the well-documented beneficial effects of radiation in reducing locoregional recurrences.) A report of three randomized adjuvant trials from the Stockholm Breast Cancer Group shows that radiation has had a 10-year impact of approximately 5% on overall survival in early breast cancer patients. Statistical significance in overall improval was not indicated for node-negative patients (RUTQVIST et al. 1989). Similarly, recent information from the Milan Institute shows a 10-year overall survival increase from 59.4% to 65% (approximately 5.5% improval) in patients treated without and with chemotherapy (CASCINELLI et al. 1991). These authors also found that improvement in survival was not statistically significant for node-negative patients. They also found this to be true for node-positive patients with primary tumors of 2 cm or less in maximum diameter and for patients with four or more nodes. Improvement in survival was only indicated in patients with lesions greater than 2 cm in maximum diameter. The results of these two studies showing that adjuvant therapies have little effect on overall survival in breast cancer patients are similar to those found in the SEER data (NATIONAL CANCER INSTITUTE 1973–1988).

Controversy over the use of adjuvant radiation and chemotherapy due to results such as these need to be placed in a context – that is, we need to carefully evaluate the clinical trials from which the results are obtained. To do this we must look at how randomized clinical trials are performed and how the data compiled from them are analyzed and reported. The rest of this chapter is devoted to evaluating trials that have had an impact on the treatment of breast cancer.

8.2 "Is It Too Much to Expect that Cancer Trials Should Be Well-Designed, Appropriately Conducted, and Honestly Presented" (Tobias and Tattersall 1985)?

8.2.1 Randomized Clinical Trials

Clinical trials in which the treatment allocation is random are critical to adequately assessing new therapies as randomization is the only method that makes it possible to reliably identify moderate differences in outcome that are related to the tested treatment. Conversely, studies based on nonrandomized control patients cannot avoid the risk of spurious differences due to an imbalance in prognostic factors. Known prognostic factors can be controlled. However, in oncology many prognostic factors are still unknown and can, therefore, not be controlled. Conclusions based on historical or concurrent nonrandomized controls can, at best, only be tentative until later verified in a prospective randomized trial. Randomized clinical trials therefore are necessary to adequately test new treatments.

Treating early breast cancer with radiation therapy occasioned one of the earliest randomized clinical trials in breast cancer. The trial, performed by Paterson at Manchester in the early 1950s (Paterson 1958, 1962; Paterson et al. 1958, 1959), compared the use of adjuvant radiation on postmastectomy patients to a watch policy and found no improvement in survival for patients who were watched. Critical analysis of this early study, however, as well as other studies conducted in the early years of randomized testing, revealed numerous flaws in how the trials were conducted, including inadequate radiation and randomization techniques (Levitt and McHugh 1977; Levitt et al. 1976). From these studies we learned a great deal about the importance of conducting careful randomized trials to secure accurate results. The tremendous advances seen in the performance of randomized trials today attests to the lessons learned from those early trials.

Even with these advances, however, difficulties remain in developing sound clinical trials and contribute greatly to the controversy over treating early breast cancer. Much of the controversy is based on differing assessments of the performance of clinical trials. Indeed, examining how a trial is conducted has become critical to assessing accurately the results obtained. The findings of a particular trial are then debated based on the differing evaluations of trial performance.

Analysis and accurate reporting of the trial data are also critical in the evaluation of clinical trials. In a brilliant article by Baar and Tannock (1989) the methods used to analyze and interpret clinical trials in chemotherapy were evaluated in a hypothetical trial in which patients with metastatic cancer were treated with chemotherapy. The article gave examples of differences in methodologic techniques that led to different conclusions based on a single set of data. The authors' findings that errors in reporting and omission led to erroneous evaluations clarifies the need for responsible clinical performance as well as for responsible evaluation of that performance. This need is further clarified in a recent article by Mueller and Lesperance (1991) showing that when the National Surgical Adjuvant Breast and Bowel Project (NSABP) trial was properly evaluated, different results than originally claimed were found that revealed statistical flaws in the trial.

A recent study conducted at the University of Minnesota showed how inadvertent or advertent mistakes in statistical technique can affect the results of any trial (Levitt et al., manuscript submitted). Both inadvertent errors (such as transcription and data entry errors) and advertent or systemic classification errors were introduced into real data from a retrospective study on Hodgkin's disease; the data was then re-analyzed to evaluate the impact of these errors on results. It was found that inadvertent errors (defined as random errors) usually do not cause important changes in the results unless there are too many of them or if the p value is very close to the cut-off point. However, advertent errors in systemic classification, such as unsuitable or vague definitions of end points, have an important impact on how trial results are analyzed and reported. For example, the study showed that the definition of an end point as death had a different effect on results and the determination of statistical and clinical significance than the definition of an end point as cancer death. Similarly, different definitions of patient selection affect results and create subsequent problems in assessing a meta-analysis composed of trials with the different definitions. For example, analysis of patients selected for a group defined as "intent to treat" will differ from the analysis of patients selected for a "treatment received" group. Results will differ according to the different definitions of patient selection, and subsequently affect treatment recommendations based on conclusions drawn from the analyses. The "intent to treat" analysis will provide a more realistic picture of what the new treatment will bring since it can be assumed that there will always be noncompliers among patients even in the absence of side effects. On the other hand, in a small study, inclusion of noncompliers might dilute the treatment effect so much that the treatment potential can be overlooked. Utmost care must be given to a "treatment received" analysis and the description of the patients included and excluded to avoid suspicion of data manipulation.

Another point clarified by the study was that if treatment takes risk factors into account, the outcome may no longer be dependent on those risk factors. This means that the treatment itself and the factors leading to a particular treatment choice have to be taken into account when, for instance, examining the association between survival and degree of abnormalities of tumor cells. Also, secondary risk factors may become evident when tailoring treatment to the main risk factors, indicating that risk factors are not absolute but treatment dependent.

This analysis, along with the studies previously mentioned, shows how easily data can be misinterpreted and erroneously analyzed and reported given the frequent flaws found in statistical technique and analysis.

8.2.2 Meta-Analysis

Individual randomized trials in oncology are often too small to reliably detect treatment-related benefits. Sample size estimations based on biostatistical considerations demonstrate that a moderate treatment benefit may require a trial with several hundred to more than one thousand patients. Meta-analysis developed out of the need to increase the number of events for analysis to obtain a more stable estimate of the effect of a certain therapy. By drawing together individual scientific statistical analyses from separate studies, meta-analysis is able to generate conclusions unavailable from the individual studies.

Along with providing adequate sample sizes to detect treatment effects, meta-analysis must minimize biases that may distort the real impact of therapy (Gelber and Goldhirsch 1986). While overviews of individual trials provide an estimate of treatment effect for each trial, combining individual trials to obtain an accumulated estimate provides an overall measure that is subject to less random variation than any of the individual trial data alone. Theoretically, then, the meta-analysis will be able to detect smaller real differences in treatment effect. If the reduction in random error is accompanied by an increase in systematic error, however, then the overview will be nonrepresentative of the true treatment effect.

To avoid systematic errors, Gelber and Goldhirsch (1986) point out that each trial included in a meta-analysis, including the overview, must provide an unbiased estimate of the treatment effect of interest. This implies that the treatment groups compared within individual trials are similar in all features that might influence outcome. It also implies the need for randomization in which treatment assignment is unknown to investigators before patient entry – and the requirement that all patients randomized must be included in the analysis according to the assigned group to prevent treatment-dependent patient selection and exclusion. Furthermore, all published and unpublished eligible trials must be included to avoid systemic bias due to trial selection.

Selection bias may be avoided by including all available trials of a particular treatment in the overview. This implies that the included trials will be dissimilar, e.g., in regard to the performance of the therapy used. Because of this circumstance, a "negative" overview result does not imply that the tested treatment modality invariably is ineffective. For example, inclusion of several large trials using ineffective treatment may obscure a clinically worthwhile benefit in smaller trials using adequate treatment. Overview estimates of treatment effects based on all patients in all available trials of a particular treatment modality represent a minimum estimate of what could be achieved with the best possible treatment regimen in an appropriately selected subgroup of patients.

The overview methodology does not presuppose that all patients in all trials are similar, nor that the performance of the treatment used in the various trials are the same. Rather, it is based on the observation that qualitative treatment interactions, as opposed to quantitative interactions, are unusual. This means that although a treatment may have its greatest effect in a given subset of patients, the effect in other subsets tends to go in the same direction (Wesley and Edwards 1988). Similarly, if a drug at a given dose produces some benefit, other dose levels will probably also produce some, or perhaps even greater, benefit. For instance, if a given dose of a particular cytotoxic agent is effective in postmenopausal breast cancer patients with liver metastases, it is likely to have some effect also in premenopausal patients with lung metastases even if the dose is slightly different. The effect in these two subgroups is probably not the same, but it is unlikely that there is a qualitative difference – that is, that there is no (or even a detrimental) effect in one of the subgroups and a benefit in the other. Similarly, if there is some benefit with a particular adjuvant therapy among patients aged 55–59 years of age, there is probably also some benefit among those aged 50–54 years or 60–64 years (EARLY BREAST CANCER TRIALISTS' COLLABORATIVE GROUP 1988).

Although the hypothesis may be correct that quantitative treatment interactions are more common than qualitative interactions in most instances, there are settings in which it is not. Endocrine therapy, using ovarian ablation, for advanced breast cancer only works in premenopausal patients; postmenopausal patients cannot be expected to benefit (EARLY BREAST CANCER TRIALISTS' COLLABORATIVE GROUP 1992). A radical surgical resection of colon cancer will cure a certain proportion of patients, whereas nonradical resections cannot be expected to cure anybody. Low doses of radiation will not cure any patient with Hodgkin's disease, whereas adequate doses will. In these instances, the patients may experience only the adverse effects of treatment and may actually do worse than without the treatment. Such mechanisms may explain qualitative treatment interactions.

Overviews help overcome problems with the correct interpretation of randomized clinical trials, mainly the problems related to inadequate statistical power in small individual trials. However, the significance of the performance of the treatment used may be difficult to assess in an overview of a large number of trials. One reason for this is that the overview often contains unpublished trials. This is demonstrated in the recent publications of the 5- and 10-year results of the overview of adjuvant breast cancer trials in which neither the drug doses used in the chemotherapy trials nor the treatment techniques used in the radiation trials were mentioned (EARLY BREAST CANCER TRIALISTS' COLLABORATIVE GROUP 1990). Another reason is that overviews often obscure the importance of distinguishing between statistical and clinical significance found in individual trials. The need for a large sample size to detect a statistical significant benefit should not be used as an argument against the clinical relevance of the benefit. For example, most oncologists would consider a reduction in mortality of one-third with a new therapy a major achievement. A trial designed to reliably identify such a benefit should include a total of 700–800 patients if the baseline survival is 70% (Fig. 8.1) (GEORGE 1985). Detection of a mortality reduction of one-quarter would require roughly twice that number.

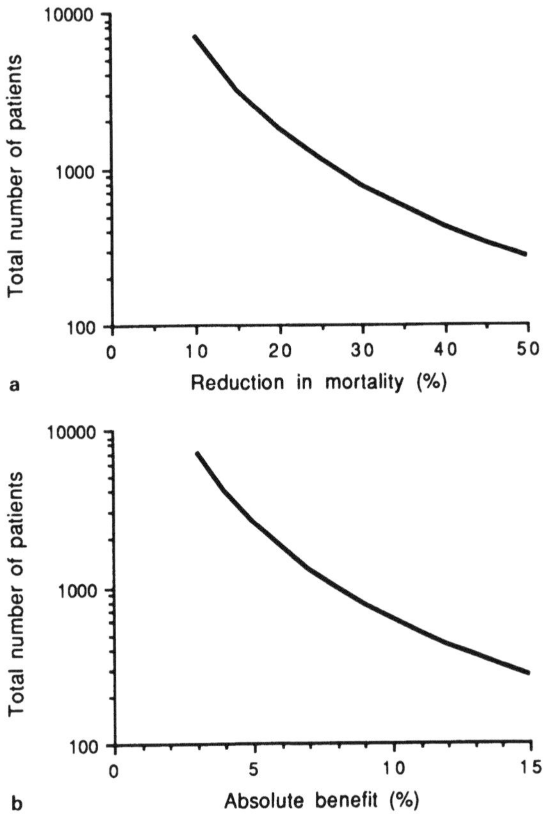

Fig. 8.1a, b. The total number of patients needed in a two-arm randomized clinical trial to ensure a reasonable statistical power to detect a given reduction of mortality (**a**) with the tested treatment or the corresponding absolute improvement of survival (**b**). The curves assume a baseline survival of 70%, a power of 80% and a two-tailed significance level of 5% (GEORGE 1985)

8.3 Adjuvant Therapies in Treating Breast Cancer: Assessing Specific Trials

8.3.1 Radiation Therapy

In analyzing the meta-analyses conducted on the use of adjuvant radiation therapy in breast cancer, it is important to emphasize that "in a meta-analysis, the methodologic rigor and scientific quality of papers to be combined should be assessed and considered in formulating recommendations. If the original methods are poor, the resulting conclusion will be less reliable" (SACKS et al. 1987). This directive provides a general rule by which to critique two major meta-analyses on radiation therapy. Our previous examination of the Stjernsward meta-analysis found inadequacies and inaccuracies in the individual trials included (LEVITT 1984, 1988; LEVITT and MCHUGH 1977; LEVITT et al. 1976, 1983). Likewise, flaws in performance and subsequent reporting were found in the individual trials included in the meta-analysis reported by CUZICK in 1987. The following examination of the findings reported by CUZICK et al. (1987a, b) illuminates the need to carefully analyze the trials used in meta-analysis in order to properly assess the results obtained.

Based on a series of pooled randomized studies, CUZICK et al. hypothesized that there was a significant excess in deaths observed among patients given adjuvant radiotherapy after 10 years. Testing the validity of Cuzick's hypothesis and meta-analysis required determining whether or not the studies met certain criteria: (a) Was the pooling of randomized tests carried out appropriately, i.e., were the studies similar in therapy delivery, patient population, and data quality? (b) Were the individual tests truly randomized and unbiased? and (c) Did the treatment pass efficacy tests, i.e., was treatment adequate and appropriate in amount delivered (dosage), areas of application, and in number of patients included to prove statistical significance (GELBER and GOLDHIRSCH 1986; SACKS et al. 1987; SIMON 1987)?

An examination of the Cuzick trials under these criteria showed that the trials were problematic for meta-analysis (LEVITT 1988). Most of the studies included were poorly designed and were carried out with many exclusions. The trials were biologically dissimilar and, in many instances, showed statistical flaws. The radiation techniques employed were also inadequate: underdosages and overdosages were applied with scant attention given to treating the appropriate fields. The results obtained from these problematic trials are therefore questionable.

Examining the Cuzick meta-analysis demonstrates the importance of carefully assessing the individual trials included in meta-analyses. If individual trials are not properly performed and rigorously evaluated, then accurate assessment of their combined results is impossible.

8.3.2 Chemotherapy

In a paper published in 1988, five clinical trials were analyzed that were used for achieving the consensus study on the use of adjuvant chemotherapy in treating breast cancer (LEVITT et al. 1988). The findings of these studies showed an improvement in overall survival in patients treated with adjuvant chemotherapy. However, problems were noted in all of these trials either in how the trials were conducted or in their statistical analyses. In studies conducted by the Milan Group (BONADONNA et al. 1976, 1977, 1985; ROSSI et al. 1981) an apparent imbalance was noted in randomization techniques, i.e., in one trial 12–13 patients were left unaccounted for by the randomization reported. Similarly, the Southwest Oncology Group Study (GLUCKSBERG et al. 1982; RIVKIN et al. 1983) showed changes in patient selection with two unaccounted for patients. Even these small shifts or losses in patient selection were shown to affect statistical significance. The other three studies – Glasgow Study (SMITH et al. 1984), Bowman Gray Study (COOPER et al. 1985), and Oslo Study (NISSEN-MEYER et al. 1978, 1984) – all showed flaws in statistical analyses, further advancing skepticism over the validity of the results obtained in these studies. These problems with the individual studies persist, a reminder that "in a meta-analysis... if the original methods are poor, the resulting conclusion will be less reliable" (SACKS et al. 1987).

A recent report by MUELLER and LESPERANCE (1991) casts doubt on the validity of another important chemotherapy trial used in the consensus study – the NSABP B-05 trial. Analysis of the results of that trial showed that adjuvant chemotherapy was recommended as a standard treatment of breast cancer based on a series of five trials using L-phenylalanine mustard and/or 5-fluorouracil. Further examination of these trials failed to show consistently improved survival outcomes for patients treated with this combination of adjuvant chemotherapy versus patients not so treated. Based on this lack of evidence of prolonged survival in premenopausal node-positive women treated with adjuvant chemotherapy, the authors emphasize the need to reconsider, and perhaps withdraw, the recommendation that adjuvant chemotherapy become the standard treatment for premenopausal node-positive women.

The recently released report updating the earlier consensus study makes an interesting point regarding the distinction between statistical significance and clinical improvement (Early Breast Cancer Trialists' Collaborative Group 1992). The study demonstrates that combining large numbers of individual randomized trials can achieve statistical significance as noted above. However, careful analysis of their data demonstrates that the differences between controls and treated are clinically quite small – survival at 10 years in polychemotherapy trials showed an improvement of 6.3% with a standard deviation of 1.4 and a logrank test of $2p < 0.00001$. The difference in node-negative survival was 3.5% for patients who underwent chemotherapy and 6.7% for node-positive patients. These later results confirm the argument made in a recent article by Henderson et al. (1990) against the use of chemotherapy in node-negative women.

One final note on the overview is that the authors found a statistically significant effect for ovarian ablation, similar to the effect of the more expensive polychemotherapy in premenopausal patients. This was found by analyzing only current trials, and is another good example of the greater accuracy in results obtained from the advances made in the performance of randomized clinical trials.

8.4 Discussion

Randomized clinical testing continues to be problematic. Flaws remain in clinical performance, statistical analysis, and reporting. Many of the conclusions are based on subset analyses. Simon noted that the reliability of subset analysis is poor due to problems of multiplicity and limitations in the numbers of patients studied (Simon 1982). This latter problem – limited number of patients – is an inherent problem in conducting randomized trials. Obtaining an adequate number of patients is difficult because physicians often fail to refer patients and patients often resist being randomized to an unknown treatment. In addition, if some patients do not comply with their assigned treatment (as always occurs in clinical practice) an increase in sample size is needed as the inclusion of noncompliers diminishes the statistical power of a trial. For example, if 10% of the randomized patients in each of two treatment groups in a trial do not comply with their assigned treatment, the total number of patients required in the trial to achieve the same statistical power increases by as much as 50%–60% (Wesley and Edwards 1988). Consequently, the statistical power of studies in which there are noncompliers may be considerably lower than suggested by the total number of included patients.

Multi-institutional studies have been carried out to overcome the problem of obtaining adequate sample sizes. However, these studies are problematic in themselves due to problems with quality control (Horiot et al. 1988; Johansson et al. 1986, 1987; Schaake-Koning et al. 1991; Vantongelen et al. 1991).

The European Organization for Research and Treatment of Cancer (EORTC) studies demonstrate the problems with quality control in developing randomized tests. In a recent report from that group looking at quality control of radiotherapy and chemotherapy in treating inoperable nonmetastatic, non-small-cell lung cancer, various therapies were compared: radiation alone, radiotherapy with cisplatinum, radiotherapy with 30 mg/m^2 cisplatinum once a week, and radiotherapy with 6 mg/m^2 daily (Schaake-Koning et al. 1991). A review team, consisting of a data manager, diagnostic radiologist, chest physician, and two radiotherapists, reviewed entry criteria, treatment data, tumor response, recurrences, and late toxicity of 177 patients. Only departments that entered more than 5% were visited. The following problems were noted: There was a 15% difference in T-staging of the patients and a 17% discrepancy in N-staging. The field sizes were insufficient in 15% of the eligible patients and in another 17% of the patients the tumor-free margin was less than 1 cm. Radiation dosages were incorrectly given to 7% of the patients, and the dose of cisplatinum deviated in 10% of the patients treated with combined modalities. Also, in the interpretation of chest X-rays, computer tomography showed important differences in tumor response, tumor recurrence, and late toxicity.

The EORTC also did a quality assurance analysis of their head and neck cancer treatment trial (Johansson et al. 1987). There were 17 participating radiotherapy departments, all above standard and well-equipped, with competent medical and physics staff. Each of them belonged to a leading national or regional tumor institute or university hospital. All of them participated in the study on a voluntary basis and devoted time and personal involvement to the preparation and practice of the intercomparisons. All had some experience treating patients according to the head and neck protocol procedures of a cooperative group. The dose delivered to the primary tumor was reasonably close to the prescribed dose, and the measurements made on the phantom were also in good agreement with the doses stated by the majority of the institutions.

Despite all of these favorable points, several problems were detected. First, there were insufficient margins around the tumor and nodes, which reflected an underestimation of primary target volume and nodal target volume, patient motions, absorbed dose gradients, as well as the inaccuracy of the machines. Although recommendations were given based on a precise protocol, different technical choices resulted in too much deviation from the expected optimal dose distribution in the various target volumes for demonstrable and microscopic disease. The same doses delivered on both sides resulted in an undesirably high dose to contralateral normal tissues. Homogeneous dose distribution to the homolateral neck resulted in a higher risk of complication or risk of failure in the posterior upper neck and underestimation of the risk of contralateral microscopic spread in both subdigastic and upper posterior neck.

8.5 Conclusion

Properly performed randomized clinical trials remain the best method of evaluating the results of treatment. Although the EORTC studies show that even dedicated institutions continue to struggle with problems developed in conducting clinical trials, these studies also reflect the great advancement in the performance and interpretation of clinical trials from earlier older trials. Continual critical appraisal of these older trials as well as current trials will further expand the usefulness and validity of results obtained from randomized clinical trials.

Meta-analysis, useful in obtaining necessary data not accessible from the individual trials, must also be critically analyzed. The recent report of the overview of breast cancer adjuvant therapies showing the benefits of adjuvant and systemic treatment demonstrates the need to critically appraise overviews, and the individual trials included in the overviews, to obtain accurate results. The benefits derived from hormonal manipulation in premenopausal patients, for example, have only become apparent with the use of the most recent overview and utilization of more recent and well-performed trials.

The challenge to rectify the problems found in the performance and interpretation of randomized clinical trials and meta-analyses is a challenge to all institutions that conduct randomized trials as well as to all who evaluate those trials. Clinicians and researchers are responsible for critically analyzing trials to improve the quality and quality control methods so that treatments can be modified and provide greater benefit to the cancer patient. Journal editors and readers must insist on standards of the highest quality from clinicians and researchers who conduct trials: editors must demand rigorous research from institutions, while readers must demand from editors a strict adherence to publishing only studies of the highest quality. Journal editors and referees have an additional responsibility to ensure that the many inherent problems in conducting a meta-analysis are critically reviewed prior to publication. Follow-up critiques of published meta-analyses, as suggested in a recent editorial (Anderson and Harrington 1992), would also help to ensure that all important trials are included in the overview and are interpreted correctly, as well as to ensure that the methodology is sound and the presentation clear. It is indeed the responsibility of us all to continually improve the performance and interpretation of randomized clinical trials and the more recent use of meta-analyses. We must also be open to the possibility that, as Hellman and Hellman point out in a recent editorial in *The New England Journal of Medicine* (1991), "techniques appropriate in the laboratory may not be applicable to humans. We must develop and use alternative methods for acquiring clinical knowledge."

Here lies our further challenge, to continually seek to develop and use alternative methods for acquiring clinical knowledge.

References

Anderson JW, Harrington D (1992) Meta-analyses need new publication standards. J Clin Oncol 10(6): 878–880

Baar J and Tannock I (1989) Analyzing the same data in two ways: a demonstration model to illustrate the reporting and misreporting of clinical trials. J Clin Oncol 7(7): 969–978

Bonadonna G, Brusamolino E, Valagussa P et al (1976) Combination chemotherapy as an adjuvant treatment in operable breast cancer. N Engl J Med 294: 405–410

Bonadonna G, Rossi A, Valagussa P et al (1977) The CMF program for operable breast cancer with positive axillary lymph nodes: updated analysis on the disease-free interval, site of relapse and drug tolerance. Cancer 39: 2904–2915

Bonadonna G, Valagussa P, Rossi A et al (1985) Ten-year experience with CMF-based adjuvant chemotherapy in resectable breast cancer. Breast Cancer Res Treat 5: 95–115

Cascinelli N, Greco M, Morabito A et al (1991) Comparison of long-term survival of 1986 consecutive patients with breast cancer treated at the National Cancer Institute of Milano, Italy (1971 to 1972 and 1977 to 1978). Cancer 68: 427–434

Cooper MR, Rhyne AL, Muss HB et al (1985) A randomized comparative trial of chemotherapy and irradiation therapy for stage II breast cancer. Cancer 47: 2833–2839

Cuzick J, Stewart H, Peto R et al (1987a) Overview of randomized trials of postoperative adjuvant radiotherapy in breast cancer. Cancer Treat Rep 71(1): 15–25

Cuzick J, Stewart H, Peto R et al (1987b) Overview of randomized trials comparing radical mastectomy without radiotherapy against simple mastectomy with radiotherapy in breast cancer. Cancer Treat Rep 71(1): 7–14

Early Breast Cancer Trialists' Collaborative Group (1988) Effects of adjuvant tamoxifen and of cytotoxic therapy on mortality in early breast cancer. N Engl J Med 319: 1681–1692

Early Breast Cancer Trialists' Collaborative Group (EBCTOCG) (1990) Treatment of early breast cancer. Worldwide evidence in 1985–1990. A systemic overview of all available randomized trials in early breast cancer of adjuvant endocrine and cytotoxic therapy. Oxford University Press, Oxford (Treatment of early breast cancer, vol 1)

Early Breast Cancer Trialists' Collaborative Group (1992) Systemic treatment of early breast cancer by hormonal, cytotoxic, or immune therapy, 133 randomized trials involving 31,000 recurrences and 24,000 deaths among 75,000 women. Lancet 339: 1–15, 71–85

Gelber RD, Goldhirsch A (1986) A concept of an overview of cancer clinical trials with special emphasis on early breast cancer. J Clin Oncol 4(11): 1696–1703

George SL (1985) The required size and length of a phase III clinical trial. In: Buyse ME, Staquet MJ, Sylvester RJ (eds) Cancer clinical trials: methods and practice. Oxford Medical, Oxford, pp 289–293

Glucksberg H, Rivkin S, Rasmussen S et al (1982) Combination chemotherapy (CMFVP) versus L-phenylalanine mustard (L-PAM) for operable breast cancer with positive axillary nodes (a Southwest Oncology Group Study). Cancer 50: 423–434

Henderson IC, Hayes DF, Parker LM et al (1990) Adjuvant systemic therapy for patients with node-negative tumors. Cancer 65: 2132–2147

Hellman S, Hellman D (1991) Sounding board: of mice but not men. N Engl J Med 324(22): 1585–1589

Horiot JC, Johansson KA, Gonzalez DG et al (1988) Quality assurance control in the EORTC cooperative group of radiotherapy. 1. Assessment of radiotherapy staff and equipment. Radiother Oncol 6: 275–284

Johansson KA, Horiot JC, Van Dam J et al (1986) Quality assurance control in the EORTC cooperative group of radiotherapy. 2. Dosimetric intercomparison. Radiother Oncol 7: 269–279

Johansson KA, Horiot JC, van der Schueren E (1987) Quality assurance control in the EORTC cooperative group of radiotherapy. 3. Intercomparison in an anatomical phantom. Radiother Oncol 9: 289–298

Levitt SH (1984) Controversies in the treatment of breast cancer: a need for return to the three R's in clinical research. Am J Clin Oncol 7: 583–591

Levitt SH (1988) Is there a role for post-operative adjuvant radiation in breast cancer? beautiful hypothesis versus ugly facts: 1987 Gilbert H. Fletcher Lecture. Int J Radiat Oncol Biol Phys 14: 787–796

Levitt SH, McHugh RB (1977) Radiotherapy in the postoperative treatment of operable cancer of the breast: Part I. Critique of the clinical and biometric aspects of the trials. Cancer 39: 924–932

Levitt SH, Khan FM, Boen JR et al (1983) Multimodal therapy in the treatment of breast cancer. Am J Clin Oncol 6: 387–391

Levitt SH, McHugh RB, Song SW (1976) Radiotherapy in the postoperative treatment of operable cancer of the breast: Part II. A reexamination of Stjernsward's application of the Mantel-Haenszel statistical method. Evaluation of the effect of the radiation on immune response and suggestions for postoperative radiotherapy. Cancer 39: 933–940

Levitt SH, Potish RA, Aeppli D, Lindgren B (1988) The consensus statements on adjuvant chemotherapy in breast cancer: fact or artifact. Am J Clin Oncol (CCT) 11(1): 73–76

Mueller CB, Lesperance ML (1991) NSABP trials of adjuvant chemotherapy for breast cancer: a further look at the evidence. Ann Surg 214: 206–212

National Cancer Institute (1973–1988) SEER Data. Cancer Statistics Review, National Institute of Health 91-2789, Bethesda, MD

Nissen-Meyer R, Host H, Kjellgren K, Musson B, Norin T (1984) Clinical results I: experience of randomized trials with surgical controls – Scandinavian trials with a short postoperative course versus a 12-cycle course. Recent Results Cancer Res 96: 48–54

Nissen-Meyer R, Kjellgren K, Malmio K et al (1978) Surgical adjuvant chemotherapy. Cancer 41: 2088–2098

Paterson R (1958) Clinical trials in malignant disease: part I. Principles of random selection. J Fac Radiol 9: 80–83

Paterson R (1962) Breast cancer – a report of two clinical trials. J R Coll Surg Edinb 7(4): 243–254

Paterson R, Russell MH (1958) Clinical trials in malignant disease: part II. Breast cancer: value of irradiation of the ovaries. J Fac Radiol 9: 130–133

Paterson R, Russell MH (1959) Clinical trials of malignant disease: Part III. Breast cancer: evaluation of postoperative radiotherapy. Clin Radiol 10(4): 175–180

Rivkin SE, Glucksberg H, Foulkes M (1983) Adjuvant chemotherapy for operable breast cancer with positive axillary nodes: a comparison of CMFVP versus L-PAM (Southwest Oncology Group Study). In: Jones SE, Salmon SE (eds) *Adjuvant therapy of cancer IV*. Grune and Stratton, Orlando, pp 209–215

Rossi A, Bonadonna G, Valagussa P, Veronesi U (1984) Multimodal treatment in operable breast cancer: 5-year results of the CMF programme. BMJ [Clin Res] 282: 1427–1431

Rutqvist LE, Cedermark B, Glas U et al (1989) Radiotherapy, chemotherapy, and tamoxifen as adjuncts to surgery in early breast cancer: a summary of three randomized trials. Int J Radiat Oncol Biol Phys 16: 629–639

Sacks HS, Berrier J, Reitman D et al (1987) Meta-analysis of randomized controlled trials. N Engl J Med 316: 450–455

Schaake-Koning C, Kirkpatrick A, Kroger R et al (1991) The need for immediate monitoring of treatment parameters and uniform assessment of patient data in clinical trials: a quality control study of the EORTC radiotherapy and lung cancer cooperative groups. Eur J Cancer 27(5): 615–619

Simon R (1987) Overviews of randomized clinical trials. Cancer Treat Rep 71(1): 3–5

Simon R (1982) Patient subsets and variation in therapeutic efficacy. Br J Clin Pharmac 14: 473–482

Smith DC, Crawford D, Dykes EH et al (1984) Adjuvant radiotherapy and chemotherapy in breast cancer. In: Jones SE, Salmon SE (eds) *Adjuvant therapy of cancer IV*. Grune and Stratton, Orlando, pp 283–289

Tobias JS, Tattersall MHN (1985) "Doing the Best for the Cancer Patient." Lancet i(8419): 35–37

Vantongelen K, Steward W, Blackledge G et al (1991) EORTC joint ventures in quality control: treatment-related variables and data acquisition in chemotherapy trials. Eur J Cancer 27(2): 201–207

Wesley MN, Edwards BK (1988) Statistical considerations in the design and interpretation of clinical trials. In: Lippman ME, Lichter I, and Danforth DN (eds) Diagnosis and management of breast cancer. Saunders, Philadelphia, pp 525–548

9 What Have We Learned from the Stockholm Trials on Adjuvant Radiation Therapy in Early-Stage Breast Cancer?

LARS-ERIK RUTQVIST

CONTENTS

9.1	Introduction	83
9.2	The First Stockholm Trial: Adjuvant Radiation Therapy Versus Surgery Alone	83
9.2.1	Joint Analysis of the First Stockholm and Oslo-II Trial	84
9.2.2	False-Negative Radiation Therapy Overviews?	86
9.2.3	Adjuvant Radiation Therapy and Long-Term Local Control	86
9.3	Cardiovascular Side Effects of Radiation Therapy?	87
9.4	The Second Stockholm Trial: Adjuvant Radiation Therapy Versus CMF Chemotherapy	89
9.5	Conclusion	90
	References	92

9.1 Introduction

In the middle of the 1970s, both American and European research groups reported significant benefits with adjuvant chemotherapy in terms of recurrence-free survival for patients with early-stage breast cancer (FISHER et al. 1975; BONADONNA et al. 1976). Since then there has been a continued emphasis on the use of adjuvant systemic therapy in the primary management of breast cancer. Unfortunately, advocates for this type of treatment have sometimes underrated the importance of local control of disease through the use of adjuvant radiation, thereby ignoring the fact that locoregional recurrences usually decrease the quality of life significantly and shorten disease-free survival. The fact that many radiation therapy studies have failed to show an overall survival benefit is often used as an argument against radiation therapy. However, an unbiased assessment of the role of adjuvant radiation in the primary management of early-stage breast cancer should acknowledge the fact that many of the radiation trails reported in the literature used outdated treatment techniques that are irrelevant to current medical practice (LEVITT 1986, 1988).

In 1971, the Stockholm Breast Cancer Study Group started a program for the diagnosis, treatment, and follow-up of women with primary breast cancer. This management program – which is still ongoing – includes two randomized radiation therapy trials with a total of more than 2000 patients. The principle aim of the trials is to evaluate the role of adjuvant radiation in the primary management of operable breast cancer. All radiation treatment in the trials is individually planned and administered with modern megavoltage techniques. The first Stockholm trial was initiated in 1971 and compared pre- or postoperative radiation therapy with surgery alone. The second trial started in 1976 and compared adjuvant chemotherapy with postoperative radiation therapy (RUTQVIST et al. 1989).

Several Swedish population-based registers – such as the National Cause-of-Death Registry and the National Cancer Registry – rely on a personal identification number to uniquely identify all registered individuals. Follow-up of the patients in both trials has been more than 99% due to using this number.

9.2 The First Stockholm Trial: Adjuvant Radiation Therapy Versus Surgery Alone

The details of the first Stockholm trial were published previously (DE SCHRYVER 1976; STRENDER et al. 1981). In summary, during 1971–1976 a total of 960 pre- and postmenopausal patients with operable stages I–III breast cancer were randomized to pre- or postoperative radiation therapy (45 Gy/4.5 weeks), or to surgery alone. About one-third of the patients were histologically node-positive. The surgery was a modified radical mastectomy in all cases. The radiation therapy was individually planned and was given with megavoltage techniques. The target volume included the chest wall (and breast in the preoperative cases) and the regional lymph

LARS-ERIK RUTQVIST, M. D., Ph.D.; on behalf of the Stockholm Breast Cancer Study Group Oncologic Center, Karolinska Hospital, 104-01 Stockholm, Sweden nodes in the axilla, supraclavicular fossa, and the internal mammary nodes. The mean follow-up time was 16 years.

The results for all patients showed a significant benefit in terms of locoregional recurrences for those treated with radiation therapy. There were also differences of borderline significance in favor of the irradiated patients in terms of distant metastases, total deaths, and deaths due to breast cancer (Table 9.1). There were no significant differences between the pre- and postoperative treatment groups. When the results were analyzed by nodal status, only node-positive patients benefited from radiation therapy. In that subset of patients there was a significant benefit ($p < 0.05$) of using postoperative radiation in terms of decreased incidence of distant metastases and deaths due to breast cancer. No such benefit was found among the node-negative patients. The preoperative cases were not included in the analysis because the radiation obscured the histologic nodal status.

Node-positive breast cancer often is described in the literature as a systemic disease already at the time of diagnosis in most patients. According to this hypothesis, prevention of distant dissemination can be achieved only with systemic therapy. However, this contention is not substantiated by current results. On the contrary, current results suggest that distant metastases can originate from uncontrolled local deposits of tumor cells. Local undertreatment thus may be deleterious in subgroups of patients with a high risk of locoregional residual disease after primary surgery.

9.2.1 *Joint Analysis of the First Stockholm and Oslo-II Trial*

In 1987, Cuzick et al. published two overviews (meta-analysis) that included selected radiation therapy studies (Cuzick et al. 1987a, b). No overall survival benefit with radiation was observed during

Table 9.1. Analysis of events among patients included in the first Stockholm trial[a]

Nodal Status	Preoperative RT ($n = 316$)	Postoperative RT ($n = 323$)	Surgery alone ($n = 321$)	Relative hazard[b]	Log-rank p-Value
Type of event	(%)	(%)	(%)		
pN0:					
Locoregional recurrence	–	5	23	0.25	<0.001
Distant metastases	–	26	25	1.02	0.94
Death due to breast cancer	–	23	22	1.05	0.80
All deaths	–	33	22	0.87	0.40
pN +					
Locoregional recurrence	–	15	48	0.29	<0.001
Distant metastases	–	52	69	0.66	<0.05
Death due to breast cancer	–	50	68	0.70	<0.05
All deaths	–	61	70	0.82	0.21
All patients					
Locoregional recurrence	11	9	33	0.27	<0.001
Distant metastases	37	35	42	0.82	0.07
Deaths due to breast cancer	35	33	40	0.83	0.09
All deaths	47	43	51	0.84	0.09

RT, radiotherapy
[a] The preoperative radiation obscured the modal status so this group was only included in the total results.
[b] Irradiated versus surgery alone patients.

the first 10 years of follow-up. It was even suggested that the radiation therapy used in the trials had an adverse effect on survival after 10–15 years. These results were interpreted to support the assumption that adjuvant radiation therapy does not prevent distant dissemination and that a survival benefit can be achieved only with systemic treatments aimed at eradicating distant micrometastases. However, the overviews have been criticized because they included several trials using inadequate treatment techniques, e.g., orthovoltage radiation (LEVITT 1986, 1988). The overviews therefore may obscure the clinically worthwhile benefit with radiation demonstrated in the more recent trials that used modern megavoltage techniques. Additionally, several studies included in the overview had methodological flaws such as biased methods of treatment allocation.

Due to these errors found in the overviews, we decided to separately analyze two of the trials included in the overviews: the Stockholm and Oslo-II trials. These studies differed from the other trials in the overviews in several important respects: they both used modern megavoltage radiation techniques, treatment included regional nodal areas, tumor dose was appropriate (45–50 Gy/4–5 weeks), and the design of the trials permitted an unconfounded, unbiased evaluation of the treatment effect by histologic nodal status. The analysis was focused on the potential effects of radiation on distant metastasis-free and overall survival, as well as on the potential treatment interactions with nodal status and tumor location. Recurrence-free survival was not used as an end point since it was well-established that radiation therapy was able to prevent locoregional recurrences. The treatment effect was evaluated by calculating the relative risk (RR) of distant metastasis or death for the radiation therapy group versus the control group. The RR was estimated with Cox's proportional hazards model stratified by treatment center (AUQUIER et al. 1992).

The Oslo-II trial included 541 pre- and postmenopausal patients randomized during 1968–1972 (HÖST and BRENNHOVD 1977). The surgery was a radical mastectomy. All patients were treated with a radiologic castration. The patients were randomly allocated to postoperative radiation therapy (Cobalt-60) or to surgery alone. The target volume included the internal mammary nodes, the supra- and infraclavicular regions and the apex of the axilla. The treatment was given with two anterior fields. The chest wall was not irradiated. The protocol dose was 50 Gy at 3 cm depth given with daily fractions of 2.5 Gy 5 days a week for a total treatment time of about 4 weeks. The mean follow-up was 16 years.

In the joint analysis of the two trials there was a significant benefit with radiation for all patients in terms of distant metastasis-free survival ($p < 0.01$). The RR of distant metastasis for irradiated versus control patients was 0.75 (95% confidence interval, 95% C.I., 0.61–0.92). However, there was no significant overall survival benefit with radiation: the RR of death for the irradiated patients was 0.92 (95% C.I., 0.77–1.10). There was a significant interaction ($p < 0.05$) between treatment and nodal status: the irradiated node-positive patients had a RR of distant metastasis of 0.63 (95% C.I., 0.48–0.83; $p < 0.001$) versus 0.97 (95% C.I., 0.70–1.33; not significant) for the irradiated node-negative patients. There was also an overall survival difference in favor of the irradiated node-positive patients ($p = 0.06$) with a 0.78 (95% C.I., 0.61–1.00) RR of death. This corresponds to a 22% relative reduction of deaths. In contrast, there was no survival benefit with radiation among the node-negative patients: the RR of death was 1.10 (95% C.I., 0.85–1.43).

Eradicating the metastases in lymph nodes along the internal mammary vessels has been suggested as a way to improve survival by using radiation therapy (ARRIAGADA et al. 1988). This would be most effective in medially located node-positive tumors, since these tumors have the highest incidence of such metastases. To study this hypothesis, RRs of distant metastasis in the node-positive subgroup were calculated according to tumor location. The RR for medial tumors (0.51) was lower than that for central or lateral tumors (0.72). However, the Cox analysis indicated no significant interaction between treatment and tumor location.

In summary, the joint analysis showed a favorable effect of radiation therapy on distant metastasis-free survival of node-positive patients and a survival difference corresponding to a 22% relative reduction of death. The effect of radiation was numerically larger among node-positive patients with inner and central tumors compared to those with lateral tumors, but there was no statistically significant interaction between treatment and tumor location. This analysis suggested that all types of locoregional residual disease – irrespective of the location – may compromise overall survival.

9.2.2 *False-Negative Radiation Therapy Overviews?*

The rationale and methodology for overviews of randomized clinical trials were previously described (EARLY BREAST CANCER TRIALISTS' COLLABORATIVE GROUP 1988). One aim of overviews is to obtain a more stable estimate of the effect of a certain therapy by increasing the number of patients available for analysis. An overview might also aim at avoiding selection bias by including all available trials of a particular treatment modality. In practice, this implies that the included trials will be dissimilar, e.g., in regard to the performance of the therapy used. Therefore, a "negative" overview result does not imply that the tested treatment modality is invariably ineffective. For instance, the overviews of radiation therapy trials included large, old trials that used orthovoltage X-rays. As previously mentioned, this may have obscured a clinically worthwhile benefit in the more recent radiation therapy trials that used adequate megavoltage treatment techniques. The results of the first Stockholm trial and the joint analysis of the Stockholm and Oslo-II trial suggest such an interpretation. As part of the international overview process including all available trials of primary treatment of early-stage breast cancer, an updated overview of all unbiased, unconfounded radiation therapy trials is currently underway. This overview will include an in-depth analysis of the significance of treatment technique.

9.2.3 *Adjuvant Radiation Therapy and Long-Term Local Control*

It has been suggested that radiation therapy should be deferred until a locoregional relapse is diagnosed so that patients who do not develop such a recurrence are spared the inconvenience and potential hazards of radiation therapy. However, such a treatment policy is based on the assumption that the eventual control rate – that is, after salvage treatment – will be the same as with a policy of giving adjuvant radiation treatment. This hypothesis was studied among patients included in the first Stockholm trial. Among those patients who developed a locoregional recurrence, the response to salvage treatment was evaluated using UICC/WHO criteria (HAYWARD et al. 1977). Treatment after recurrence was decided individually by the responsible clinician.

There was no significant difference between the two radiation therapy groups compared with the surgery alone group in the best response to salvage treatment (Table 9.2) (RUTQVIST et al., manuscript submitted). About 70% in the radiation therapy groups achieved an objective response (complete or

Table 9.2. Local tumor control according to allocated adjuvant treatment among patients in the first Stockholm trial who developed a locoregional recurrence

	Pre- and postoperative radiotherapy[a] n (%)		Surgery alone[b] n (%)	
Number with a locoregional recurrence	64	10	105	33
Best response to salvage treatment[c]				
Complete remission	32/63	51	67/101	66
Partial remission or disease stabilization	12/63	19	12/101	12
Progressive disease	19/63	31	22/101	22
Number with progressive disease after an initial objective response of disease stabilization	16/44	36	36/79	46
Number with uncontrolled local disease at death or at last follow-up[d]	39/639	6	50/314	16[e]

[a] $n = 639$
[b] $= 321$
[c] One irradiated and four surgery alone patients were unevaluable.
[d] Seven surgery alone patients were unevaluable.
[e] Irradiated versus surgery alone patients: $p < 0.01$.

partial remission) or disease stabilization compared with 78% in the surgery alone group. Similarly, there was no significant difference in the proportion of patients who developed progressive disease after an initial response to treatment. The total proportion of patients who eventually showed progressive disease was high in both the irradiated group and the surgery alone group: 66% compared with 68%. The long-term outcome of salvage treatment was thus poor irrespective of the initially allocated adjuvant therapy. However, since the total number of locoregional failures was greater in the surgery alone group, the overall proportion of patients with uncontrolled locoregional disease present at death or at last follow-up was significantly greater in that group than in the irradiated group (16% versus 6%; $p < 0.01$).

These results indicate that a policy of deferred treatment only for those who actually develop a locoregional recurrence will eventually result in a higher incidence of patients with uncontrolled local disease than will a policy of prevention of locoregional recurrences by the use of adjuvant radiation therapy.

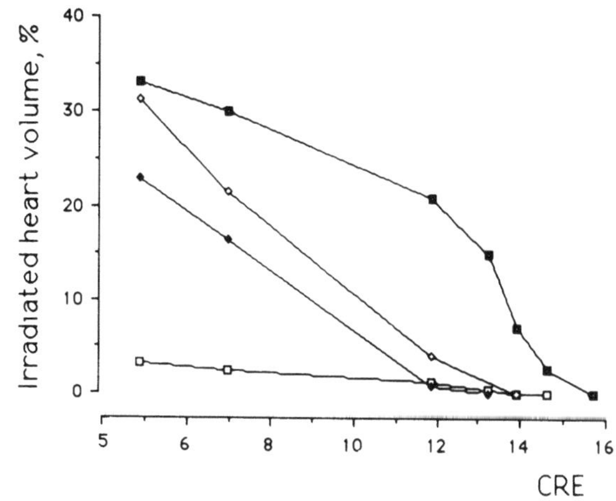

Fig. 9.1. Results of an analysis of the radiation dose to the myocardium with the different treatment techniques used in the first Stockholm trial. The curves show the relationship between the cumulative biologic dose of radiation – expressed as cumulative radiation effect (CRE) – and irradiated heart volume according to tumor laterality and treatment technique. The results relate to a model patient with an intermediate chest wall thickness (100% heart volume = 1080 cm^3). On the basis of these results the treatment techniques were classified as giving a high dose-volume (left-sided tumors, tangential cobalt-60 fields, *black squares*), intermediate dose-volume (electron techniques irrespective of tumor laterality; *white rhombus*, left-sided; *black rhombus*, right-sided), or a low dose-volume in the myocardium (right-sided, tangential cobalt-60 fields, *white squares*)

9.3 Cardiovascular Side Effects of Radiation Therapy?

One concern with radiation therapy is that it may be associated with cardiovascular side effects. Analyses of cause-specific mortality in individual radiation trials (Höst et al. 1986; Haybittle et al. 1989) and one population-based cohort study (Rutqvist and Johansson 1990) have shown an increase in mortality due to ischemic heart disease associated with radiation. However, dose–effect relationships and the significance of treatment technique were not evaluated in these studies.

To assess the potential cardiovascular effects of radiation therapy used in the first Stockholm trial, cumulative dose-volumes in the myocardium were estimated for each of the techniques used in the study since it seemed reasonable to assume that any adverse cardiac effect of radiation should be correlated with both the dose and the irradiated volume (Rutqvist et al. 1992). The long-term outcome in terms of the pattern of cause-specific mortality in subgroups of patients was then evaluated according to the estimated myocardial dose-volume. Figure 9.1 shows the relationship between cumulative radiation effect (CRE) and irradiated volume in a model patient according to treatment technique and tumor laterality. The internal mammary nodes, chest wall, and breast in patients who underwent preoperative irradiation were generally treated with tangential cobalt-60 beams. In patients treated postoperatively, the chest wall was treated with 7–15 MeV electrons. The choice of energy depended on the individually measured chest wall thickness. The consistently highest maximum CRE and largest irradiated volume were obtained with left-sided tangential cobalt-60 fields. The consistently smallest dose-volume was obtained with right-sided tangential cobalt-60 fields. Irrespective of the laterality of the tumor, the electron techniques resulted in intermediate dose-volumes.

Table 9.3 shows an analysis of cause-specific mortality by allocated treatment and estimated radiation dose-volume. With increasing dose-volume, there was no significant trend in mortality due to breast cancer, other types of cancer, cardiovascular diseases other than ischemic heart disease, miscellaneous causes, or all causes. However, mortality due to ischemic heart disease was significantly higher in the high dose-volume subgroup (that is, patients with left-sided tumors treated with tangential cobalt-60 fields) than in the

Table 9.3. Cause-specific mortality by allocated treatment and estimated radiation dose volume in the myocardium among patients in the first Stockholm trial[a]

Cause of death	Surgery alone		Radiation dose-volume[b] Low		Intermediate		High		Trend-test
	D/1000WY	RH	D/1000WY	RH[c]	D/1000WY	RH[c]	D/1000WY	RH[c]	
Breast cancer	33.9	1.0	26.1	0.8	25.6	0.8	31.2	0.9	n.s
Other cancers	4.2	1.0	3.6	0.9	3.6	0.8	1.6	0.4	n.s
Ischemic heart disease	2.3	1.0	1.5	0.7	2.2	1.0	7.1	3.2	$p < 0.05$
Other cardiovascular disease	2.8	1.0	2.6	0.9	2.5	0.9	1.6	0.6	n.s
Miscellaneous causes	2.5	1.0	2.0	0.8	3.0	1.2	3.3	1.3	n.s
All causes	45.7	1.0	35.8	0.8	36.9	0.8	44.9	1.0	n.s

D/1000 WY, deaths per thousand woman-years; RH, relative hazard.
[a] The "high" dose-volume group included patients with left-sided tumors whose chest wall was treated with tangential photons, the "intermediate" group included all patients treated with electrons, and the "low" group included patients with right-sided tumors treated with tangential photons (see Fig. 9.1).
[b] Preoperative and postoperative radiotherapy.
[c] Irradiated patients versus surgery alone group.

surgical controls: 7.1/1000 woman–years at risk (WYR) versus 2.3/1000 WYR ($p < 0.05$), although there was no difference in total mortality (44.9/1000 WYR versus 45.7/1000 WYR).

Figure 9.2 shows the cumulative mortality due to ischemic heart disease in the high dose-volume subgroup compared with that in the surgical controls. The difference between the groups emerged after 4–5 years and appeared to increase with longer follow-up. In the low and intermediate dose-volume subgroups, the mortality due to ischemic heart disease – 1.5 and 2.2/1000 WYR respectively – was similar to that among the surgical controls.

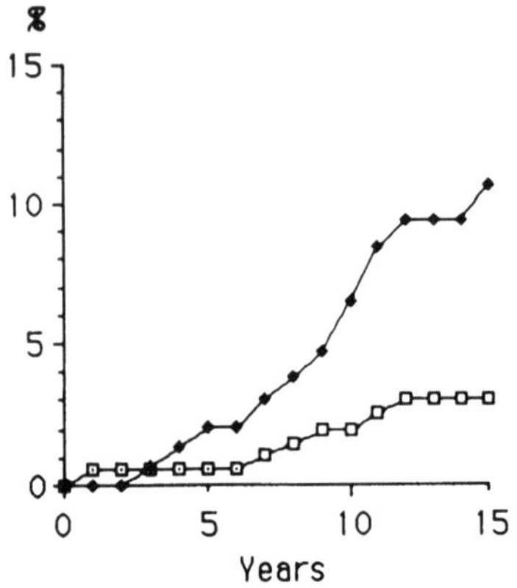

Fig. 9.2. Cumulative incidence of deaths due to ischemic heart disease. The data concern patients included in the first Stockholm trial who were treated with tangential cobalt-60 photons because of a left-sided tumor (i.e., patients receiving a high dose-volume in the myocardium; *black squares*) and untreated patients in the surgery-alone group (*white squares*)

There was thus no overall increase in cardiovascular mortality among the irradiated patients. However, cardiac mortality was significantly related to the distribution of biologic dose of radiation in the myocardium. An increase in cardiovascular mortality was not found to be associated with treatment of right-sided tumors with either tangential cobalt-60 beams or electrons nor with treatment of left-sided tumors with electrons. However, tangential photon fields including the internal mammary nodes should probably be avoided in patients with left-sided tumors for whom electrons appear to be a more attractive alternative. The current results illustrate that an increased cardiovascular mortality related to radiation therapy can be avoided by the use of appropriate treatment techniques and avoiding excessive treatment. However, individual treatment planning is necessary to assess the dose distribution in the myocardium.

The internal mammary nodes are located close to the myocardium. If they are included in the target volume the dose-volume in the myocardium will invariably increase, provided all other treatment-related factors are the same. Is it then important to treat these nodes? Randomized trials of superradical surgery, including dissection of the internal mammary nodes versus less radical surgery, have not produced evidence of any significant survival benefit with the more extensive surgery. Also, there are no randomized radiation trials that have studied the relevance of internal mammary node treatment. The only data available are based on retrospective analyses. As previously mentioned in the joint analysis of the Stockholm and Oslo-II trials, the metastasis-free survival benefit with radiation according to tumor location suggested a greater benefit for patients with medial tumor (who are more likely to have involved internal mammary nodes) than those with lateral or central tumors (AUQUIER et al. 1992). Also, in a retrospective evaluation of more than 1200 patients from the Institut Gustave-Roussy, ARRIAGADA et al. (1988) showed that treatment of the internal mammary nodes – either with surgery or radiation – was associated with a significant overall survival benefit. The available data thus suggest that uncontrolled metastases in these nodes may compromise survival. The current analysis showed that radiation treatment including these nodes can be given without increasing the risk of cardiovascular mortality provided excessive treatment to the myocardium is avoided. Also, since metastases in the internal mammary nodes are most frequent in the first three costal interspaces, the treatment fields covering these nodes may not have to be extended down to the xyphoid in all cases.

9.4 The Second Stockholm Trial: Adjuvant Radiation Therapy Versus CMF Chemotherapy

In the middle of the 1970s, preliminary results from the Oslo-II and the first Stockholm trial showed significant improvements in recurrence-free survival with adjuvant megavoltage radiation. Around this same time, results from Milan and National Surgical Adjuvant Breast and Bowel Project (NSABP) groups showed significantly improved recurrence-free survival with adjuvant chemotherapy in women with node-positive breast cancer (FISHER et al. 1975; BONADONNA et al. 1976). Because of these observations, the second Stockholm trial was designed to directly compare postoperative radiation therapy with adjuvant cyclophosphamide, methotrexate, and 5-fluorouracil (CMF) chemotherapy. The rationale was that before adjuvant chemotherapy could be accepted as a standard treatment, it should be compared with the best possible alternative – postoperative radiation.

The trial included both pre- and postmenopausal patients. The patients were required to have either histologically verified lymph node metastases or a tumor diameter exceeding 30 mm (measured on the surgical specimen). For the postmenopausal subgroup, the study also included a randomized comparison of tamoxifen (40 mg daily for 2 or 5 years) versus no adjuvant endocrine treatment (RUTQVIST et al. 1989). The patients were thus randomized among postoperative radiation therapy, radiation therapy plus tamoxifen, chemotherapy, or chemotherapy plus tamoxifen. Due to a temporary shortage of radiation treatment capacity in the Stockholm area, the randomization between radiation therapy and chemotherapy was deliberately unbalanced during 1982–1984: two-thirds of the patients were randomized to chemotherapy and one-third to radiation therapy. This explains the differences in the number of patients included in the two treatment groups. As in the first Stockholm trial, all radiation therapy was given with high-voltage techniques. The tumor dose was 46 Gy/4.5 weeks. The target volume included the chest wall, axilla, supraclavicular fossa, and the ipsilateral internal mammary nodes. A total of more than 1200 patients have been included in the trial. The results presented here were based on a preliminary analysis of those 706 patients randomized during 1976–1984. Their mean follow-up was 7 years.

The recurrence-free survival by allocated treatment is shown in Fig. 9.3. There was no significant difference between radiation therapy and chemotherapy for all patients. However, postmenopausal patients fared better in terms of recurrence-free survival with a gain of 21% at 7 years (57% versus 36%; $p < 0.01$). Among premenopausal patients, there was no significant difference between the treatment groups. There was an overall survival difference in favor of the chemotherapy group among the premenopausal patients (68% versus 62%) and in favor of the radiation therapy group among the postmenopausal patients (62% versus 54%), but these differences were not significant.

Figure 9.4 illustrates that distant metastases were reduced to a greater extent with chemotherapy among the premenopausal patients ($p = 0.08$) and with radiation therapy among the postmenopausal patients ($p = 0.02$). In both pre- and postmenopausal patients, locoregional recurrences were reduced to a greater extent with radiation therapy. Among the postmenopausal patients, those treated with adjuvant chemotherapy alone fared the worst (Fig. 9.5). The addition of tamoxifen to chemotherapy increased the recurrence-free survival to a level similar to that achieved with radiation therapy ($p < 0.01$). The best result in terms of recurrence-free survival was observed among those treated with radiation therapy plus tamoxifen, but there was no significant difference between this

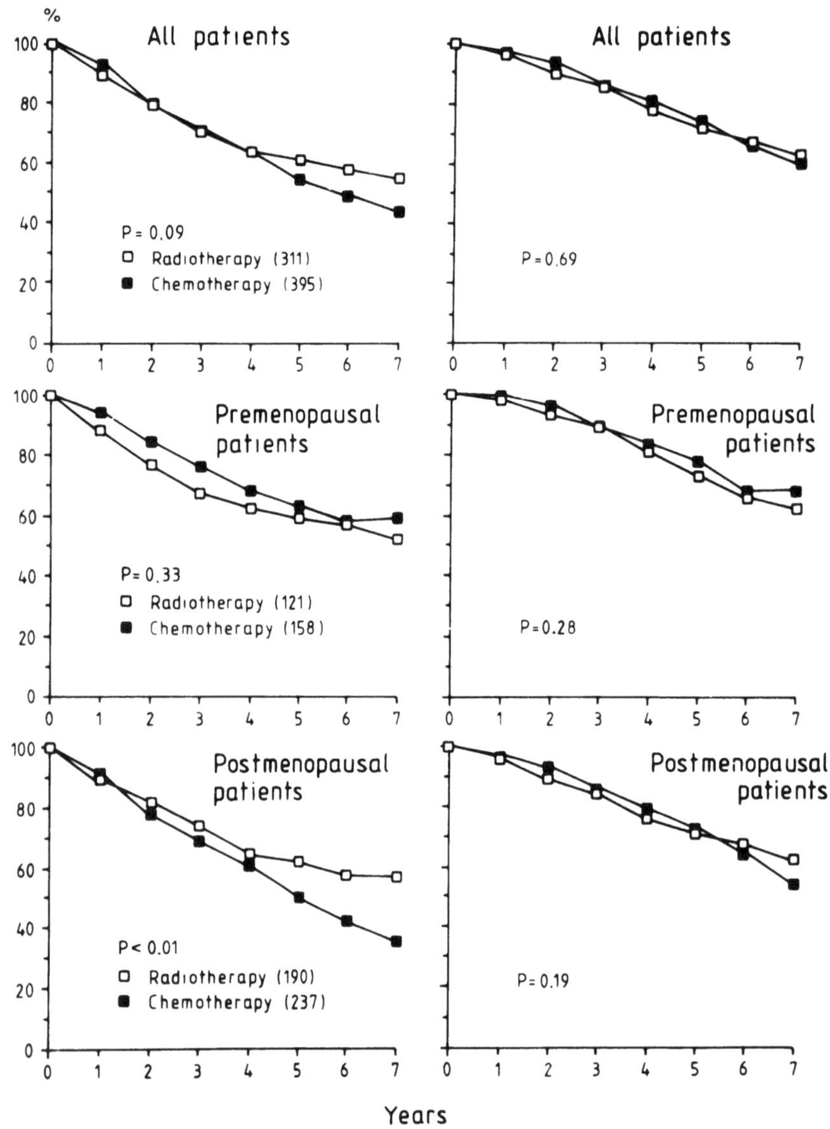

Fig. 9.3. Recurrence-free (*left traces*) and overall (*right traces*) survival for patients included in the second Stockholm trial of postoperative radiation therapy versus adjuvant cyclophosphamide, methotrexate, and 5-fluorouracil chemotherapy. Note that the uneven number of patients in the treatment groups was due to the unbalanced randomization. Log-rank *p* values are indicated

group and those treated with radiation therapy alone.

In summary, radiation therapy was superior to chemotherapy in terms of locoregional recurrences, distant metastases, and recurrence-free survival in postmenopausal patients. This result agrees with the conclusions from the first Stockholm trial and provides further support for the hypothesis that adjuvant megavoltage radiation can prevent distant dissemination in subgroups of patients. On the other hand, the results tended to be better with adjuvant chemotherapy among premenopausal patients, except for locoregional recurrences, which were reduced to a greater extent with radiation therapy.

9.5 Conclusion

The first Stockholm trial showed that adjuvant radiation therapy is an effective treatment for the prevention of locoregional recurrence. In addition, node-positive patients allocated to radiation therapy had fewer distant metastases and a decreased mortality due to breast cancer compared with the surgery alone group. As a result of poor long-term results of salvage therapy, the policy of deferred

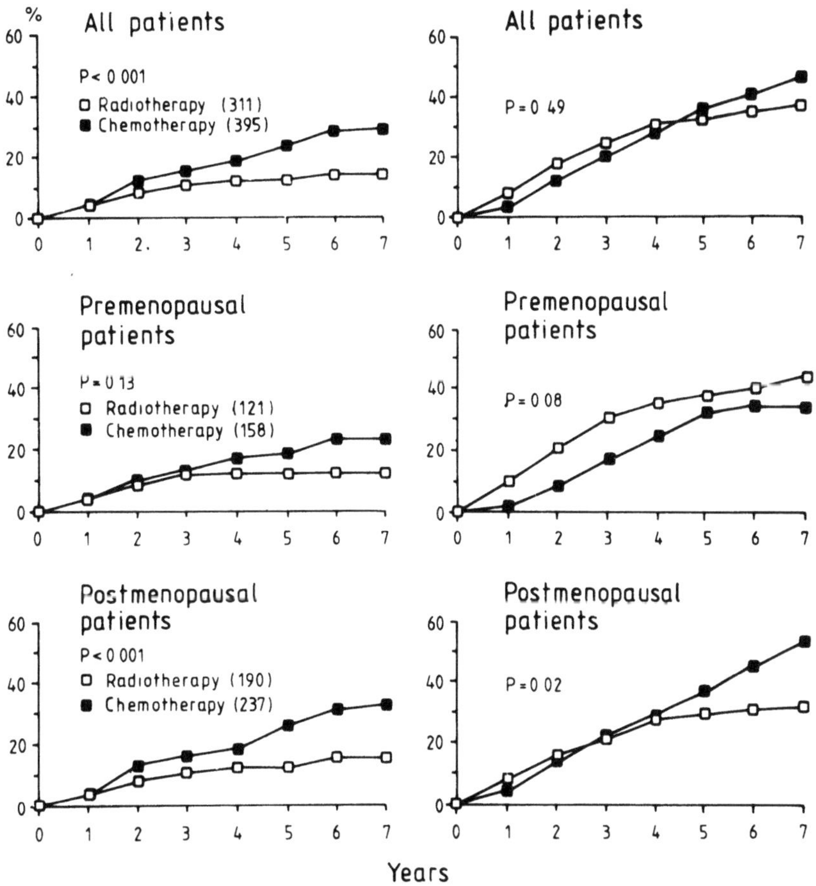

Fig. 9.4. Cumulative incidence of locoregional recurrence (*left traces*) and distant metastasis (*right traces*) among patients included in the second Stockholm trial

local treatment – as in the surgery alone group – resulted in a significantly higher incidence of patients who eventually developed uncontrolled local disease.

It is well-established that radiation can have significant adverse effects in normal tissues with a close three-dimensional association with the target volume, as in the lungs. Because of late radiation-induced effects in the myocardium, an increased cardiovascular mortality could possibly offset the benefit with radiation therapy. However, the analysis of cause-specific mortality according to treatment technique in the first Stockholm trial illustrated that such adverse effects can be avoided through the use of techniques aimed at lowering the dose to the myocardium. These observations highlight the importance of appropriate radiation treatment techniques and the significance of local tumor control in the primary management of breast cancer.

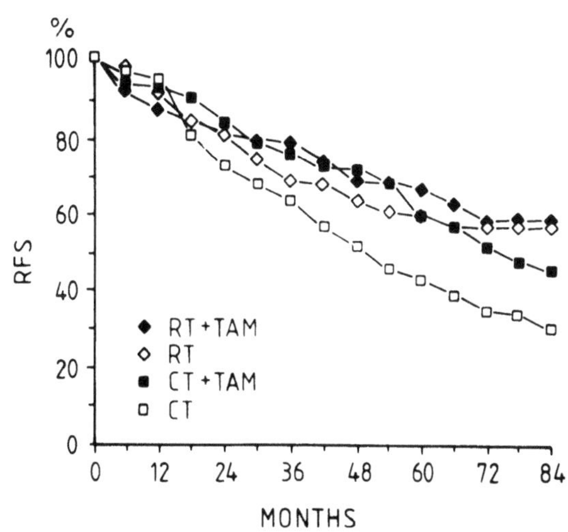

Fig. 9.5. Recurrence-free survival among postmenopausal patients included in the second Stockholm trial. Log-rank comparisons indicated that the only significant difference between the curves was that the chemotherapy-alone arm was significantly worse than all three other arms ($p < 0.01$; *RT*, radiotherapy; *CT*, chemotherapy; *TAM*, tamoxifen)

The second Stockholm trial showed that for postmenopausal patients with high-risk disease, postoperative radiation therapy was a better treatment option than adjuvant chemotherapy in terms of prevention of locoregional recurrences and improvement of recurrence-free survival. The best result in terms of recurrence-free survival was achieved with radiation therapy plus tamoxifen, but there was no significant difference between this group and the group who received radiation therapy alone. These observations concur with the results of the international overview of all available trials of adjuvant systemic therapy in early-stage breast cancer, which showed little, if any, effect of adjuvant chemotherapy among women aged above 50 years, and a moderate, although highly statistical significant, survival benefit with tamoxifen (Early Breast Trialists' Collaborative Group 1988). The overview also showed a significant benefit among women under 50 years with adjuvant chemotherapy. Our results concur with this observation in showing a trend toward a decreased incidence of distant metastases with adjuvant chemotherapy among the premenopausal women. However, radiation therapy was also more effective in preventing locoregional recurrences in these young women.

In summary, the results of the Stockholm trials indicate that radiation therapy should continue to play an important role in the primary management of early-stage breast cancer, either as the only adjunct to surgery in patients who cannot be expected to benefit from systemic treatment, or in combination with adjuvant chemotherapy or tamoxifen in selected subsets of patients. We believe that refinements in currently available radiation therapy techniques – for example based on three-dimensional treatment planning, multi-leaf collimation, and new electron techniques – may further improve the results of treatment and decrease the risk of adverse side effects. Also, a more sophisticated use of prognostic factors will probably in the near future permit a more accurate selection of patients who potentially could benefit from radiation therapy.

Acknowledgements. The studies were supported by the King Gustaf V Jubilee Fund, the Stockholm Cancer Society, and the Swedish Cancer Society.

References

Arriagada R, Le MG, Mouriesse H et al (1988) Long-term effect of internal mammary chain treatment. Results of a multivariate analysis of 1204 patients with operable breast cancer and positive axillary nodes. Radiotherapy and Oncology 11: 213–222

Auquier A, Rutqvist LE, Höst H et al (1992) Postmastectomy megavoltage radiation: the Oslo and Stockholm trials. Eur J Cancer 28: 433–437

Bonadonna G, Brusamolino E, Valagussa P et al (1976) Combination chemotherapy as an adjuvant treatment in operable breast cancer. N Engl J Med 294: 405–410

Cuzick J, Stewart H, Peto R (1987a) Overview of randomised trials comparing radical mastectomy against simple mastectomy with radiotherapy in breast cancer. Cancer Treat Rep 71: 7–14

Cuzick J, Stewart H, Peto R (1987b) Overview of randomised trials of postoperative adjuvant radiotherapy in breast cancer. Cancer Treat Rep 71: 15–29

de Schryver A (1976) The Stockholm breast cancer trial: preliminary report of a randomized study concerning the value of preoperative or postoperative radiotherapy in operable disease. Int J Radiat Oncol Biol Phys 1: 601–609

Early Breast Cancer Trialists' Collaborative Group (1988) Effects of adjuvant tamoxifen and of cytotoxic therapy on mortality in early breast cancer. N Engl J Med 319: 1681–1692

Fisher B, Carbone P, Economou SG et al (1975) L-phenylalanin mustard (L-PAM) in the management of primary breast cancer: a report of early findings. N Engl J Med 292: 117–122

Haybittle JL, Brinkley D, Houghton J et al (1989) Postoperative radiotherapy and late mortality: evidence from the Cancer Research Campaign trial for early breast cancer. BMJ 298: 1611–1614

Hayward JL, Carbone PP, Hausson J-C (1977) Assessment of response to therapy in advanced breast cancer. Eur J Cancer 13: 89–94

Höst H, Brennhovd IO (1977) The effect of postoperative radiotherapy in breast cancer. Int J Radiat Oncol Biol Phys 2: 1061–1067

Höst H, Brennhovd I, Loeb M (1986) Postoperative radiotherapy in breast cancer – long-term results from the Oslo study. Int J Radiat Oncol Biol Phys 12: 727–732

Levitt SH (1986) The role of radiation therapy as an adjuvant in the treatment of breast cancer. Int J Radiat Oncol Biol Phys 12: 843–844

Levitt SH (1988) Is there a role for postoperative adjuvant radiation in breast cancer? Beautiful hypothesis versus ugly facts: 1987 Gilbert H. Fletcher lecture. Int J Radiat Oncol Biol Phys 14: 787–796

Rutqvist LE, Johansson H (1990) Mortality by laterality of the primary tumour among 55000 breast cancer patients from the Swedish Cancer Registry. Br J Cancer 61: 866–868

Rutqvist LE, Cedermark B, Glas U et al (1989) Radiotherapy, chemotherapy and tamoxifen as adjuncts to surgery in early breast cancer: a summary of three randomized trials. Int J Radiat Oncol Biol Phys 16: 629–639

Rutqvist LE, Lax I, Fornander T, Johansson H (1992) Cardiovascular mortality in a randomized trial of adjuvant radiation therapy versus surgery alone in primary breast cancer. Int J Radiat Oncol Biol Phys (in press)

Strender LE, Wallgren A, Arndt J, et al (1981) Adjuvant radiotherapy in operable breast cancer. Correlation between dose in internal mammary nodes and prognosis. Int J Radiat Oncol Biol Phys 7: 1319–1326

10 Pathologic Factors Predictive of Local Recurrence in Patients with Invasive Breast Cancer Treated by Conservative Surgery and Radiation Therapy

STUART J. SCHNITT

CONTENTS

10.1	Introduction	93
10.2	General Considerations	93
10.3	Pathologic Features Predictive of Local Recurrence	94
10.3.1	Microscopic Margins of Excision	94
10.3.2	Extensive Intraductal Component	97
10.4	Other Histologic Features	100
10.4.1	Histologic Tumor Type	100
10.4.2	Histologic Grade	101
10.4.3	Lymphatic Vessel Invasion	101
10.4.4	Necrosis	101
10.4.5	Mononuclear Cell Reaction	101
10.4.6	Tumor Size and Axillary Nodal Status	101
10.5	Conclusion	101
	References	102

10.1 Introduction

The combination of breast-conserving surgery and radiotherapy has been established as an alternative to mastectomy for many women with early-stage invasive breast cancer. In fact, participants at the National Institutes of Health (NIH) Consensus Conference on Early-stage Breast Cancer in June 1990 concluded that the breast-conserving approach is "preferable" since it provides survival rates equivalent to those of mastectomy while preserving the breast (NIH CONSENSUS CONFERENCE 1991).

Although high levels of local tumor control are obtained when employing careful patient selection and surgical and radiotherapeutic techniques, a small proportion of patients treated with the breast-conserving approach will develop a recurrence in the treated breast. In most series, this risk for local recurrence is approximately 1.5%–2% per year for at least the first 10 years after treatment (HARRIS et al. 1984; RECHT et al. 1988a; FOWBLE et al. 1991b). In recent years, attention has focused upon factors that may be associated with such local recurrences. The purpose of this research is to further reduce the risk of local recurrence either by improved patient selection or by improvements in treatment.

A number of treatment-related factors appear to be important determinants of local tumor control in patients treated with conservative surgery and radiotherapy. For example, a high rate of local recurrence is generally observed when a tumor is not grossly excised prior to radiotherapy (BEDWINEK et al. 1980; CHU et al. 1984; RECHT et al. 1986; VAN LIMBERGEN et al. 1987). Also, the rate of local recurrence appears to be lower when a very wide resection of breast tissue is performed than when a more limited excision of the tumor is employed (VERONESI et al. 1990a). In addition, the use of adjuvant chemotherapy is associated with a lower incidence of local recurrence, implying an additive or synergistic effect between radiation and chemotherapy on local tumor control (FISHER et al. 1989; FOWBLE et al. 1991a; ROSE et al. 1989; VERONESI et al. 1990b). Patient factors also are associated with the risk of local recurrence. For example, a number of investigators have identified young patient age as an important risk factor for local recurrence (FOURQUET et al. 1989; KURTZ et al. 1990a; RECHT et al. 1988b). Finally, many investigators have demonstrated that certain pathologic characteristics of the tumor are important prognostic factors for recurrence in the treated breast.

This chapter reviews the current knowledge on pathologic risk factors for local recurrence after conservative surgery and radiotherapy for early-stage invasive breast cancer, and the clinical implications of these risk factors.

10.2 General Considerations

Investigators from a number of institutions have reported results of their analyses of pathologic predictors of local recurrence after conservative

STUART J. SCHNITT, M. D., Associate Professor of Pathology, Harvard Medical School, Pathologist, Beth Israel Hospital, 330 Brookline Avenue, Boston, MA 02215, USA surgery and radiotherapy. However, direct comparisons among these studies are difficult because of interinstitutional differences in a variety of parameters. These include the criteria used for patient selection, the extent of surgical resection of the primary tumor (simple gross excision versus excision with a predefined margin of "normal" tissue – wide excision – versus quadrantectomy), techniques and dose of radiation therapy (including the use of a boost to the primary site), and the length of follow-up. In addition, some investigators base their conclusions on the original surgical pathology reports only, whereas others performed detailed examinations of the histologic slides. Finally, some of the studies differ with regard to the histologic features evaluated, the criteria used to define the various histologic features, examination of possible interactions between histologic features, and the methods used for data analysis and presentation (crude versus actuarial data, univariate versus multivariate analyses). In the subsequent discussion of pathologic risk factors for local recurrence, interinstitutional differences will be highlighted that may explain apparent discrepancies in results.

10.3 Pathologic Features Predictive of Local Recurrence

A variety of pathologic features of the primary tumor have been assessed as possible risk factors for tumor recurrence in the breast after conservative surgery and radiotherapy. The two factors receiving the greatest attention to date are the microscopic margins of excision and the presence of an extensive intraductal component (EIC) in the initial excision specimen. Other factors include the histologic tumor type, tumor grade, lymphatic vessel invasion, necrosis, and mononuclear cell reaction to the tumor.

10.3.1 Microscopic Margins of Excision

A number of studies clearly demonstrate that a complete gross excision of the primary tumor prior to radiotherapy is the minimum surgical procedure required to provide acceptable levels of local tumor control (Bedwinek et al. 1980; Chu et al. 1984; Recht et al. 1986; van Limbergen et al. 1987); however, the extent of surgical resection necessary beyond a complete gross excision remains a matter of debate. Although in some series more extensive breast surgery (i.e., wide excision or quadrantectomy) is associated with a lower risk of local recurrence than a simple gross excision of the tumor, the more extensive surgical procedures adversely affect the cosmetic results (de la Rochefordiere et al. 1991; Veronesi et al. 1990a). In recent years, there has been increasing interest in identifying markers that might predict the likelihood of residual tumor in the breast following breast-conserving surgery – markers therefore useful for assessing the adequacy of breast surgery before proceeding to radiation therapy. One method receiving considerable attention is the use of "inked" margins of excision. In this method, the outer surfaces of a breast excision specimen are painted with a dye that forms an insoluble precipitate on the specimen surface and can be identified on subsequent histologic sections. A variety of commercially available products are suitable for this purpose, including India ink and tattoo dyes. However, there are a number of important limitations in the evaluation of microscopic margins of breast excision specimens. These relate to both technical factors and to the growth pattern of breast cancers.

There are several technical difficulties in the evaluation of microscopic margins of breast excision specimens. First, if a breast excision is submitted to the pathologist in two or more fragments, it is usually not possible to accurately evaluate the microscopic margins unless the orientation of the specimens to each other is indicated by the surgeon. Second, there is a tendency of ink, placed on the surface of the specimen, to track down into the substance of the specimen through defects in the surface. This may create difficulties in defining the true margin of excision on microscopic examination. In addition, the surfaces of the breast excisions are highly complex and irregular, and the surface area may be quite large. Therefore, any method used to examine the specimen (i.e., sections taken through the equatorial plane, shaved or peeled margins) is necessarily a sampling process and subject to sampling error. Unfortunately, there are no generally accepted guidelines for the sampling of margins and the extent of sampling varies widely among different institutions. One recent study suggested that a useful adjunct to evaluating breast excision margins is the use of imprint cytology that may, to some extent, overcome the sampling error associated with the use of histologic sections (Cox et al. 1991).

A further problem in the evaluation of margins is the lack of uniformly accepted definitions of "positive," "negative," and "close" margins. Pathologists generally agree that tumor present at an inked surface of the specimen represents a positive margin. However, the definition of a negative margin is more problematic. Some authors believe that the margin should be considered negative unless the tumor is identified directly at the inked surface. For example, in the National Surgical Adjuvant Breast and Bowel Project (NSABP) B-06 protocol, the presence of a few adipocytes or collagen fibers betwen the tumor and the inked surface was sufficient to render a margin negative (FISHER et al. 1986). Others require that there be some arbitrary minimum distance (e.g., 5 mm) between the edge of the tumor and the inked surface to categorize a margin as negative (SCHMIDT-ULLRICH et al. 1989). However, even when pathologists at different institutions use the same criteria for categorizing margins, discrepancies are frequent. For example, in the NSABP B-06 trial, there were 52 excision specimens in which the pathologist at the original hospital categorized a margin as positive. Upon review, the pathologists at NSABP headquarters agreed with the initial interpretation in only 31% of the cases (FISHER et al. 1986).

A final technical consideration in the evaluation of margins relates to the effects of the surgical excision itself. After excision of a breast mass, a small rim of tissue at the periphery of the biopsy cavity becomes devitalized as a result of the surgery. It is likely that small areas of residual tumor at the biopsy site can be destroyed by this process of devitalization and subsequent tissue repair; this may account for some cases in which margins of the initial excision are positive, while a subsequent re-excision specimen from the biopsy site shows no identifiable tumor.

A consideration of the growth pattern of cancer within the breast is also useful in interpreting the significance of margin involvement. While recent studies demonstrate that, in most cases, tumor spread within the breast is contiguous, in some cases true multicentric foci are observed (HOLLAND et al. 1985). Thus, categorization of a margin as "negative" does not preclude the possibility of noncontiguous foci of residual cancer in the remaining breast tissue. Even in cases where tumor growth is contiguous, this contiguity may be difficult to demonstrate in some planes of section given the complex ramifying nature of the ductal system of the breast. This phenomenon may result in a "negative" margin in patients who could have considerable residual cancer at the tumor site. In addition, intraductal involvement by cancer around an invasive lesion in many cases is not randomly distributed; the ducts oriented toward the nipple are more likely to be involved than other ducts. For this reason, specimen orientation by the surgeon may be valuable in assisting the pathologist's assessment of the margins. Specimen orientation may also be useful in determining the need for further surgery. For example, if the only positive margin is a deep margin of excision abutting the pectoral fascia, removal of additional breast tissue, even by mastectomy, may not improve the margin of concern. Considering these limitations to evaluating margins, examination now can be given to the available clinical data on margins of excision.

Two types of studies have evaluated the potential significance of microscopic margins of breast excision specimens. In the first type, the status of the margins is related to the frequency of residual cancer in re-excision or mastectomy specimens (FISHER et al. 1986; FRAZIER et al. 1989; MCCORMICK et al. 1987; SCHNITT et al. 1987; SOLIN et al. 1986; WAPNIR et al. 1989; WAZER et al. 1991). These results, summarized in Table 10.1, indicate that residual tumor is identified more frequently in patients with positive margins (45%–69%) than in patients with negative margins (12%–33%). It

Table 10.1. Percentage of cases with residual tumor in re-excision or mastectomy specimens related to microscopic margins of excision specimen

		Status of microscopic margins			
Study	No. of patients	Positive	Unknown	Close	Negative
SOLIN et al. (1986)	185	60	49	–	–
FISHER et al. (1986)	52	67	–	–	12
MCCROMICK et al. (1987)	33	55	–	–	–
SCHNITT et al. (1987)	29	69	64	–	33
FRAZIER et al. (1989)	87	53	–	32	26
WAPNIR et al. (1989)	60	45	–	–	28
WAZER et al. (1991)	104	57	43	–	–

should be stressed, however, that positive margins do not guarantee the presence of residual tumor and negative margins do not preclude it. Inter-institutional differences in the extent of the initial surgical excision, the extent of sampling of the margins, definitions used for "positive," "negative," and "close" margins, and the extent of sampling of re-excision and mastectomy specimens may account for at least some of the variability in these results. It is also important to emphasize that, in most studies, neither the extent of margin involvement (focally versus extensively positive), the nature of tumor at the margins (in situ or invasive), nor the nature and extent of tumor in the re-excision or mastectomy specimens is reported.

In the second type of study, the relationship between microscopic margins and the frequency of tumor recurrence in the breast has been analyzed (BARTELINK et al. 1988; CLARKE et al. 1985; KURTZ et al. 1990a, PEZNER et al. 1988; SCHMIDT-ULLRICH et al. 1989; SOLIN et al. 1991; VERONESI et al. 1990a). In most of these studies, the presence of positive microscopic margins is not associated with a significantly increased risk of local recurrence as shown in Table 10.2. This might partially be explained by the fact that in several of these series the total radiation dose to the primary site was determined by the status of the microscopic margins, so that patients with close or positive margins received a higher dose than patients with negative margins. BARTELINK et al. (1988) found a higher rate of local recurrence for patients with positive margins than for patients with negative margins (6% versus 2% at 6 years). However, only eight local recurrences were seen in patients with evaluable margins in this series, and these authors considered completeness of excision to be of "only minor importance." In the series of KURTZ et al. (1990a), the prognostic significance of positive margins was seen only in post-menopausal patients. In addition, in that series, the resection margins had not been inked and were evaluated retrospectively. Thus, the results of most studies suggest that when a boost is employed, microscopically positive margins do not significantly increase the risk of local recurrence.

The results from two studies suggest that the risk of local recurrence for patients with negative margins treated without a boost is comparable to that of patients with positive margins treated with a boost. FISHER et al. (1991) reported a 9-year 12% actuarial rate of recurrence in the breast of patients in the NSABP B-06 Trial who received whole breast irradiation without a boost following an excision with "negative" microscopic margins. In a smaller retrospective series, PEZNER et al. observed no local recurrences at four years among 54 patients with "negative" margins treated without a boost (PEZNER et al. 1988).

It should be clear from the foregoing discussion that the status of the microscopic margins of breast excision specimens is neither an absolute predictor of residual tumor in the vicinity of the primary, nor highly predictive of local recurrence after excision and radiotherapy. Given these observations, should the microscopic margins of breast excisions be evaluated? Until further data are available, it seems reasonable to continue the evaluation of microscopic margins for a number of reasons. In some

Table 10.2. Incidence of breast tumor recurrence related to status of microscopic margins[a]

Reference	Follow-up (years)	Status of microscopic margins: Positive		Unknown		Close		Negative		*p*
		%	*n*	%	*n*	%	*n*	%	*n*	
CLARKE et al. (1985)	5 (mean)	10	80					5	282	NS
BARTELINK et al. (1988)	6 (actuarial)	6	32			4	95	2	242	0.02
PEZNER et al. (1988)	4 (actuarial)	14	8	13	28			17	9	NS
SCHMIDT-ULLRICH et al. (1989)	5 (median)	0	0			0	0	0	0	NS
KURTZ et al. (1990)	5 (actuarial)	23	50					6	277	< 0.001
VERONESI et al. (1990a)	3 (minimum)									
QUART		0	7					2	169	NS
TART		13	46					6	237	NS
SOLIN et al. (1991)	4.8 (median)	2	57	9	346	11	37	7	257	NS

QUART, Quadrantectomy, axillary dissection and radiation therapy; TART, Tumorectomy, axillary dissection and radiation therapy; NS, not significant

[a] Analysis limited to patients treated with whole breast irradiation and a radiation boost after tumor excision.

breast cancers, the extent of the tumor cannot be accurately determined on physical examination, surgical exploration, or even on gross pathologic examination. Included in this group are many cases of pure ductal carcinoma in situ, many infiltrating lobular carcinomas, and infiltrating ductal carcinomas that have an EIC (see Sect. 10.3.2). Evaluation of the microscopic margins in such cases may be extremely useful in assessing the adequacy of the excision. In addition, most investigators recommend the use of a boost to the primary site when there is focal involvement of the microscopic margins.

In conclusion, the evaluation of microscopic margins appears to be of some value but should not be used as an absolute guide to determine the adequacy of the surgical excision. As will be discussed below, certain microscopic features of the primary tumor may be more highly predictive of residual tumor burden near the primary site than the status of margins; these features also need to be considered in planning the extent of surgical resection.

10.3.2 Extensive Intraductal Component

Most infiltrating breast cancers have an associated in situ component and the extent of this in situ component appears to have prognostic significance. Almost two decades ago, SILVERBERG and CHITALE demonstrated that, in patients treated with mastectomy, tumors with a higher proportion of intraductal carcinoma were associated with a higher survival rate (SILVERBERG and CHITALE 1973). More recent studies indicate that the extent and distribution of intraductal carcinoma in association with an invasive cancer is also important in determining the risk of local recurrence in breast cancer patients treated with conservative surgery and radiation therapy. Investigators at the Joint Center for Radiation Therapy (JCRT) were the first to report an association between an EIC in the primary tumor and an increased risk of local recurrence following local excision and radiation therapy (HARRIS et al. 1983; SCHNITT et al. 1984). As defined by this group, tumors with an EIC are infiltrating ductal carcinomas that show the simultaneous presence of prominent intraductal carcinoma within the tumor *and* intraductal carcinoma beyond the edges of the invasive tumor. Also included among the EIC-positive cases are tumors that are predominantly intraductal carcinomas with one or more microscopic foci of stromal invasion.

In the most recent analysis from the JCRT, patients with EIC-positive tumors comprised 28% of patients with infiltrating ductal carcinoma and had a 5-year actuarial local recurrence rate of 24%. In contrast, patients with EIC-negative tumors had a local recurrence rate of 6% ($p = 0.0001$) (BOYAGES et al. 1990). Most of the local recurrences in EIC-positive patients are at or near the primary site (BOYAGES et al. 1990; JACQUEMIER et al. 1990). In the JCRT series, 89% of recurrences in EIC-positive patients were true recurrences (directly at the primary site) or marginal misses (immediately adjacent to the boost area), and only 4% were elsewhere in the breast. In contrast, only 55% of recurrences in EIC-negative patients were categorized as true recurrences or marginal misses, while 28% were elsewhere ($p = 0.004$) (BOYAGES et al. 1990). Of note, the risk of local recurrence is higher for EIC-positive than for EIC-negative tumors, regardless of the tumor size (EBERLEIN et al. 1990). Osteen et al. further divided the JCRT EIC-positive cases into two groups: "macro," in which the surgeon and pathologist detected a clearly defined tumor and the cancer was limited to the palpable lesion; and "micro," in which a clearly defined tumor was not appreciated. The local recurrence rates were significantly higher for cases in the "micro" group (27% at 5 years and 71% at 8 years) than for those in the "macro" group (18% at 5 and 8 years). The macroscopic differences in these two groups of EIC-positive lesions correspond to microscopic differences: histologically, tumors in the "micro" group were predominantly intraductal carcinomas with focal invasion (microinvasion), whereas those in the "macro" group were predominantly invasive cancers (OSTEEN et al. 1987).

It is important to emphasize that the JCRT data were obtained from a patient population treated between 1968 and 1982 during which time breast surgery, prior to irradiation, in most cases consisted of a simple local excision of the tumor without the routine evaluation of the microscopic margins. In addition, preoperative mammography was not routinely performed in this patient population. Subsequent studies demonstrated that the risk of local recurrence in EIC-positive cases may be reduced by the use of wider excisions (VICINI et al. 1991) and that about two-thirds of EIC-positive cases can be suspected on preoperative mammograms by the presence of widespread microcalcifications or a soft tissue density with microcalcifications within and adjacent to it (HEALEY et al. 1989).

A number of other investigators also have evaluated the relationship between an EIC and local recurrence after conservative surgery and radiotherapy (BARTELINK et al. 1988; FOURQUET et al. 1989; JACQUEMIER et al. 1990; KURTZ et al. 1990a; LINDLEY et al. 1989; LOCKER et al. 1989; YEH et al. 1991). These data, along with the JCRT data, are summarized in Table 10.3. Despite variations in the proportion of patients with EIC-positive tumors and the overall risk of local recurrence, these studies consistently demonstrate an increased risk of local recurrence for EIC-positive tumors compared with EIC-negative lesions. The proportion of EIC-positive tumors in these series ranges from 8% to 28%. This in part is related to different definitions of EIC used at various institutions, but patient selection may also be a factor. For example, the very small proportion of EIC-positive cases in the series from the University of Pennsylvania may be related to the use of preoperative mammography and assessment of margins in many of these patients and the exclusion of patients with widespread microcalcifications or prominent margin involvement (YEH et al. 1991). The local recurrence rates in EIC-positive patients also vary in these studies from 9% to 50%, with most series reporting recurrence rates in the range of 20%–25% at 5 years. Variations in the definition of EIC, patient selection, the extent of the surgical resection of the primary tumor, and the technique and dose of irradiation may account for these differences. The presence of an EIC retained its prognostic significance in multivariate analyses in the JCRT and Marseille series (BOYAGES et al. 1990, KURTZ et al. 1990a), but did not remain a significant predictor of local recurrence in the multivariate analyses in the Nottingham and Curie series (LOCKER et al. 1989; FOURQUET et al. 1989). Of note, EIC-positive tumors are not associated either with an increased risk of distant metastases (BOYAGES et al. 1990; JACQUEMIER et al. 1990) or with contralateral breast cancer (HARRIS and RECHT 1991). The presence of an EIC is also not associated with an increased local recurrence rate in patients treated with mastectomy (ROSEN et al. 1986).

Several authors report not finding an association between an intraductal component and an increased risk of local recurrence. However, in all of these series the intraductal component was scored only as present or absent with no attempt to evaluate its extent or distribution (CLARKE et al. 1985; FISHER et al. 1986; MATE et al. 1986; VAN LIMBERGEN et al. 1987). In addition, in the NSABP B-06 trial, patients with positive microscopic margins of excision were excluded from the breast-conserving arms of the study (FISHER et al. 1986). Since most EIC-positive patients have positive microscopic margins after a local excision (SCHNITT et al. 1987), it is likely that many EIC-positive patients were excluded from the conservative treatment arms of that trial.

Studies from several institutions show that EIC-positive tumors are more frequent in younger women. However, the magnitude of this association varies depending upon the age groups compared. For example, EIC-positive tumors in the JCRT series were seen in 31% of patients 34 years of age

Table 10.3. Relationship between an extensive intraductal component (EIC) and local recurrence

Reference	Location of study	Number of patients	Surgical Procedure	Percentage with EIC	Follow-up (years)	Local recurrence EIC + (%)	EIC − (%)	p
BOYAGES et al. (1990)	JCRT	584	LE	28[a]	5 (actuarial)	24	6	0.0001
LOCKER et al. (1989)	Nottingham	263	LE	15[d]	5 (actuarial)	50	25	<0.01
JACQUEMIER et al. (1990)	Marseilles	496	WE	21[a]	5 (actuarial)	18	8	<0.001
LINDLEY et al. (1989)	Westminster	293	WE	20[b]	2 (minimum)	22	10	<0.05
BARTELINK et al. (1988)	Netherlands	585	WE	16[b]	6 (actuarial)	9	2	0.006
FOURQUET et al. (1989)	Curie	434	WE	15[c]	10 (actuarial)	23	5	0.03
YEH et al. (1991)	Pennsylvania	275	LE/WE	8[a]	5 (actuarial)	22	4	0.03

LE, local excision, WE, wide excision
[a] Intraductal carcinoma comprising at least 25% of tumor areas plus any intraductal carcinoma adjacent to tumor.
[b] Intraductal carcinoma comprising more than 25% of tumor area.
[c] Intraductal carcinoma comprising more than 25% of tumor area plus more than 25% of adjacent area.
[d] Intraductal carcinoma involving four quadrants adjacent to tumor.

or younger, in 33% of patients 35–50 years old, in 27% of patients 51–65 years old, and in only 18% of patients older than 65 years of age (HARRIS and RECHT 1991). In the Institut Curie series, EIC-positive tumors were present in 37% of patients 45 years of age or younger and in 19.5% of patients 46 years of age or older (FOURQUET et al. 1989). In the series from Marseille, EIC-positive tumors were seen in 28% of premenopausal women and in 15.5% of postmenopausal women (JAQUEMIER et al. 1990). In the JCRT series, the presence of an EIC was strongly associated with an increased risk of local recurrence for patients 35–65 years of age and was relatively less important in patients aged over 65 years (HARRIS and RECHT 1991). In contrast, an adverse effect of an EIC on local tumor control was seen only in premenopausal patients in the study from Marseille (JAQUEMIER et al. 1990; KURTZ et al. 1990a). KURTZ et al. suggested that the higher risk of local recurrence observed in younger women reflects a higher prevalence of adverse histologic findings (such as an EIC) in this subgroup of patients, and that young age per se is not an independent risk factor for local recurrence (KURTZ et al. 1990b). In the JCRT series, however, the adverse prognostic influence of young age on local recurrence was independent of the presence of an EIC (BOYAGES et al. 1990).

A number of studies have attempted to determine the reason for an association between EIC-positive tumors and an increased risk of local recurrence after conservative surgery and radiotherapy. In a study of patients who underwent a re-excision of the primary site following an initial gross excision in which there were positive or close margins, investigators at the JCRT found that the likelihood of residual cancer was significantly higher in EIC-positive cases than in EIC-negative cases (88% versus 48%; $p = 0.002$). Moreover, for patients in the EIC-positive group this residual tumor was composed primarily of intraductal carcinoma and was often widespread. Prominent residual intraductal cancer was seen in the re-excision specimen in 44% of EIC-positive cases compared with only 2% of patients in the EIC-negative group ($p < 0.0001$). In contrast, the residual tumor found in the EIC-negative patients typically consisted of only scattered microscopic foci of infiltrating and/or intraductal cancer. Additionally, the presence of an EIC was more highly predictive of the residual tumor burden in the re-excision specimen than was the presence of positive microscopic margins in the initial excision specimen, since patients with EIC-negative tumors and positive margins rarely had considerable residual cancer (SCHNITT et al. 1987).

In a more recent study of specimens from patients treated by mastectomy, HOLLAND et al. used a correlated radiologic-pathologic mapping technique to relate the presence or absence of an EIC in the primary tumor to the type and extent of residual tumor in the remainder of the breast. In this study, patients with EIC-positive tumors were significantly more likely than those with EIC-negative lesions to have residual intraductal cancer in the breast (71% versus 28%; $p = 0.00001$). Furthermore, in about 30% of patients with EIC-positive tumors, this residual intraductal carcinoma was prominent and extended at least 2 cm beyond the edge of the primary tumor. In patients with EIC-negative tumors, however, such extensive residual intraductal tumor was seen in only 2% of the patients ($p < 0.0001$) (HOLLAND et al. 1990). The results of these two studies suggest that EIC-positive tumors are lesions in which the associated intraductal involvement is often more extensive than can be appreciated clinically or at the time of surgery. Therefore, EIC-positive patients who undergo a limited resection of the clinically evident tumor frequently have considerable residual subclinical intraductal cancer in the vicinity of the tumor site. The most likely explanation for the high risk of local recurrence observed in EIC-positive patients is that the residual tumor burden in such patients is too large to be eradicated by cosmetically acceptable doses of radiation. It is also possible that this residual intraductal cancer contains a hypoxic compartment that renders it relatively radioresistant (MAYR et al. 1991).

Results from a recent study from the JCRT offer additional support for the hypothesis that a large residual burden of intraductal cancer is responsible for the high local recurrence rate seen in EIC-positive patients. If this hypothesis was correct, one would anticipate that the risk of local recurrence in EIC-positive patients could be reduced by the use of wider resections of breast tissue. A study by Vicini et al. confirms this expectation. In a study relating the volume of resected breast tissue to the likelihood of local recurrence, Vicini et al. found that for both T1 and T2 tumors larger resections were associated with a substantially lower risk of local recurrence in patients with EIC-positive tumors (Table 10.4) (VICINI et al. 1991).

In summary, EIC-positive tumors represent a subcategory of infiltrating ductal carcinomas that

Table 10.4. Five-year actuarial local recurrence rates in relation to the extent of breast resection in patients with EIC-postive tumors

Extent of breast resection[a]	Tumor size T1 ($n = 83$) (%)	T2 ($n = 78$) (%)
Smallest	29	36
Intermediate	22	26
Largest	10	9

[a] For patients with T1 tumors, the volumes of resected breast tissue were <13 cm^3, 13–48 cm^3, and >48 cm^3 for smallest, intermediate, and largest resections, respectively. For patients with T2 tumors, the volumes of resected breast tissue were <35 cm^3, 35–74 cm^3, and 74 cm^3 for smallest, intermediate, and largest resections, respectively. (Adapted from VICINI et al. 1991)

are more common in younger women and characterized by a high frequency of subclinical intraductal involvement in the vicinity of the primary tumor. In some cases, this involvement may extend for large distances from the primary site. The presence of an EIC can be frequently suspected preoperatively based upon mammographic findings. Clinical studies indicate that patients with EIC-positive tumors have an increased risk of local recurrence when treated with a limited excision prior to radiotherapy. There is also evidence suggesting that it may be possible to reduce this risk by the use of wider resections in these EIC-positive cases. These studies further indicate that for the majority of infiltrating ductal cancers that are EIC-negative, a limited breast resection prior to irradiation results in acceptably low rates of local recurrence. Therefore, assessment of the presence or absence of an EIC is a useful method for guiding the extent of breast surgery required prior to radiotherapy (HARRIS et al. 1985).

10.4 Other Histologic Features

10.4.1 Histologic Tumor Type

Since approximately 80% of patients with invasive breast cancer have infiltrating ductal carcinomas, factors predictive of outcome in consecutive series of patients treated with conservative surgery and radiotherapy largely reflect those of infiltrating ductal cancers. There is considerably less experience with the use of breast-conserving treatment for other histologic types. Experience to date indicates that the risk of local recurrence is acceptably low for patients with medullary carcinomas treated with conservative surgery and radiotherapy. In one study of 27 patients with medullary carcinoma, the 5-year actuarial local recurrence rate was 4% (KURTZ et al. 1989). In another study of 41 patients with medullary carcinoma, the 6-year actuarial local recurrence rate was 14% (FOURQUET et al. 1987). There is even less experience with mucinous (colloid) carcinoma. KURTZ et al. observed no local recurrences at 5 years among 11 patients with mucinous carcinoma treated with conservative surgery and radiotherapy (KURTZ et al. 1989).

Slightly more information is available for patients with infiltrating lobular carcinomas, the second most common type of invasive breast cancer. MATE et al. found that patients with infiltrating lobular histology had a higher local recurrence rate than patients with infiltrating ductal cancers. However, in that series there were only 12 patients with infiltrating lobular tumors and a significant difference in local recurrence rates was seen only in patients with stage II lesions (MATE et al. 1986). Kurtz et al. studied 67 patients with infiltrating lobular carcinoma. The 5-year actuarial local recurrence rate was slightly higher in these patients than it was in patients with infiltrating ductal cancers (13.5% versus 8.8%; $p = 0.11$) (KURTZ et al. 1989). Investigators at the JCRT found that for 49 patients with infiltrating lobular carcinomas, the 5-year actuarial risk of local recurrence was similar to that of patients with infiltrating ductal carcinomas when the latter were considered as a single group (12% versus 11%). However, the 12% 5-year actuarial local recurrence rate in patients with infiltrating lobular carcinoma was higher than that of patients with EIC-negative infiltrating ductal carcinomas (5%), but lower than that of patients with EIC-positive infiltrating ductal lesions (23%) (SCHNITT et al. 1989). In addition, there is a tendency for local recurrences in patients with infiltrating lobular carcinoma to occur later than those in patients with infiltrating ductal carcinoma (SCHNITT et al. 1989). This may be related to the fact that upon physical examination, infiltrating lobular carcinomas, both as primary tumors and recurrent lesions in the breast, often present with subtle changes such as vague areas of induration or thickening, rather than as discrete masses. Therefore, more time may elapse before the recurrences in these cases are detected clinically.

10.4.2 Histologic Grade

Nine studies have assessed the impact of histologic grade on local recurrence after conservative surgery and radiotherapy. In five studies, high tumor grade was associated in univariate analysis with a significantly increased risk of local recurrence (CLARKE et al. 1985; KURTZ et al. 1990a; LINDLEY et al. 1989; LOCKER et al. 1989; YEH et al. 1991). In one of these studies, grade remained significant in multivariate analysis (CLARKE et al. 1985), and in another study a significant relationship between high grade and local recurrence was seen in multivariate analysis only in postmenopausal women (KURTZ et al. 1990a). In the third study, grade did not remain a significant predictor for local recurrence in multivariate analysis (LOCKER et al. 1989), and in the remaining two studies, multivariate analysis was not performed (LINDLEY et al. 1989; YEH et al. 1991). High tumor grade was not significantly associated with local recurrence in the four other studies (BOYAGES et al. 1990; FISHER et al. 1986; FOURQUET et al. 1989; MATE et al. 1986).

10.4.3 Lymphatic Vessel Invasion

In three studies, lymphatic vessel invasion (LVI) was a significant predictor of local recurrence in univariate analysis (BOYAGES et al. 1990; FOURQUET et al. 1989; LOCKER et al. 1989). In two other studies, an adverse effect of LVI on local recurrence was of borderline significance (FISHER et al. 1986; LINDLEY et al. 1989). However, in only two studies (FOURQUET et al. 1989; LOCKER et al. 1989) did this factor remain significant in multivariate analysis. In the JCRT series, the effect of LVI on local recurrence was confounded by the presence of an EIC. In patients with EIC-negative tumors, the presence of LVI did not significantly increase the local recurrence rate. The 5-year actuarial local recurrence rate for EIC-negative/LVI-positive tumors was 9% compared with 5% for EIC-negative/LVI-negative tumors (not significant). In contrast, patients with EIC-positive tumors with LVI had a significantly higher local recurrence rate than those with EIC-positive tumors without LVI (34% versus 20%; $p = 0.0001$) (BOYAGES et al. 1990).

10.4.4 Necrosis

Two studies have reported an association between tumor necrosis and a significantly increased risk of local recurrence (MATE et al. 1986; LINDLEY et al. 1989). However, in one series the significance was related to necrosis in the invasive component (MATE et al. 1986), while in the other it was associated with necrosis in the intraductal component (LINDLEY et al. 1989).

10.4.5 Mononuclear Cell Reaction

A prominent mononuclear inflammatory cell reaction (MCR) to the tumor has been reported to be associated with an increased risk of local recurrence in two studies (KURTZ et al. 1990a; LINDLEY et al. 1989). In one of these studies, however, the adverse effect of MCR was seen only in premenopausal patients (KURTZ et al. 1990a). In a third study, there was no relationship between MCR and local recurrence (MATE et al. 1986). A fourth study showed that the absence of an inflammatory response rather than a prominent MCR was associated with a higher local recurrence rate (YEH et al. 1991).

10.4.6 Tumor Size and Axillary Nodal Status

Although both larger tumor size and involved axillary lymph nodes are associated with an increased risk of local recurrence (as well as distant metastases) in patients treated with mastectomy, these factors have not been found to be significantly associated with an increased local recurrence rate in patients treated with conservative surgery and radiotherapy (FOWBLE et al. 1991b). In fact, in two large prospective series patients with positive axillary lymph nodes have had a lower risk of recurrence in the breast than patients with negative nodes (FISHER et al. 1989; VERONESI et al. 1990b). This in part may be related to the use of adjuvant chemotherapy in node-positive patients.

10.5 Conclusion

On the basis of available data, it can be concluded that certain pathologic features of the tumor should be taken into consideration, along with the clinical and mammographic findings, in selecting patients for and implementing breast-conserving therapy. Although none of the pathologic features discussed here should be considered an absolute contraindication to breast-conserving treatment, the assessment of some of these parameters is useful in determining the details of treatment, such as the extent of surgery prior to radiotherapy.

It is clear that performing an adequate excision of the tumor before irradiation is essential to obtain acceptable levels of local tumor control. Careful mammographic and pathologic evaluation are both important to accomplish this objective. Mammography facilitates identifying additional foci of cancer away from the index lesion and may also be helpful in identifying lesions that may be associated with a large subclinical tumor burden at the primary site after a simple gross excision (i.e., EIC-positive cases). While the evaluation of microscopic margins of excision is likely to be important in some cases, the status of the margins should not be used as an absolute guide and needs to be interpreted in the context of the histologic features of the tumor. For example, the presence of focally positive microscopic margins does not appear to be associated with either a large residual tumor burden or with a high risk of local recurrence when a radiation boost is employed for patients with EIC-negative tumors treated with a limited gross excision. In such patients a simple gross excision is usually adequate surgical treatment. In contrast, patients with EIC-positive tumors usually have positive microscopic margins after a simple gross excision and the presence of an EIC is frequently associated with a considerable residual tumor burden. Therefore, in these patients a wider resection may be necessary to obtain acceptable local control rates.

In practice, patients at our institution typically undergo a total gross excision of the tumor with a small rim of adjacent grossly normal tissue as the initial surgical procedure. For patients with EIC-negative tumors, this limited excision is usually adequate. If the microscopic margins are extensively involved, a re-excision of the biopsy site is recommended. For patients with EIC-positive tumors, a re-excision of the biopsy site is typically recommended to assess the presence and extent of residual tumor. If the re-excision specimen shows prominent residual tumor with involvement of the new margins of excision, a mastectomy is usually recommended. If there is little or no residual tumor and the margins appear to be clear, radiation therapy is considered a reasonable option. The approach to patients with infiltrating lobular carcinomas is similar to that used for EIC-positive infiltrating ductal cancers since these lesions may also have more extensive tumor spread in the vicinity of the primary site than can be appreciated clinically or at the time of surgery. At this time there are insufficient data on the relative importance of the other pathologic features discussed here to alter patient management based upon their presence.

References

Bartelink H, Barger JH, van Dongen JA et al (1988) The impact of tumor size and histology on local control after breast-conserving therapy. Radiother Oncol 11: 297–303

Bedwinek JM, Perez CA, Kramer S et al (1980) Irradiation as the primary management of stage I and II adenocarcinoma of the breast. Cancer Clin Trials 3: 11–18

Boyages J, Recht A, Connolly JL et al (1990) Early breast cancer: predictors of breast recurrence for patients treated with consecutive surgery and radiation therapy. Radiother Oncol 19: 29–41

Chu AM, Cope O, Russo R et al (1984) Patterns of local recurrence and results in stages I and II breast cancer treated by irradiation following limited surgery. Am J Clin Oncol 7: 221–229

Clarke DH, Le MG, Sarrazin D et al (1985) Analysis of local-regional relapses in patients with early breast cancers treated by excision and radiotherapy: experience of the Institut Gustave-Roussy. Int J Radiat Oncol Biol Phys 11: 137–145

Cox CE, Ku NN, Reintgen DS et al (1991) Touch preparation cytology of breast lumpectomy margins with histologic correlation. Arch Surg 126: 490–493

de la Rochefordiere A, Abner A, Silver B et al (1991) Are cosmetic results following conservative surgery and radiotherapy dependent on technique? Int J Radiat Oncol Biol Phys 21 [Suppl 1]: 133

Eberlein TJ, Connolly JL, Schnitt SJ et al (1990) Predictors of local recurrence following conservative breast surgery and radiation therapy: the influence of tumor size. Arch Surg 125: 771–777

Fisher ER, Sass R, Fisher B et al (1986) Pathologic findings from the National Surgical Adjuvant Breast Project (Protocol 6). II. Relation of local breast recurrence to multicentricity. Cancer 57: 1717–1724

Fisher B, Redmond C, Poisson R et al (1989) Eight-year results of a randomized clinical trial comparing total mastectomy and lumpectomy with or without irradiation in the treatment of breast cancer. N Engl J Med 320: 822–828

Fisher B, Anderson A, Fisher ER et al (1991) Significance of ipsilateral breast tumor recurrence after lumpectomy. Lancet 338: 327–331

Fourquet A, Vilcoq JR, Zafrani B et al (1987) Medullary breast carcinoma: the role of radiotherapy as primary treatment. Radiother Oncol 10: 1–6

Fourquet A, Campana F, Zafrani B et al (1989) Prognostic factors of breast recurrence in the conservative management of early breast cancer: a 25-year follow-up. Int J Radiat Oncol Biol Phys 17: 719–725

Fowble BL, Solin LJ, Schultz DJ et al (1991a) Ten-year results of conservative surgery and irradiation for stage I

and II breast cancer. Int J Radiat Oncol Biol Phys 21: 269–277
Fowble B, Solin LJ, Shultz DJ (1991b) Conservative surgery and radiation for early breast cancer. In: Fowble B, Goodman RL, Glick JH, Rosato EF (eds) Breast cancer treatment. A comprehensive guide to management. Mosby Year Book, St. Louis, pp 105–149
Frazier TG, Wong RWY, Rose D (1989) Implications of accurate pathologic margins in the treatment of primary breast cancer. Arch Surg 124: 37–38
Harris JR, Recht A (1991) Conservative surgery and radiotherapy. In: Harris JR, Hellman S, Henderson IC, Kinne DW (eds) Breast diseases, 2nd edn. Lippincott, Philadelphia, pp 388–419
Harris JR, Connolly JL, Schnitt SJ et al (1983) Clinical-pathologic study of early breast cancer treated by primary radiation therapy. J Clin Oncol 1: 184–189
Harris J, Recht A, Amalric R et al (1984) Time course and prognosis of local recurrence following primary radiation therapy for early breast cancer. J Clin Oncol 2: 37–41
Harris JR, Connolly JL, Schnitt SJ et al (1985) The use of pathologic features in selecting the extent of surgical resection necessary for breast cancer patients treated by primary radiation therapy. Ann Surg 201: 164–169
Healey EA, Osteen RT, Schnitt SJ et al (1989) Can the clinical and mammographic findings at presentation predict the presence of an extensive intraductal component in early stage breast cancer? Int J Radiat Oncol Biol Phys 17: 1217–1221
Holland R, Veling SH, Mravunac M et al (1985) Histologic multifocality of Tis, T1-2 breast carcinomas: implications for clinical trials of breast-conserving surgery. Cancer 56: 979–990
Holland R, Connolly JL, Gelman R et al (1990) The presence of an extensive intraductal component following a limited excision correlates with prominent residual disease in the remainder of the breast. J Clin Oncol 8: 113–118
Jacquemier J, Kurtz JM, Amalric R et al (1990) An assessment of extensive intraductal component as a risk factor for local recurrence after breast-conserving therapy. Br J Cancer 61: 873–876
Kurtz JM, Jacquemier J, Torhorst J et al (1989) Conservation therapy for breast cancers other than infiltrating ductal carcinoma. Cancer 63: 1630–1635
Kurtz JM, Jacquemier J, Amalric R et al (1990a) Risk factors for breast recurrence in premenopausal and postmenopausal patients with ductal cancers treated by conservative therapy. Cancer 65: 1867–1878
Kurtz JM, Jacquemier J, Amalric R et al (1990b) Why are local recurrences after breast-conserving therapy more frequent in younger patients? J Clin Oncol 8: 591–598
Lindley R, Bulman A, Parsons P et al (1989) Histologic features predictive of an increased risk of early local recurrence after treatment of breast cancer by local tumor excision and radical radiotherapy. Surgery 105: 13–20
Locker AP, Ellis IO, Morgan DAL et al (1989) Factors influencing local recurrence after excision and radiotherapy for primary breast cancer. Br J Surg 76: 890–894
Mate TP, Carter D, Fischer DB et al (1986) A clinical and histopathologic analysis of the results of conservation surgery and radiation therapy in stage I and II breast carcinoma. Cancer 58: 1995–2002
Mayr NA, Staples JJ, Robinson RA et al (1991) Morphometric studies in intraductal breast carcinoma using computerized image analysis. Cancer 67: 2805–2812
McCormick B, Kinne DW, Petrek J et al (1987) Limited resection for breast cancer: a study of inked specimen margins before radiotherapy. Int J Radiat Oncol Biol Phys 13: 1667–1671
NIH Consensus Conference (1991) Treatment of early-stage breast cancer. J Am Med Assoc 265: 391–395
Osteen RT, Connolly JL, Recht A et al (1987) Identification of patients at high risk for local recurrence after conservative surgery and radiation therapy for stage I and II breast cancer. Arch Surg 122: 1248–1252
Pezner RD, Lipsett JA, Desai K et al (1988) To boost or not to boost: decreasing radiation therapy in conservative breast cancer treatment when "inked" tumor resection margins are pathologically free of cancer. Int J Radiat Oncol Biol Phys 14: 873–877
Recht A, Connolly JL, Schnitt SJ et al (1986) Conservative surgery and radiation therapy for early breast cancer: results, controversies, and unsolved problems. Semin Oncol 13: 434–449
Recht A, Silen W, Schnitt SJ et al (1988a) Time-course of local recurrence following conservative surgery and radiotherapy for early stage breast cancer. Int J Radiat Oncol Biol Phys 15: 255–261
Recht A, Connolly JL, Schnitt SJ et al (1988b) The effect of young age on tumor recurrence in the treated breast after conservative surgery and radiotherapy. Int J Radiat Oncol Biol Phys 14: 3–10
Rose MA, Henderson IC, Gelman R et al (1989) Premenopausal breast cancer patients treated with conservative surgery, radiotherapy, and adjuvant chemotherapy have a low risk of local failure. Int J Radiat Oncol Biol Phys 17: 711–717
Rosen PP, Kinne DW, Lesser M et al (1986) Are prognostic factors for local control of breast cancer treated by primary radiotherapy significant for patients treated by mastectomy? Cancer 57: 1415–1420
Schmidt-Ullrich R, Wazer DE, Tercilla O et al (1989) Tumor margin assessment as a guide to optimal conservative surgery and irradiation in early stage breast carcinoma. Int J Radiat Oncol Biol Phys 17: 733–738
Schnitt SJ, Connolly JL, Harris JR et al (1984) Pathologic predictors of early local recurrence in stage I and II breast cancer treated by primary radiation therapy. Cancer 53: 1049–1057
Schnitt SJ, Connolly JL, Khettry U et al (1987) Pathologic findings on re-excision of the primary site in breast cancer patients considered for treatment by primary radiation therapy. Cancer 59: 675–681
Schnitt SJ, Connolly JL, Recht A et al (1989) Influence of infiltrating lobular histology on local tumor control in breast cancer patients treated with conservative surgery and radiotherapy. Cancer 64: 448–454
Silverberg SG, Chitale AR (1973) Assessment of significance of proportions of intraductal and infiltrating tumor growth in ductal carcinoma of the breast. Cancer 32: 830–837
Solin LJ, Fowble B, Martz K et al (1986) Results of re-excisional biopsy of the primary tumor in preparation for definitive irradiation of patients with early stage breast cancer. Int J Radiat Oncol Biol Phys 12: 721–725
Solin LJ, Fowble BL, Schultz DJ et al (1991) The significance of the pathology margins of the tumor excision on the outcome of patients treated with definitive irradiation for early stage breast cancer. Int J Radiat Oncol Biol Phys 21: 279–287
van Limbergen E, van der Bogaert W, van der Schueren E et al (1987) Tumor excision and radiotherapy as primary treatment of breast cancer: analysis of patient and

treatment parameters and local control. Radiother Oncol 8: 1–9

Veronesi U, Volterrani F, Luini A et al (1990a) Quadrantectomy versus lumpectomy for small size breast cancer. Eur J Cancer 26: 671–6473

Veronesi U, Salvadori B, Luini A et al (1990b) Conservative treatment of early breast cancer. Long-term results of 1232 cases treated with quadrantectomy, axillary dissection and radiotherapy. Ann Surg 211: 250–259

Vicini FA, Eberlein TJ, Connolly JL et al (1991) The optimal extent of resection for patients with stages I and II breast cancer treated with conservative surgery and radiotherapy. Ann Surg 214: 200–205

Wapnir IL, Bancila E, Devereux DF et al (1989) Residual tumor and breast biopsy margins. Breast Dis 2: 81–86

Wazer DE, Sinesi M, Schmidt-Ullrich R et al (1991) Importance of surgical and pathologic determinants of tumor margin status for breast conservation therapy. Breast Dis 4: 285–292

Yeh I, Fowble B, Viglione MJ et al (1991) Pathologic assessment and pathologic prognostic factors in operable breast cancer. In: Fowble B, Goodman RL, Glick JH, Rosato FF (eds) Breast cancer treatment. A comprehensive guide to management. Mosby Year Book, St. Louis, pp 167–208

11 What Is the Optimal Technique of Irradiation in Breast-Conserving Treatment?

TATIANA I. LINGOS and JAY R. HARRIS

CONTENTS

11.1 Introduction 105
11.2 General Considerations 105
11.2.1 Selecting the Treatment Volume 106
11.2.2 Reproducing the Daily Set-Up 106
11.2.3 Minimizing Dose to Critical Structures 107
11.2.4 Achieving Dose Homogeneity. 108
11.3 Special Considerations 110
11.3.1 Tumor Bed Boost. 110
11.3.2 Regional Nodal Irradiation 111
11.3.3 Techniques of Nodal Irradiation 112
11.4 Future Directions. 113
References 114

11.1 Introduction

Over the last two decades irradiation, in conjunction with breast-conserving surgery, has been found to offer breast cancer patients equivalent disease-free and overall survival rates in the vast majority of cases (BADER et al. 1987; BARTELINK and VAN DONGEN 1989; BLEICHERT-TOFT et al. 1988; FISHER et al. 1989; SARRAZIN et al. 1989; VERONESI 1987). As these data have accumulated and as breast cancer has been diagnosed at earlier stages, more and more women are opting for conservative treatment of their disease (NIH CONSENSUS CONFERENCE 1990). The use of this breast-conserving therapy is growing and currently more than 35% of patients with breast cancer are treated in this manner (LEVITT 1990).

The ultimate goal of breast-conserving therapy is to provide patients with effective treatment of their cancer without the psychological trauma of mastectomy. Certain criteria must be met for this to succeed: survival must not be compromised; the risk of local recurrence must be low; the cosmetic result must be aesthetically pleasing and physically satisfying for the patient; and the incidence of complications must be low. The technique of irradiation is therefore of great importance. In this chapter, we address the salient points of optimizing the radiation technique for localized breast cancer: selecting treatment volumes and boundaries; achieving reproducibility of treatments on a daily basis; minimizing dose to lung and heart; maximizing homogeneity of dose; and avoiding overlap of fields. Additionally, we discuss the role of radiation as having a systemic component in some breast cancer patients.

Before focusing on the specifics of irradiation technique, it should be stressed that optimal management and outcome in patients with breast cancer stems from a multidisciplinary approach. A close working relationship between the radiation oncologist, medical oncologist, and surgeon is important for optimal patient care. The cosmetic outcome and, to some degree, local control is dependent on the type and extent of resection, the location of the incision, and the type of closure. In addition, a decision regarding the use and timing of any adjuvant systemic treatment may also have a bearing on the final outcome (RECHT et al. 1991a). These issues are dealt with elsewhere in this text.

11.2 General Considerations

The goal of irradiation in stage I and stage II breast cancer is to treat the breast to a homogeneous tumoricidal dose with minimal dose to surrounding structures and tissues. This is accomplished with supervoltage equipment and coplanar opposed tangential fields designed to limit the amount of lung and heart irradiated (HARRIS and RECHT 1991; FOWBLE et al. 1991; MARCIAL 1990). A dose of 45–50 Gy (4500–5000 rads) is considered necessary to sterilize subclinical disease. Fraction size is important in that the likelihood of long-term sequelae is directly related to the daily dose. The policy at the Joint Center for Radiation Therapy (JCRT)

TATIANA I. LINGOS, M. D., Instructor of Radiation Oncology; JAY R. HARRIS, M. D., Professor of Radiation Oncology; Joint Center for Radiation Therapy, Harvard Medical School, 50 Binney Street, Boston, MA 02115, USA is to administer 180–200 cGy (the former if the patient is to receive chemotherapy or has large breasts) for 23–25 fractions to a total dose of 45–46 Gy to the whole breast over 4.5–5 weeks. Doses in excess of this range to the entire breast may result in undesirable fibrosis and retraction (HARRIS et al. 1979). A minimum weekly dose of at least 800 cGy is necessary if one is to avoid an increased risk or failure within the breast (KURTZ et al. 1983; OSBORNE et al. 1984). A higher dose to the tumor bed, in the manner of a "boost", has been traditionally utilized to administer a tumoricidal dose to the area most likely to contain residual tumor cells. If the draining lymph nodes are to be treated, an additional field will be used. The value of these last two points is controversial and will be discussed in further detail below.

11.2.1 Selecting the Treatment Volume

The target volume is the entire breast with a margin of surrounding normal tissue to allow for patients' breathing, slight variation in daily set-up, and the penumbra of the beam. The superior and inferior margins must therefore be 1–1.5 cm beyond the breast, with a 1–2 cm clearance of light field anteriorly above the highest part of the breast. The lateral border of the tangential field is usually 1 cm beyond the breast at the mid-posterior axillary line. Medially, the border should be adequate to cover the breast, typically at the midline. If the internal mammary nodes are to be included, the medial border is determined by lymphoscintigraphy or computed tomography scan (see Sect. 11.3.3). The superior border of the field is generally at the lower edge of the head of the clavicle. These borders must be individualized to allow for the location of the scars, the shape of the breast, and the chest wall contour. The posterior field edges are made coincident to eliminate unnecessary divergence through normal tissue (HARRIS and RECHT 1991; MARCIAL 1990; FOWBLE et al. 1991).

11.2.2 Reproducing the Daily Set-Up

Daily treatments over 5.5–6 weeks must be reproducible if they are going to be effective and safe. Small variations in patient position, particularly in the ventral direction, can affect the treatment volume and amount of normal tissue irradiated, particularly of the lung (PHOTON TREATMENT PLANNING COLLABORATIVE WORKING GROUP 1991). The first step towards assuring accuracy of daily set-up is simulation using fluoroscopy. At the JCRT, patients are planned in the supine position, lying on a styrofoam cast with a cut-out area for their head and arm. Their head is turned slightly to the contralateral side to project the midline structures out of the beam. Both arms are raised above the head, resting in a flexed position, to permit full exposure of the superior portion of the breast. If draining lymph nodes are to be irradiated, only the ipsilateral arm is raised, positioned just greater than perpendicular to the patient's body, thus minimizing excessive skin folds in the supraclavicular-axillary region. In some centers, individualized alpha-cradle forms are custom-made for each patient. Occasionally a wooden tilt board/angle board is needed to adjust for a steep sternal angle, thereby aligning the chest wall in a horizontal plane. If a patient has very large or pendulous breast, netting (e.g., Dressinet) is used at the JCRT to immobilize the breast and avoid overlap of skin surfaces. Taping open redundant skin folds will help to decrease acutc and chronic reactions.

To ensure consistency of set-up on a daily basis, permanent skin marks, tattoos, are placed at the time of simulation. At the JCRT, we put tattoos at the superior and inferior corners of the medial tangential entrance beam, the central axis and inferior corner of the lateral tangent entrance beam, and the medial edge of the field. These tattoos also serve as a record of the patient's treatment volume should additional treatment be considered. Photographs of the patient in the treatment position with accurate documentation of all details by the simulator radiation therapist are essential. During treatment, portal films are taken on the first day and subsequently on a regular basis, usually once a week, with corrections made as necessary.

At the Netherlands Cancer Institute, the radiotherapy department is developing more sophisticated methods of guaranteeing reproducibility of treatment. Data are generated with on-line electronic portal imaging devices (EPID) with ionization chambers housed in a cassette attachable to existing radiotherapy equipment. A dedicated microcomputer measures the currents of the chambers, and restores and processes the images with quality comparable to film (VAN HERK and MEERTENS 1988). This provides images that are available within a few seconds after the start of treatment, thus permitting immediate decisions regarding patient set-up. A portal imaging study utilizing the device was performed on 12 patients receiving tangential field irradiation to measure the interfraction variation (i.e., reproducibility of daily set-up) and intrafraction variation (i.e., alterations in patient position during one treatment session) during therapy. Multiple images of the patients during the treatment were obtained with the EPID as well as with hard copy films. Variations of set-up parameters of central lung distance (CLD), central beam edge distance to skin distance (CBESD), central irradiated width (CIW), field length (FL), field width (FW), and craniocaudal distance (CCD) were measured and were found to vary about 1 mm during one fraction. The difference between simulation and daily treatments (interfraction variation) of all fractions was 2–3 mm for CLD and CBESD. This confirmed that daily treatment was highly reproducible and that the patient's respiration did not have a significant impact on the treatment volume (VAN TIENHOVEN et al. 1991). It is likely that quality control will assume an even greater role in radiotherapy and that daily verification using this approach may become standard.

11.2.3 Minimizing Dose to Critical Structures

In delivering tangential field irradiation, it is important to minimize the risk of lung and cardiac toxicity. The use of central lung distance, as described by BORNSTEIN et al. (1990) from the JCRT, is a method by which the amount of ipsilateral lung included in a tangential field can be estimated from simulation films. The CLD is the perpendicular distance from the posterior field edge to the posterior part of the anterior chest wall at the center of the field. Linear regression analysis indicated a coefficient of determination $r^2 = 0.799$ between CLD and the percent ipsilateral lung volume on computed tomography scan. Thus, a CLD of 1.5 cm predicts that approximately 6% of the ipsilateral lung is included in the tangential field, a CLD of 2.5 cm about 16% of ipsilateral lung, and a CLD of 3.5 cm about 26% of the ipsilateral lung (BORNSTEIN et al. 1990). It is not clear what is the tolerable amount of lung irradiated in tangential fields, but most centers as a rule allow a maximum CLD of 3 cm. In patients who are to be receiving adjuvant chemotherapy, many prefer a maximum CLD of 2.5 cm. A case-control study looking at the risk of radiation pneumonitis in over 1600 patients treated at the JCRT did not find an increased incidence over a limited range of CLD, but did note a higher incidence of radiation pneumonitis in chemotherapy patients. Therefore, the more limited volume of lung in these patients seems justifiable (LINGOS et al. 1991).

Late cardiac toxicity from irradiation of left-sided lesions has been demonstrated in clinical trials from Manchester and the Cancer Research Campaign (CRC) (BRINKLEY et al. 1984; HAYBITTLE et al. 1989), but patients in these trials were treated by irradiation techniques that would now be considered suboptimal. In both studies, orthovoltage equipment was used with multiple fields resulting in significant cardiac irradiation. The Oslo-II trial of postoperative irradiation also had increased mortality from cardiac causes (HOST et al. 1986), but the techniques used gave a significant dose to the coronary arteries with large fraction sizes. RUTQVIST et al. (1992) recently examined the cardiovascular mortality of 960 patients treated for primary breast cancer in a randomized trial in which pre- or postoperative radiation therapy was administered to the breast/chest wall, axilla, supraclavicular fossa, and internal mammary nodes. Surgery consisted of modified radical mastectomy. Preoperative patients were treated with tangential ^{60}Co fields to a total dose of 45 Gy, 1.8 Gy daily, 5 days a week for approximately 5 weeks. Postmastectomy patients were treated with oblique electron fields utilizing 7.5–15 MeV electrons determined by the depth of the internal mammary nodes and chest wall thickness. There was an overall survival difference of borderline significance favoring the irradiated patients ($p = 0.09$), and no overall increase in intercurrent mortality due to any cause was noted. Of great interest, however, was the fact that the subset of patients who were treated with left-sided tangential ^{60}Co fields, which delivered a large dose to the heart, had a significantly increased risk of death due to ischemic heart disease compared to surgical controls (relative hazard: 3.2; $p < 0.05$). This was not seen in patients treated with electrons or those with right-sided tumors. The authors concluded that cardiovascular mortality associated with radiation therapy for early breast cancer correlated directly with the radiation dose to the heart and that this can be minimized by appropriate irradiation techniques (RUTQVIST et al. 1992).

The concern for cardiac toxicity may be greater in patients treated with adjuvant chemotherapy, especially Adriamycin (doxorubicin). An increased incidence of cardiac effects in patients treated for left-sided lesions was noted by VALAGUSSA et al. (1992). Among a group of 798 patients of whom 483 received doxorubicin to a maximum cumulative dose of 300 mg/m^2, 347 received concomitant breast irradiation (50 Gy, with an additional 10 Gy boost in 4–6 weeks) without dose modifications. Ninety-four patients (11.8%) were found to have cardiac disturbances. In women who had irradiation to the left breast, 17.7% had cardiac abnormalities. If these women had concomitant doxorubicin, the incidence rose to 31.2%. This effect was more frequent in women over the age of 55. Electrocardiographic abnormalities, manifested as ST-T wave changes, were also seen more frequently in those women whose left breasts were treated (11.3%). If doxorubicin was utilized, the incidence was 15.6% compared with only 3.2% if cyclophosphamide, methotrexate, and 5-fluorouracil (CMF) were utilized. The abnormalities resolved in 92% of the patients (Valagussa et al. 1992). The details of the irradiation are not provided in this study. Buzzoni et al. (1991) described the results of the prospectively randomized study from the same institution in which women with three or more positive nodes received either doxorubicin followed by CMF or alternating regimens of CMF and doxorubicin. In those patients treated with breast-conserving procedures, irradiation consisted of 50 Gy plus a boost of 10 Gy in 4–6 weeks, administered concomitantly with adjuvant chemotherapy. Of the 361 patients in the study population, four developed congestive heart failure while on treatment. All had received irradiation to the left breast. One patient died as a result of cardiac toxicity and two were still requiring medical therapy. The fourth patient fully recovered (Buzzoni et al. 1991). These data stress the importance of minimizing dose to the heart in patients receiving adjuvant doxorubicin and suggest that radiation and concomitant doxorubicin should not be utilized.

11.2.4 Achieving Dose Homogeneity

Homogeneity of radiation dose with a 10% or less variation throughout the breast is another goal of treatment in order to have satisfactory cosmetic results and minimal complications. Breast irradiation in early-stage breast cancer should provide an adequate dose to the superficial portion of the breast while sparing the skin to maintain the cosmetic result. There are options in machine energy and beam characteristics that can be optimally chosen to suit the size of a patient's breast and separation. As the energy of the beam increases, so does dose homogeneity, thus decreasing the inevitable "hot spots" at the lateral edges of the tangential fields. But the use of higher energy also has a more skin-sparing effect and a lower dose to the subcutaneous tissues, which may not always be desirable in treatment of breast cancer. Measurements using breast phantoms and photon beams of ^{60}Co, 4 MV, 6 MV, and 8 MV by Chin et al. demonstrated a 100% isodose from the skin surface of 0.1–0.4 cm for ^{60}Co, to 0.5–1.4 cm for 8 MV (Chin et al. 1989). In most patients, 6 MV appears to provide the best compromise with regard to dose homogeneity and superficial dose. In patients with smaller separations, ^{60}Co and 4 MV will be satisfactory. Patients with larger separations may benefit from treatment on higher energy machines, although it may be advisable to use bolus or a beam 'spoiler' periodically to increase the skin dose. The use of bolus, however, to shift the location of the 100% isodose will increase the skin dose and may not be desirable on a daily basis.

Other factors affecting dose homogeneity are the underlying lung with its low-density tissue and the changing external contour of the target volume. To compensate for the conical shape of the breast, wedges are used in most cases as tissue compensators. This can be done with small wedges on both the medial and lateral fields, or a single larger wedge on the lateral field only. The latter reduces the scatter dose to the contralateral untreated breast, which is increased by the presence of a medial wedge (Fraass et al. 1985). This may be useful in younger patients given the concern of increased risk of contralateral radiogenic breast cancer as described by Boice et al. (1992). This approach, however, results in an asymmetric dose within the treated breast.

The presence of lung results in an increased dose to the underlying tissue and accentuates the "hot spots" at the edges of the tangential fields. This effect may lead to increased problems with respect to morbidity and unsatisfactory cosmetic results. It is now possible to determine dose distribution accounting for lung density and the varying contours along the longitudinal axis of the patient. A study from the Netherlands Cancer Institute investigated whether or not lung homogeneity corrections should be made during tangential breast irradiation. The authors concluded that lung tissue in the tangential field increases dose between 3% and 7% and is slightly overpredicted in the commercially available systems. However, this occurs in the already high dose regions and therefore they recommend that inhomogeneity corrections be applied during tangential field irradiation to minimize the effect (MIJNHEER et al. 1991).

Utilizing three-dimensional computed tomography planning with inhomogeneity correction algorithms incorporating lung density, FRAASS et al. (1988) studied the influence of lung volume on dose distribution in 34 patients using differing photon energies and determining what portion of the breast actually received more than 110% of the prescribed dose. For treatment with ^{60}Co, 32% of the breast may receive more than 110% of the prescribed dose, for 4 MV it was 24% of the breast, for 6 MV it was 19%, and for 10 MV it was 11% (FRAASS et al. 1988). Thus, inhomogeneity of as much as 20% is possible, particularly when large-breasted women are treated on low energy machines. A study at the JCRT investigated the effect of lung volume by studying the three-dimensional dose distributions calculated for an "average" breast phantom for ^{60}Co, 4 MV, 6 MV, and 8 MV photon beams. The hot spots were at the breast periphery near the posterior plane and near the apex of the breast, with the highest dose (as much as 125%) occurring at the inferior margin for lower energy photons. Factoring in lung corrections revealed an increased dose at the left margin of lung volumes. For the average breast phantom (lung density 0.31 g/cm^3), correction factors were energy-dependent and were found to be between 1.03 and 1.06, and were less for higher energy machines. To correct for this effect would require three-dimensional compensators for each patient (CHIN et al. 1989).

An in vivo dosimetric study of the potential advantage of three-dimensional dose distribution during tangential field irradiation was performed at the Netherlands Cancer Institute utilizing 8 MV photons and a two-dimensional treatment planning system. Diodes were placed at the central beam axes and peripheral high-dose regions and measured the actual dose delivered. A comparison of the dose delivery and the calculated dose revealed that the delivered dose was 2% less at the isocenter and 5.7% more at points behind the lung. Limitations in the dose calculation algorithms and dose calculation procedures were measured and were found to compensate for each other at the isocenter. The authors concluded that a two-dimensional treatment planning system was an adequate method for dose calculation. Greater accuracy would require an estimation of the lack of scatter due to missing tissue, the changes in dose distribution due to oblique incident beams, and incorporation of the actual output of the treatment machine (HEUKELOM et al. 1991). Thus the three-dimensional system has not yet been shown to have a clinical advantage over the two-dimensional treatment planning now utilized by most institutions and, since it is much more time-consuming and expensive, is not widely used.

The use of a wedge as a tissue compensator does not account for variations of the patient in the longitudinal direction. MAYLES et al. (1991) from the Royal Marsden Hospital assessed the potential for enhancing the dose distribution in 37 patients by basing the treatment plan on multilevel data and by utilizing a tissue compensator designed on the basis of "radiological thickness" (i.e., the path length through the breast corrected for tissue density). With standard two-dimensional treatment planning, for 6 MV the dose along the central slice ranged from +15% to −10% of the midtarget dose. With a compensator that corrected transverse and longitudinal breast contour, reduced lung attenuation and also differences in SSD between medial and lateral tangential fields, dose variation was reduced to +4% to −11%. This analysis revealed how three-dimensional tissue compensators can achieve improvements in dose distribution (primarily by reducing the high dose regions) if compensation for the effect of lung density is included. Many institutions are investigating the possibility of producing three-dimensional compensators cheaply and reliably. Of concern with the use of three-dimensional compensators is the need for even greater patient immobilization to ensure a precise matching of compensator and target volume on a daily basis. At this time, two-dimensional compensators are standard at most institutions.

The location at which the dose is prescribed (normalization point) varies from institution to institution. The National Surgical Adjuvant Breast and Bowel Project (NSABP) prescribes the dose of up to 5300 cGy at a depth two-thirds the distance between the skin overlying the breast and the base of the tangential fields at midseparation (FISHER et al. 1985). The Cancer and Leukemia Group B (CALGB) calculates dose at a point two-thirds the distance from the apex of the breast to the baseline (i.e., the line connecting the posterior edge of the two tangential fields) at the midseparation of the beams, with variation in dose from the base of the breast to its apex not to exceed 15%. In the studies described above from the Royal Marsden, the edge of the target volume was defined at the

92% point of the beam (Mayles et al. 1991). At the JCRT, the normalization point is 1.5 cm anterior to the deep edge of the field along a perpendicular through the isocenter (Harris and Recht 1991). This point was chosen because a JCRT phantom study found that the dose varied by less than 1% in a 1 cm radius hemisphere anterior to and centered at the perpendicular bisector and anterior lung contour. The minimum target dose was therefore chosen to be 1 cm more anterior to this point (Chin et al. 1989). This isodose level concurs with that chosen by Fraass et al. (1988) via a separate analysis.

11.3 Special Considerations

There are a number of topics for which there is a divergence of opinion and these are discussed below.

11.3.1 Tumor Bed Boost

Whether or not the tumor bed requires a supplemental dose of irradiation to minimize risk of local failure is an issue that has not been resolved. The rationale behind the "boost" is that the largest amount of malignant cells remaining following limited surgery is in the region of the original tumor. Holland et al. (1985) systematically examined 264 mastectomy specimens with invasive carcinoma using a correlated histologic and radiographic technique for the presence of residual disease. These specimens contained tumors which were 4 cm or less and deemed suitable candidates for breast-conserving treatment. Only 39% of the specimens were free of tumor foci beyond the primary tumor (group A). Twenty percent of specimens had residual disease restricted to the immediately surrounding 2 cm around the reference tumor (group B). Forty-one percent of the specimens contained foci of malignancy beyond the 2 cm perimeter, including 27% in which the residual disease was entirely intraductal (group C) and 14% harboring both invasive and intraductal tumor (group D) (Holland et al. 1985). This study demonstrated that additional foci of malignant cells are frequently present in the vicinity of the tumor and may be a source of local recurrences within the breast. Clinically, the majority of failures within the breast following conservative surgery and irradiation are within the area that would be encompassed in the boost volume. In a study from the JCRT, 48 of the 67 failures (72%) were at or near the primary tumor site (Recht et al. 1988a). Similar results have been observed by other institutions.

The indications for a boost should be considered in relation to the extent of surgical resection, the presence of tumor at the margins of resection, and the histologic characteristics of the tumor. Since the likelihood of residual disease diminishes as the distance from the primary tumor increases (Holland et al 1985), it seems probable that the boost may be more important following simple excision than after a quadrantectomy or wide local excision. The results of the NSABP B-06 trial demonstrated a 11% local failure rate with a median follow-up of 81 months in patients who had undergone excisional biopsy with "negative margins" (Fisher et al. 1989). In patients with focal margin involvement, a boost is generally recommended. In patients treated by wide resection with clearly negative margins, the need for a boost is uncertain and can reasonably be omitted (Pezner et al. 1988).

One histologic finding that may require special consideration with respect to the need for a boost is the presence of an extensive intraductal component (EIC) of a ductal carcinoma in situ in association with the primary tumor (Holland et al. 1990). Higher local failure rates have been noted in these patients suggesting that boost irradiation may be even more important in these women. Given the segmental pattern of these tumors as demonstrated by mammography and ductography, it is reasonable that the boost should follow these anatomic ductal paths.

The majority of series that utilized conservative surgery and irradiation for early stage breast cancer incorporated a boost dose of 10–15 Gy and found little morbidity and minimal alteration in cosmetic outcome with either interstitial or external beam irradiation. The type of irradiation used for boosting the tumor bed has evolved over the years. Most centers are currently utilizing electrons because of their greater convenience, equal efficacy, and possibly improved long-term cosmetic result compared with implant. At the JCRT, interstitial iridium implants were routinely used from 1970 to 1981, but, beginning in 1982, electron beam boosts became available to us. A recent analysis by de la Rochefordiere et al. (1992) from the JCRT indicated that both boost techniques offered excellent local control and that there was little difference in the long-term cosmetic result. Other centers have compared boost techniques and found similar results (FOWBLE et al 1986). At the JCRT, nearly all patients are treated with a boost to the primary site, since the extent of surgery performed here is typically limited, and this approach has resulted in excellent local control and cosmetic result.

Standard boost treatment at the JCRT consists of en face electrons for an additional 16 Gy in eight fractions. The field is used to treat the tumor bed, which is determined by reviewing the surgeon's notes, the initial mammogram, and the patient's description. It must be stressed that in some cases, the scar is not an accurate indication of the location of the tumor bed. Daily reproducibility is accomplished by the use of a clear film template placed over the patient's skin onto which anatomic landmarks and tattoos are transferred. The patient is positioned to provide a flat surface and is photographed. The electron energy chosen depends on the depth of the tumor bed and the thickness of the breast tissue, and is typically determined by ultrasonography. Another option is for the surgeon to place opaque clips at the margins of the tumor bed (usually placed medial, lateral, cephalad, caudad, and at the base of the surgical bed posteriorly), at the time of excisional biopsy, thus allowing visualization of the tumor bed at the time of simulation (SOLIN et al. 1985). The anterior border is taken as the skin margin, since the entire surgical bed is considered to be contaminated by the tumor. The depth is determined by the use of a series of parallel link chains placed over the tumor bed. Orthogonal films and/or rotational stereo shift films are obtained on the simulator and the depth of the clips is determined by their relationship to the link chains on the skin surface. The appropriate electron energy can then be determined to cover the target volume (SOLIN et al. 1987).

11.3.2 Regional Nodal Irradiation

While most people agree that treatment to the breast is beneficial, the management of the draining lymph nodes – axillary, internal mammary, and supraclavicular – is more controversial. The unanswered question regarding regional nodal irradiation is whether or not it has any effect on survival (HARRIS and OSTEEN 1985). The available information indicates that any benefit, if present, is small. Axillary dissection has traditionally been used in the management of patients with clinically nondisseminated breast cancer as it is effective in reducing axillary failure and provides useful prognostic information. In the past, the results were used to guide the utilization of adjuvant systemic therapy. Nowadays, however, increasing numbers of patients are being treated with systemic therapy regardless of nodal status and the value of surgically staging the axilla is less clear-cut. In patients who present initially with bulky axillary adenopathy, management should include axillary dissection followed by irradiation, since the dose of irradiation necessary to sterilize gross disease would be much higher than that required for microscopic residual and the risk of complications far greater.

When making a judgement whether or not to irradiate the adjacent lymph nodes, one must judge the risk of subsequent failure in that region in relation to the morbidity of treatment including the risk of arm edema, brachial plexopathy, and radiation pneumonitis. This decision must also be considered in conjunction with the extent of surgery performed. At the JCRT, axillary surgery typically consists of a level I–II axillary dissection in which the adventitial tissue from the axillary vein is not removed. This has led to a much lower incidence of arm edema (LARSON et al. 1986), without compromising local control or the ability to assess prognosis. In patients who have undergone axillary dissection and have been found to have no axillary nodes involved, the risk of regional nodal failure is very small. RECHT et al. (1991b) from the JCRT found that only 9 out of 420 patients (2.1%) failed in the axilla following treatment with only tangential field irradiation. In this same group of patients, only 1.9% failed in the supraclavicular region. Even in those women whose axillary dissection yielded one to three positive lymph nodes, and who had received only tangential field irradiation, the rate of failure in the axilla was 2.1% (1/47 patients). The incidence of supraclavicular failure in these two populations was 1.9% (8/420) and 0% (0/47) (RECHT et al. 1991b). Therefore, at our institution, for patients who have had a level I–II dissection and who have zero to three positive lymph nodes, radiation treatment with tangents only is routinely used.

The randomized studies from Milan and the NSABP B-06 compared mastectomy with conservative surgery and irradiation, which was directed to the breast alone. The satisfactory results achieved in these trials establishes breast irradiation alone as one reasonable treatment option. Although irradiation only to the breast is considered adequate in any patient who has undergone axillary dissection, there are some patients who should be considered candidates for regional nodal irradiation. In patients who have undergone a level I–II axillary dissection (without stripping of the axillary vein) and have been found to have four or more positive nodes, treatment to the full axilla should be considered. This would pertain especially to patients who had involvement of more than half of the nodes sampled, had extracapsular extension of tumor into fat, or had involvement of the highest node sampled. In addition, in those patients who have axillary nodal involvement or lesions in the medial portion of the breast (particularly if axillary nodes are involved), it is reasonable to consider treatment to the internal mammary as well as supraclavicular nodes, provided morbidity can be kept to a minimum. The technique for treating the internal mammary nodes is described below.

In patients who do not undergo axillary dissection, irradiation to the draining lymph nodes can be accomplished with excellent clinical results and minimal morbidity. This is the current treatment approach at the JCRT until a subpopulation of patients with very small risk of nodal involvement can be identified. In the JCRT study described above, failure rates in the axilla and supraclavicular regions following three-field irradiation without axillary dissection were 0.8% (3/355) for N0 and 2.9% (1/35) for N1 clinical disease (Recht et al. 1991b).

Long-term complications related to nodal irradiation in patients treated at the JCRT have been found to be uncommon. Arm edema in those who received three-field irradiation without axillary dissection occurred at a rate of 4% in 235 patients compared with 13% for the 240 patients who had axillary surgery ($p = 0.006$) (Larson et al. 1986). The incidence of radiation pneumonitis in patients treated with three-field irradiation was 0.6% (5/788) if no chemotherapy was given and increased to 3.3% (11/328) in patients who had received chemotherapy ($p = 0.001$). In the chemotherapy group of patients, the incidence was 1.3% (3/236) if the drugs were administered sequentially compared with 8.8% (8/92) if they were given concurrently with the irradiation ($p = 0.002$) (Lingos et al. 1991). Brachial plexopathy was seen in 20/1624 (1.2%) women treated between 1968 and 1985 at the JCRT and was related to the use of a third field to irradiate the draining lymph nodes. The incidence was then 1.8% (20/1117). No cases of brachial plexopathy were seen in patients treated with tangents only. If chemotherapy was administered with three-field irradiation, the incidence rose to 4.5% (15/330) compared with 0.6% (5/787) without chemotherapy ($p = 0.0001$). The dose to the axilla also had an effect on the incidence of brachial plexopathy, with a rate of 1.3% (13/991) if total axillary dose was less than 50 Gy compared with 5.6% (7/125) with an axillary dose of more than 50 Gy. The median time to its occurrence was 10.5 months (range 1.5–77 months) and the brachial plexopathy completely resolved in 80% of the cases (Pierce et al. 1992).

There are some patients in whom it may be desirable to only treat the lower axillary nodes by including them in tangential fields, utilizing a higher than usual superior border. This will incorporate the lower axillary nodes, but will not irradiate significant amounts of normal tissue nor require the extra time, effort, and potential morbidity of three-field irradiation. This approach is considered in patients with small primary tumors who are clinically N0, particularly if they are elderly or have lung disease.

11.3.3 Techniques of Nodal Irradiation

The use of three-field irradiation for breast carcinoma requires attention to detail if one is to accomplish the goals of aesthetically pleasing results, excellent local control, and minimal toxicity. One must achieve a nearly perfect geometric match between the tangential fields and the anterior nodal field in order to avoid "hot" or "cold" spots in the dose distribution, the former leading to matchline fibrosis and the latter to a potential decrease in local tumor control. Siddon et al. (1983) described a technique for accomplishing this, currently used at the JCRT, which involves three steps: (1) a shielding block (half-field or central axis block) is used to cover the caudal half of the supraclavicular field to eliminate divergence, resulting in a vertical transverse plane to which the tangential fields are matched; (2) small corner blocks are used on the cephalic edges of the tangential fields to produce the vertical edge for matching to the anterior field, thus eliminating overlap regardless of gantry and collimator position; and (3) the couch is rotated in opposite directions for each tangential field to eliminate divergence along the superior border (Siddon et al. 1983; Svensson et al. 1980. A beam alignment device (protractor) with pegs that project onto the light field along the matchline help facilitate daily set-up and ensure accuracy (Buck et al. 1985).

The anterior supraclavicular–axillary field is angled 10–15° from vertical to avoid direct irradiation of the spinal cord. The superior border of the field is typically placed at the top of the first rib to avoid "flash" on the skin in the supraclavicular region. The lateral border of the field varies depending on the amount of axilla to be treated. If full axillary irradiation is indicated, the border is placed at two-thirds the medial to lateral distance of the humeral head. If only the axillary apex and supraclavicular nodes are to be treated, it is placed at the lateral edge of the coracoid process at the insertion of the pectoralis minor. When the full axilla is treated the dose is calculated to a depth of 5 cm below the surface of the skin; for the supraclavicular nodes only, a depth of 3 cm is used. A dose of 45 Gy–46 Gy is given in 23–25 fractions.

There are occasions when the axilla requires a dose above 46 Gy. This is generally accomplished at the JCRT with an en face axillary boost (EAB) in which the beam is angled from the axilla towards the supraclavicular nodes by moving the couch, gantry, and collimator. In this technique, the anterior edge of the field is at the midportion of the pectoralis major thus sparing the portion of that muscle which received the highest dose from the anterior supraclavicular field. The dose is calculated at 5 cm. An additional two to five fractions of 200–250 cGy are administered depending on the clinical situation, extent of disease, and extent of surgical resection (HARRIS and RECHT 1991). In most situations in which a boost is used, the axilla is taken to a dose of approximately 50 Gy. Alternatively, the posterior axillary boost (PAB) may be utilized. The boundaries of the PAB are as follows: superior border parallel to the clavicle, inferior border at the superior border of the tangential field, medial border approximately 2 cm into the lung along the chest wall and the lateral border at the middle of the humeral head. The dose is calculated from the posterior skin surface to a depth of the separation minus 5 cm. At the University of Pennsylvania, the axilla is boosted with a posterior axillary field delivered at 100 cGy per fraction with two to three fractions per week as required – on average a total of 800–1000 cGy – per patient (FOWBLE et al. 1991).

When a clinical decision has been made to irradiate the internal mammary nodes it is generally accomplished in one of two ways. The first is with an anterior field ("hockey stick") overlying the internal mammary and supraclavicular nodes matched with tangential fields. The second utilizes isocentric opposed tangential fields encompassing the breast, chest wall, and the internal mammary nodes, adding a second en face field for the supraclavicular nodes. Using the anterior field, it is very difficult to avoid overlap or underdosage with the medial tangential border to minimize matchline fibrosis or marginal failure. Another drawback of this technique is that more lung and heart (in left-sided lesions) is included in these treatment fields than with wide tangents. Electrons can also be used to irradiate the internal mammary nodes but, again, it is difficult to match with the medial tangential field and avoid over- or undertreatment. The technique used at the JCRT is to attempt to include the internal mammary nodes in the tangential fields while avoiding inclusion of a significant amount of myocardium or lung. Many institutions have used a general guideline of 3 cm beyond the midline as the entry point for the medial tangential field to irradiate the internal mammary nodes. This approach was evaluated at the JCRT utilizing radionuclide lymphoscintigraphy (SIDDON et al. 1983) to localize the internal mammary nodes. In this population of 167 patients, the 3 cm guideline would have excluded at least one node in 17% and would have overshot the node by 1 cm in 66% and by 2 cm in 48%. Thus, excessive lung and/or heart would have been irradiated in two-thirds of the patients (RECHT et al. 1988b). Computed tomography can also be used to determine location of these nodes. Following localization of their position, it is possible to use metal markers on the chest wall to identify their position and to make a clinical decision at simulation whether or not the amount of additional normal tissue to be irradiated warrants their inclusion. Given the current uncertainties regarding the survival benefit of such treatment, the internal mammary nodes are included at our institution only in patients with significant risk of involvement in which their inclusion does not result in excessive heart or lung irradiation.

11.4 Future Directions

Techniques of surgery and the criteria for patient eligibility for conservative treatment are evolving. More attention is being paid to placement of scars and the volume of resection. Patients with larger tumors, involvement of the nipple, or with limited skin involvement are no longer automatically recommended for mastectomy. Radiologists are correlating mammographic findings with the pathologists' histologic results, which will help identify patients who may be at risk for local failure. This will hopefully lead to clearer guidelines regarding the use of boost fields. The increase in screening mammography has led to a marked improvement in the diagnosis of early stage disease. This has implications for identifying which patients may be candidates for treatment to less than the entire breast or would perhaps safely be able to avoid irradiation altogether. The increasing numbers of patients receiving adjuvant systemic therapy will require close scrutiny of what factors contribute to long-term morbidity and how these can be minimized. Technological advancements with equipment will make three-dimensional treatment planning, customized individual compensators, and on-line portal imaging devices readily available.

The current techniques described above have evolved over several years to yield results that are comparable to mastectomy in terms of survival and superior in terms of aesthetics and lifestyle. Now that the basic question of effectiveness of breast-conserving treatment has been answered, the trend is towards perfecting the techniques of treatment, identifying certain subsets of patients who may require more or less treatment, and integrating local and systemic therapy in an optimal manner. To this end, studies are in progress that will attempt to clarify these issues.

References

Bader J, Lippman M, Swain S et al (1987) Preliminary report of the NCI early breast cancer (BC) study: A prospective randomized comparison of lumpectomy (L) and radiation (XRT) to mastectomy (M) for stage I and II BC [abstr]. Int J Radiat Oncol Biol Phys 13 [Suppl]: 160

Bartelink H, van Dongen JA (1989) Randomized clinical trial to assess the value of breast conserving therapy (BCT) in stage I and stage II breast cancer. Proceedings of the 5th European Conference on Clinical Oncology (Abstract)

Bleichert-Toft M, Brincker H, Andersen JA et al (1988) A Danish randomized trial comparing breast preserving therapy with mastectomy in mammary carcinoma. Acta Oncol 27: 6471–6676

Boice JD, Harvey EB, Blettner M, Stovall M, Flannery JT (1992) Cancer in the contralateral breast after radiotherapy for breast cancer. N Engl J Med 326: 781–785

Bornstein BA, Cheng CW, Rhodes LM, Rashid H, Stomper PC, Siddon RL, Harris JR (1990) Can simulation measurements be used to predict the irradiated lung volume in the tangential fields in patients treated for breast cancer? Int J Radiat Oncol Biol Phys 18: 181–187

Brinkley D, Haybittle JL, Houghton J (1984) The Cancer Research Campaign (King's/Cambridge) trial for early breast cancer: An analysis of the radiotherapy data. Br J Cancer 57: 309–316

Buck BA, Siddon RL, Svensson GK (1985) A beam alignment device for matching fields. Int J Radiat Oncol Biol Phys 11: 1039–1043

Buzzoni R, Bonadonna G, Valagussa P, Zambetti M (1991) Adjuvant chemotherapy with doxorubicin plus cyclosphosphamide, methotrexate, and fluorouracil in the treatment of resectable breast cancer with more than three positive axillary nodes. J Clin Oncol 9: 2134–2140

Chin LM, Cheng CW, Siddon RL, Rice RK, Mijnheer BJ, Harris JR (1989) Three-dimensional photon dose distributions with and without lung corrections for tangential breast intact treatments. Int J Radiat Oncol Biol Phys 17: 1327–1335

de la Rochefordiere A, Abner AL, Silver B, Vicini F, Recht A, Harris JR (1992) Are cosmetic results following conservative surgery and radiation therapy for early breast cancer dependent on technique? Int J Radiat Oncol Biol Phys (in press)

Fisher B, Bauer M, Margolese R et al (1985) Five-year results of a randomized clinical trial comparing total mastectomy and segmental mastectomy with or without radiation in the treatment of breast cancer. N Engl J Med 312: 665–673

Fisher B, Redmond C, Poisson R, Margolese R et al (1989) Eight-year results of a randomized clinical trial comparing total mastectomy and lumpectomy with or without irradiation in the treatment of breast cancer. N Engl J Med 320: 822–828

Fowble B, Solin LJ, Martz KL et al (1986) The influence of the type of boost (electrons vs implant) on local control and cosmesis in patients with stage I and II breast cancer undergoing conservative surgery and radiation. Int J Radiat Oncol Biol Phys 12 [Suppl]: 150 (Abstract)

Fowble B, Solin LJ, Schultz DJ (1991) Conservative surgery and radiation for early breast cancer. In: Fowble B, Goodman RL, Glick JH, Rosato EF (eds) Breast cancer treatment – a comprehensive guide to management. Mosby Year Book, St. Louis, pp 122–149

Fraass BA, Roberson PL, Lichter AS (1985) Dose to the contralateral breast due to primary breast irradiation. Int J Radiat Oncol Biol Phys 11: 485–497

Fraass BA, Lichter AS, McShan DL et al (1988) The influence of lung density corrections on treatment planning for primary breast cancer. Int J Radiat Oncol Biol Phys 14: 179–190

Harris JR, Levene MB, Svensson G et al (1979) Analysis of cosmetic results following primary radiation therapy for stages I and II carcinoma of the breast. Int J Radiat Oncol Biol Phys 5: 257–261

Harris JR, Osteen RT (1985) Patients with early breast cancer benefit from effective axillary treatment. Breast Cancer Res Treat 5: 17–21

Harris JR, Recht A (1991) Primary treatment of breast cancer – conservative surgery and radiotherapy. In: Harris JR, Hellman S, Henderson IC, Kinne DW (eds) Breast diseases, 2nd edn. Lippincott, Philadelphia, pp 388–419

Haybittle JL, Brinkley D, Houghton J et al (1989) Postoperative radiotherapy and late mortality: evidence from the Cancer Research Campaign trial for early breast cancer. BMJ 2948: 1611–1641

Heukelom S, Lanson JH, van Tienhoven G, Mijnheer BJ (1991) In vivo dosimetry during tangential breast treatment. Radiother Oncol 22: 269–279

Holland R, Veling SH, Mravunac M et al (1985) Histologic multifocality of Tis, T1-2 breast carcinomas: Implications for clinical trials of breast-conserving surgery. Cancer 56: 979–990

Holland R, Connolly JL, Gelman R et al (1990) The presence

of an extensive intraductal component following a limited excision correlates with prominent residual disease in the remainder of the breast. J Clin Oncol 8: 113–118
Host H, Breenhovd I, Loeb M (1986) Postoperative radiotherapy in breast cancer – long-term results from the Oslo study. Int J Radiat Oncol Biol Phys 2: 727–732
Kurtz JM, Spitalier JM, Amalric R (1983) Late breast recurrence after lumpectomy and irradiation. Int J Radiat Oncol Biol Phys 9: 1191–1194
Larson D, Weinstein M, Goldberg I et al (1986) Edema of the arm as a function of the extent of axillary surgery in patients with stage I–II carcinoma of the breast treated with primary radiotherapy. Int J Radiat Oncol Biol Phys 12: 1575–1582
Levitt SH (1990) Radiation oncology. Cancer 65: 2119–2120
Lingos TI, Recht A, Vicini F et al. (1991) Radiation pneumonitis in breast cancer patients treated with conservative surgery and radiation therapy. Int J Radiat Oncol Biol Phys 21: 355–360
Marcial VA (1990) Primary therapy for limited breast cancer – radiation therapy techniques. Cancer 65: 2159–2164
Mayles WPM, Yarnold JR, Webb S (1991) Improved dose homogeneity in the breast using tissue compensators. Radiother Oncol 22: 248–251
Mijnheer BJ, Heukelom S, Lanson JH et al (1991) Should inhomogeneity corrections be applied during treatment planning of tangential breast irradiation? Radiother Oncol 22: 239–244
NIH Consensus Conference (1991) Treatment of early-stage breast cancer. JAMA 265: 391–397
Osborne MP, Ormiston N, Harmer CL et al (1984) Breast conservation in the treatment of early breast cancer. Cancer 53: 349–355
Pezner RD, Lipsett JA, Desai K et al (1988) To boost or not to boost: decreasing radiation therapy in conservative breast cancer treatment when "inked" tumor resection margins are pathologically free of cancer. Int J Radiat Oncol Biol Phys 14: 873–877
Photon Treatment Planning Collaborative Working Group (1991) Project summary. Int J Radiat Oncol Biol Phys 21: 3–8
Pierce SM, Recht A, Lingos TI et al (1992) Long-term radiation complications following conservative surgery and radiation therapy in patients with early stage breast cancer. Int J Radiat Oncol Biol Phys 23: 915–923
Recht A, Silen W, Schnitt C et al (1988a) Time-course of local recurrence following conservative surgery and radiotherapy for early stage breast cancer. Int J Radiat Oncol Biol Phys 15: 255–261
Recht A, Siddon RL, Kaplan WD et al (1988b) Three-dimensional mammary lymphoscintigraphy: Implications for radiation therapy treatment planning for breast carcinoma. Int J Radiat Oncol Biol Phys 14: 477–481
Recht A, Come SE, Gelman RS et al (1991a) Integration of conservative surgery, radiotherapy and chemotherapy for the treatment of early-stage, node-positive breast cancer: sequencing, timing, and outcome. J Clin Oncol 9: 1662–1667
Recht A, Pierce SM, Abner A et al (1991b) Regional nodal failure after conservative surgery and radiotherapy for early-stage breast carcinoma. J Clin Oncol 9: 988–996
Rutqvist LE, Lax I, Fornander T, Johansson H (1992) Cardiovascular mortality in a randomized trial of adjuvant radiation therapy versus surgery alone in primary breast cancer. Int J Radiat Oncol Biol Phys 22: 887–896
Sarrazin D, Le MG, Arriagada R et al (1989) Ten-year results of a randomized trial comparing a conservative treatment to mastectomy in early breast cancer. Radiother Oncol 14: 177–184
Siddon RL, Chin LM, Zimmerman RE et al (1982) Utilization of parasternal lymphoscintigraphy in radiation therapy of breast carcinoma. Int J Radiat Oncol Biol Phys 8: 1059–1063
Siddon RL, Buck BA, Harris JR, Svensson GK (1983) Three-field technique for breast irradiation using tangential field corner blocks. Int J Radiat Oncol Biol Phys 9: 583–588
Solin LJ, Danoff BF, Schwarz GF et al (1985) A practical technique for the localization of the tumor volume in definitive irradiation of the breast. Int J Radiat Oncol Biol Phys 11: 1215–1220
Solin LJ, Chu JCH, Larsen R et al (1987) Determination of depth for electron breast boosts. Int J Radiat Oncol Biol Phys 13: 1915–1919
Svensson GK, Bjarngard BE, Larson RD, Levene MB (1980) A modified three-field technique for breast treatment. Int J Radiat Oncol Biol Phys 6: 689–694
Valagussa P, Moliterni A, Zambetti M, Bonadonna G (1992) Long-term sequelae from adjuvant chemotherapy (in press)
van Herk M, Meertens H (1988) A matrix ionisation chamber imaging device for on-line patient setup verification during radiotherapy. Radiother and Oncol 11: 369–378
van Tienhoven G, Lanson JH, Crabeels D et al (1991) Accuracy in tangential breast treatment set-up: a portal imaging study. Radiother Oncol 22: 317–322
Veronesi U (1987) Rationale and indications for limited surgery in breast cancer: current data. World J Surg 11: 493–498

12 Which Patients Should Be Treated by Breast Conservation Surgery and Which by Modified Radical Mastectomy

TIMOTHY J. EBERLEIN and LINDA M. DOUVILLE

CONTENTS

12.1 Introduction 117
12.2 Local Recurrence in Patients Treated with Mastectomy or Conservative Surgery 117
12.3 Retrospective Studies of Primary Radiation Therapy 118
12.4 Randomized Prospective Studies of Primary Breast Radiation Therapy Versus Mastectomy 119
12.5 Cosmetic Results of Conservative Surgery and Primary Radiation Therapy 120
12.6 Complications of Conservative Surgery and Primary Radiation Therapy 121
12.7 Treatment Selection for Early Breast Cancer 122
12.8 Importance of Mammography. 123
12.9 Influencing Factors on the Extent of Breast-Conserving Surgery 123
12.10 Technical Aspects of Conservative Breast Surgery. 124
12.11 Axillary Lymph Node Dissection 126
12.12 Conclusion 127
References. 127

12.1 Introduction

Conservative surgery and primary radiation therapy is the preferred method of treatment for clinical stage I and II breast cancer. This therapy may be defined as lumpectomy, partial mastectomy, segmental mastectomy, or quadrantectomy; it is usually performed in combination with surgical staging of the axilla followed by primary radiation therapy to the entire breast with an implant or boost of radiation to the area of the tumor. In some cases, additional radiation may be administered to the draining nodal tissues. Patients treated with breast-conserving therapy have a more positive body image and less fear of recurrence of cancer than do patients who are treated with radical mastectomy (SCHAIN et al. 1983; BARTELINK et al. 1985). The goal of breast-conserving treatment is to provide highly satisfactory cosmesis without compromise of local tumor control or survival when compared with more radical surgery such as mastectomy.

In this chapter, we review the data from retrospective and prospective clinical trials that were the basis, in part, for the recommendations of the National Institutes of Health consensus conference on treatment of early-stage breast cancer (NATIONAL INSTITUTES of HEALTH CONSENSUS CONFERENCE 1991). We then examine some of the current controversies concerning patient selection and surgical technique, as well as the management of regional lymph nodes.

12.2 Local Recurrence in Patients Treated with Mastectomy or Conservative Surgery

In order to evaluate the comparison between conservative surgery and primary breast radiation therapy versus mastectomy, it is important to examine local recurrence rates in patients treated with either mastectomy or conservative surgery alone without radiation therapy.

The incidence of locoregional recurrence following mastectomy is due to several factors. The most important of these factors appears to be whether or not the axillary lymph nodes are pathologically involved with tumor. The chance of locoregional recurrence following radical surgery for a patient with pathologically negative axillary lymph nodes is approximately 3%–8%. However, this rate of recurrence increases to 19%–27% if the axillary lymph nodes are pathologically involved with tumor (DONEGAN et al. 1966; HAAGENSEN 1971; VALAGUSSA et al. 1985). Among all patients with

TIMOTHY J. EBERLEIN, M.D., Associate Professor of Medicine, Harvard Medical School, Chief, Division of Surgical Oncology, Brigham and Women's Hospital, 75 Francis Street, Boston, MA 02115, USA; LINDA M. DOUVILLE, R.N., Clinical Coordinator, Biologic Cancer Therapy Program, Division of Surgical Oncology, Brigham and Women's Hospital, 75 Francis Street, Boston, MA 02115, USA locoregional recurrence, one-third of the recurrences are also associated with distant metastases while two-thirds of them occur as isolated recurrences. These isolated instances of locoregional recurrence are difficult to treat, since almost all of these patients will eventually develop distant metastases even when the local recurrences are eradicated. In a recent series, the 5-year survival rate for patients with isolated locoregional diseases ranges from approximately 35% to 50%, with only 20% –30% having a disease-free survival (Bedwinek et al. 1981; Toonkel et al. 1983; Aberizk et al. 1986; Beck et al. 1983). Thus, locoregional recurrence is associated with a poor prognosis.

The National Surgical Adjuvant Breast Project (NSABP) B-06 trial is one of the only published randomized studies comparing conservative surgery alone with either conservative surgery and radiation therapy or with mastectomy alone. All of the patients in this study underwent axillary dissection and, if they had positive lymph nodes, received adjuvant chemotherapy. All of the patients who underwent conservative surgery had negative margins. If margins were involved (approximately 10%), the patients were treated with mastectomy. As seen in Fig. 12.1a, there is a statistically significant increase in the local recurrence rate in patients treated with conservative surgery alone when compared with those undergoing conservative surgery and radiation therapy. This was true regardless of whether the nodes were positive or negative. However, as demonstrated in Fig. 12.1b, there was no statistically significant difference in the overall survival of these two patient groups. This trend suggests that the effectiveness of local control may in fact have an impact on patient survival, particularly for those patients with early-stage cancer. Patients with pathologically negative nodes would seem to have the greatest potential for cure by effective locoregional treatment alone. Patients with pathologically positive nodes would appear much more likely to have systemic subclinical disease at initial presentation. Therefore, the effectiveness of local treatment may have less impact on the overall survival of this patient subset.

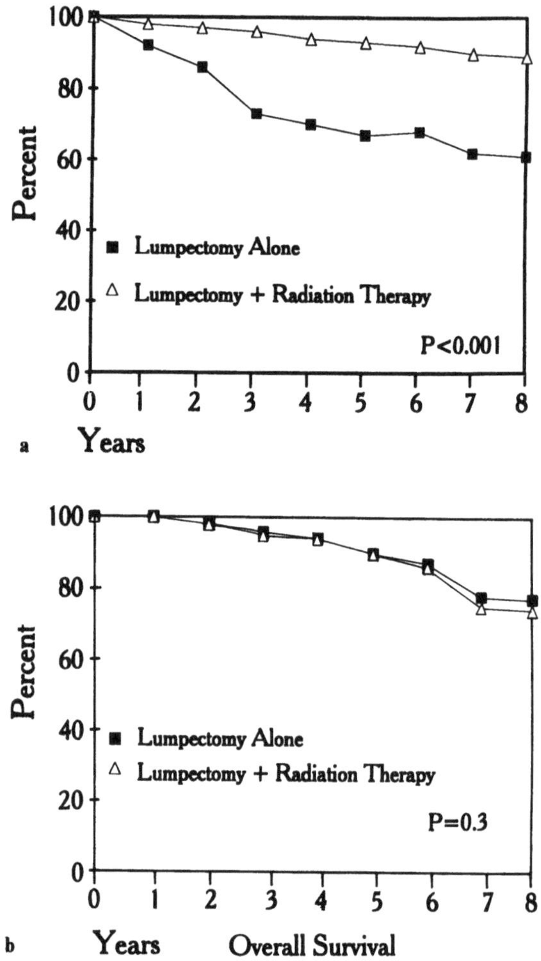

Fig. 12.1a, b. Life-table analysis of the NSABP B-06 trial demonstrates **a** the percentage of patients who remained free of breast tumor after lumpectomy alone or after lumpectomy with breast irradiation (*black squares*, 572 patients and 175 events; *white triangles*, 569 patients and 39 events). **b** Overall survival rate of this same patient population (*black squares*, 106 deaths; *white triangles*, 125 deaths). (Modified from Fisher et al. 1985, reprinted with permission)

12.3 Retrospective Studies of Primary Radiation Therapy

Since the mid-1950s, several medical centers have reported their results of primary radiation therapy as treatment for patients with clinical stage I and stage II breast cancer (Montague 1984; Harris et al. 1985b; Recht et al. 1984; Calle et al. 1983; Clarke et al. 1985; Kurtz et al. 1983; Clarke 1983).

Comparison of these various series is difficult for many reasons, such as differences in patient selection, radiation dose and dose distribution, as well as the surgical and clinical staging of patients. Similarly, the methods of data presentation and analysis employed differed. Over the course of these studies, treatment policies and techniques often changed. As an example, the Joint Center for Radiation Therapy (JCRT) treated 411 patients with excisional biopsy and radiation therapy from 1968 to 1980. In addition to excisional biopsy, patients

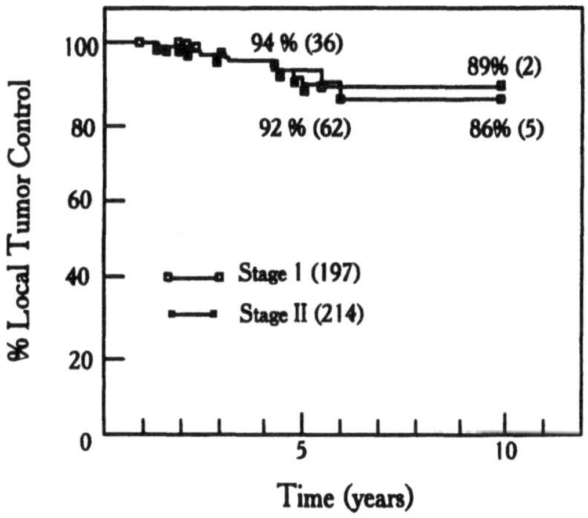

Fig. 12.2. The Joint Center for Radiation Therapy study of 411 patients treated from 1968 to 1980 demonstrates extent of local tumor control with excisional biopsy and dose to primary site of at least 6000 cGy. (Reprinted with permission from EBERLEIN et al. 1990)

received whole breast irradiation with a supplemental boost of radiation utilizing external beam or implants, thus the dose of primary radiation exceeded 6000 cGy. As seen in Fig. 12.2, the 5-year breast recurrence rate was 6% for clinical stage I and 8% for clinical stage II patients. In contrast, 211 patients with clinically uninvolved axillary lymph nodes were treated at the Royal Marsden Hospital and were found to have a crude locoregional recurrence rate of 14.5% at 5 years and 21.5% at 10 years (OSBORNE et al. 1984). Patients treated at the Royal Marsden were given an average of 4500 cGy to the breast in 20 fractions over 8 weeks followed by a boost of 1000 cGy in 5 fractions over 2 weeks. No axillary dissections were performed. The differences in the total dose and number of fractions between these institutions most likely account for the differences in results.

A very important conclusion to be drawn from such retrospective analysis, however, concerns the time to local recurrence. Most locoregional recurrences following mastectomy will occur within the first few years. Patients treated with primary radiation therapy, however, must be followed closely for local recurrence for a much longer period of time. A collaborative study of 152 patients treated before 1967 at the Institut Curie, the Marseilles Cancer Institute, or the Princess Margaret Hospital with a minimum follow-up of 15 years, retrospectively, was reviewed (HARRIS et al. 1984). While the techniques, equipment, and doses utilized in these studies were outdated when compared with current practice, the conclusions are still valid. Most breast recurrences occurred during the first 5 years after treatment, and the actual area of local recurrence was virtually constant for 14 years after primary breast irradiation. There were no local recurrences seen between 15 and 20 years after primary treatment. While the absolute risk of developing a breast recurrence may be somewhat less when utilizing modern techniques, the time to local recurrence is still valid. The salvage of patients who develop locoregional disease with subsequent surgery (usually a total mastectomy) yielded a 58% rate of freedom from distant metastases at 5 years and 50% at 10 years. Salvage rates did not vary significantly in regards to time to recurrence after primary treatment. Thus, these data suggest both the likelihood of optimum local control with higher doses of radiation therapy, as well as a higher rate of long-term salvage for patients who develop local failure after primary radiation therapy when compared with those patients who experience local recurrence following mastectomy.

12.4 Randomized Prospective Studies of Primary Breast Radiation Therapy Versus Mastectomy

Several randomized prospective trials have addressed the use of radiation therapy versus mastectomy for primary treatment of breast cancer. These trials are comparable in terms of prognostic features and have had sufficient patient numbers as well as follow-up time to adequately evaluate survival rates.

The earliest such trial was conducted in 1961 at the Guy's Hospital in London (ATKINS et al. 1972; HAYWARD 1977, 1983). All of the trial participants had T1 or T2 lesions, and all had N1 or N2 nodal disease. Premenopausal patients were excluded from the study. The patients were randomly allocated to receive either radical mastectomy or wide excision; both groups received postoperative radiation therapy. All patients prior to 1968 also received adjuvant thiotepa. None of the patients who underwent wide excision had an axillary dissection. The patients with either clinically negative axillary lymph nodes or clinically enlarged axillary lymph nodes who had received inadequate doses of radiation according to current standards experienced a significantly higher rate of locoregional recurrence. However, the incidence of freedom from distant metastases and the resulting likelihood of survival were the same in both arms for the N0 patients.

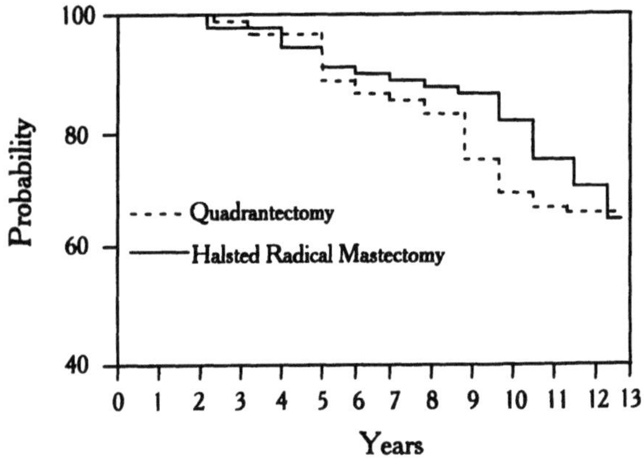

Fig. 12.3. Results of the National Cancer Institute of Milan trial of 701 patients with T1 N0 breast cancer randomized to receive either radical mastectomy or conservative surgery with axillary dissection and radiotherapy which demonstrate no statistical significance in either of the two arms. (Modified from VERONESI et al. 1981, reprinted with permission)

There was a survival advantage at 10 years for the N1 patients treated with radical mastectomy but, with further follow-up at 15 years, freedom from distant relapse was similar in these groups.

From 1973 to 1980, 701 evaluable patients with primary tumors of up to 2 cm in size and clinically uninvolved axillary lymph nodes (T1N0) were entered into the National Cancer Institute of Milan randomized study (VERONESI et al. 1981; VERONESI 1985; BONADONNA et al. 1983). Patients were randomized to receive either radical mastectomy or conservative surgery (quadrantectomy) and radiotherapy. Axillary dissection was performed in all patients. Patients receiving radiation therapy received a dose of 5000 cGy in 5 weeks with an additional 1000 cGy using orthovoltage to the site of tumor. The two arms were well-balanced with regard to age, tumor size, and axillary nodal status. As seen in Fig. 12.3, patients treated with conservative surgery and radiation fared at least as well in overall survival as patients with a standard Halsted radical mastectomy.

The NSABP initiated a three-arm randomized trial (B-06) that began in 1976 and closed to patient accrual in 1984. This trial compared mastectomy with segmental mastectomy with or without radiation therapy and is currently the largest series published (FISHER et al. 1985). Evaluable patients with clinical stage I or stage II breast cancer and a primary tumor of up to 4 cm in size were eligible. All patients underwent axillary dissection and those with positive lymph nodes received adjuvant chemotherapy. Segmental mastectomy as defined in this trial included a resection of the tumor, which included removal of enough normal tissue to ensure tumor-free margins. Approximately 10% of the patients who underwent segmental mastectomy had tumor-positive margins and therefore underwent subsequent total mastectomy. As seen in Fig. 12.4, there was no statistical difference in disease-free survival, distant disease-free survival, or overall survival when mastectomy was compared with segmental mastectomy and radiation therapy.

Another trial studied 179 patients with tumors of up to 2 cm in size with either clinically involved or uninvolved lymph nodes from 1972 through 1979 at the Institut Gustave-Roussy (SARRAZIN et al. 1984). Again, there was no statistically significant difference in either the incidence of distant metastases or the overall survival between the groups treated with mastectomy or tumorectomy plus radiation therapy.

Similar results were obtained from the National Cancer Institute in Bethesda, which randomized patients with clinical stage I or II breast cancers to receive modified radical mastectomy or conservative excision, axillary dissection and radiation therapy (FINDLAY et al. 1985). No significant difference in outcome between these two groups has been seen. Another randomized study by the Danish group reported similar results (BLICHERT-TOFT et al. 1988).

These randomized prospective trials demonstrate two important points: radiation therapy techniques significantly affect the likelihood of local recurrence which, in turn, appears likely to impact survival in some patients; and when adequate treatment techniques are utilized, no significant difference in survival exists between patients treated with radical surgery or with conservative surgery and primary radiation therapy. Thus, these randomized prospective trials confirm the previously reported retrospective studies.

12.5 Cosmetic Results of Conservative Surgery and Primary Radiation Therapy

The cosmetic results following conservative surgery and primary radiation therapy generally range from good to excellent. As seen in Fig. 12.5, the results of the JCRT are typical of the other series which utilized modern equipment and state of the art techniques (BEADLE et al. 1984a, b). Poor cosmesis is associated with doses of external beam

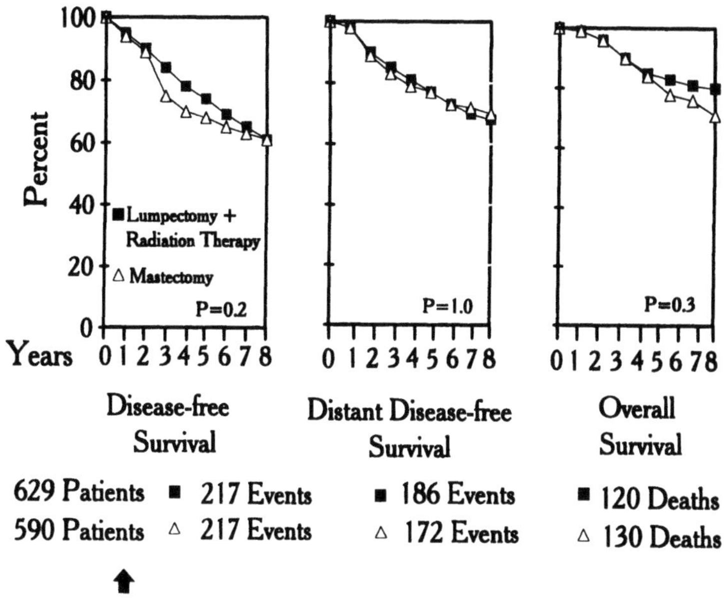

Fig. 12.4. Life table analysis of the NSABP B-06 trials which reveals no statistically significant differences in the rates of disease-free survival (217 events in both groups), distant disease-free survival (172 events in the mastectomy group versus 186 in the lumpectomy plus radiation therapy group), and overall survival (120 deaths in the mastectomy group versus 130 in the lumpectomy plus radiation therapy group) of patients treated with total mastectomy (*white triangles*; 590 patients) or lumpectomy and breast irradiation (*black squares*; 629 patients). (Modified from FISHER et al. 1985, reprinted with permission)

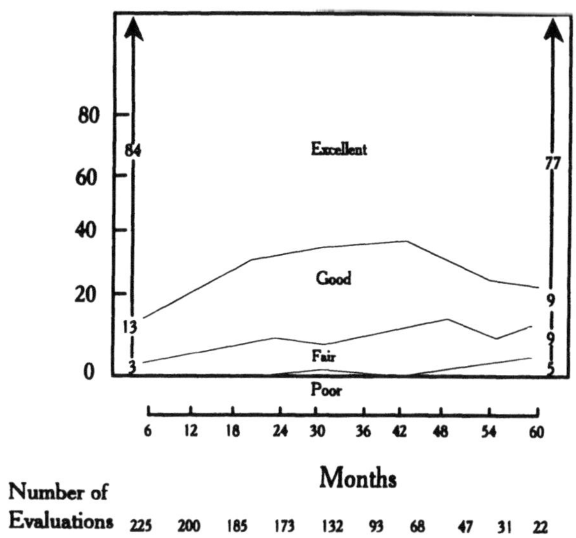

Fig. 12.5. Overall cosmetic results in 239 patients treated at the Joint Center for Radiation Therapy with radiotherapy and no chemotherapy treated from 1976 to 1980. (Reprinted with permission from BEADLE et al. 1984b)

radiation greater than 5000 cGy, which results in an increased incidence of retraction and fibrosis. Poor cosmesis also is a result of implants delivering larger doses as well as higher than usual overall doses to the primary tumor. The use of chemotherapy also appears to negatively affect the overall cosmetic result; however, further follow-up is required to prove this hypothesis.

12.6 Complications of Conservative Surgery and Primary Radiation Therapy

The short-term complications of primary radiation therapy for early breast cancer most commonly include fatigue and irradiation or erythema of the skin. The latter can occasionally result in a moist desquamation which requires temporary cessation of the radiation therapy. These complications are usually self-limiting, however, and resolve within several days to several weeks after treatment.

Development of significant long-term complications is rare. In the JCRT series, the most common complications reported were rib fracture (5%), significant arm edema (4%), and radiation pneumonitis (2%). Paresthesias or brachial plexus disorders were rarely seen. Complications such as radiation pericarditis, soft tissue necrosis, or fibrosis of the pectoral muscles occurred even more rarely.

The amount of arm edema is directly related to the extent of axillary surgery, as well as the technique and extent of axillary irradiation (LARSON et al. 1984). The risk of arm edema in patients who did not undergo axillary surgery was 4%, as compared with a risk of 13% for those patients who did have axillary dissection.

Another potential long-term complication of primary radiotherapy is carcinogenesis. In the JCRT series of 525 patients treated between 1968 and 1980, there has been only one case of acute nonlymphocytic leukemia. An increased risk in contralateral breast cancer following primary radiation is also of concern. No significant increase in contralateral breast disease has been seen to date, and it appears unlikely to occur. Similarly, sarcomas of the bones or soft tissue in the treatment fields have also been reported following primary radiotherapy. These, however, have been exceedingly rare (KURTZ et al. 1985; SVENSSON et al. 1981).

12.7 Treatment Selection for Early Breast Cancer

The indications for mastectomy are as follows:

1. Patient preference
2. Diffuse disease
3. Medical contraindications
4. Pregnancy
5. Anticipated poor cosmetic result
6. Quality of radiation therapy

In our institution the most common indication for mastectomy is patient preference. Diffuse disease or nonadjacent primaries in the same breast are also indications for mastectomy, as these patients are poor candidates for breast-conserving treatment. The cosmetic results of multiple wide excisions combined with radiation boosts are likely to be undesirable, and the patients may have other large concentrations of tumor cells within the breast. Similarly, patients whose mammograms reveal extensive microcalcifications are also poor candidates for breast-conserving surgery. As one would expect, the rate of recurrence in these patients is substantially higher, since the radiation dose delivered to the entire breast is less likely to control the large number of residual tumor cells most likely present after excisional biopsy. Scleroderma or certain collagen vascular diseases are also contraindications to breast-conserving surgery, since these predisposing medical conditions often result in more difficult follow-up after radiation therapy. Pregnancy, especially in the first two trimesters, is also a contraindication to breast-conserving surgery and primary radiation therapy. If the diagnosis is made late enough in the pregnancy, perhaps an induction of labor and premature delivery could be undertaken and subsequent primary radiation therapy administered.

One of the most frequent contraindications for breast-conserving surgery is anticipated poor cosmesis. Obviously, this is determined by several factors, such as the size of the primary tumor, the size of the breast, the location of the tumor, and the extent of the surgical margin deemed necessary. For example, in patients who have tumor involvement just behind the nipple–areola complex, the treatment would be resection of the nipple–areola complex and primary radiation therapy. The acceptance of this deforming surgery by the patient is an equally important consideration.

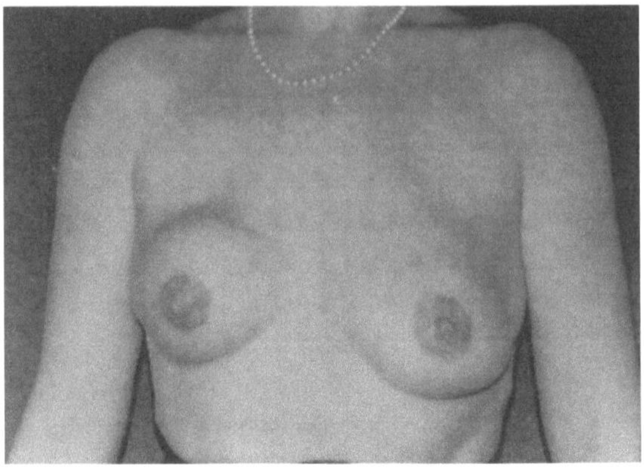

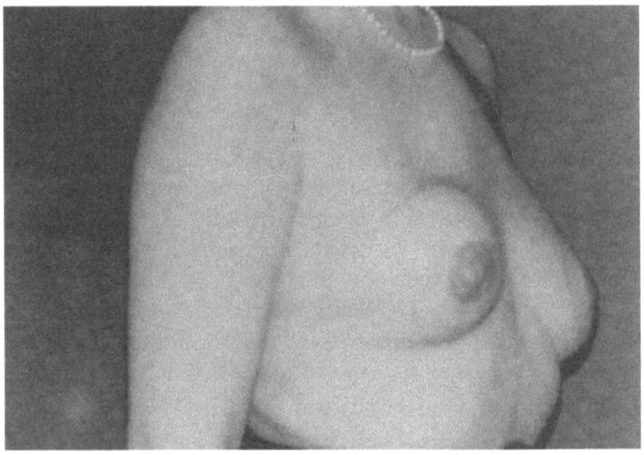

Fig. 12.6. A patient who has undergone sequential mastectomies. The left side was reconstructed with a transverse rectus abdominis musculocutaneous (TRAM) flap, and the right side was reconstructed with a latissimus dorsi musculoadipocutaneous flap (without an implant 6 months later)

Finally, the quality and availability of radiation therapy can also influence a patient's decision to choose mastectomy. While the quality of radiation therapy is steadily improving, patient accessibility to an institution with state-of-the-art equipment and techniques may be relatively limited, thereby making mastectomy a more feasible alternative.

If mastectomy is anticipated, immediate reconstruction is offered in our institution. In our recent series of over 500 mastectomies and reconstructions, a very small risk of complication was found (L.D. Crespo, personal communication). In a series of over 200 prospectively followed patients, we showed that while surgery and length of stay for immediate reconstruction, especially with autologous tissue transfer, is longer, the cosmetic result as judged by the patient is significantly better (SMITH et al. 1992) (Fig. 12.6). Immediate reconstruction is a gratifying experience for the surgeon as it demonstrates the most positive patient support.

12.8 Importance of Mammography

General consensus exists about the importance of mammography in patient selection for primary radiation therapy. Modern film screening mammography is superior to older zero-mammograms and provides critical information in the initial evaluation of patients. Optimally, mammography should be performed prior to biopsy, if possible, in order to avoid overlooking important details such as the extent of soft tissue densities or calcifications obscured by postoperative scarring or hematoma. Similarly, postbiopsy mammograms can also be very important in evaluating other potential contraindications to breast-conserving surgery and is useful in assessing the extent of residual calcifications or other abnormalities prior to definitive conservative surgery. This is particularly important when intraductal disease is present.

12.9 Influencing Factors on the Extent of Breast-Conserving Surgery

Local recurrence in the breast is clearly more frequent among patients who do not have a complete gross excision of the primary tumor. In the JCRT series, the incidence of recurrence in the breast following incisional biopsy was 31%, as compared with 7% in a group of 510 breast patients treated with excision (HARRIS et al. 1985b; RECHT et al. 1984). Higher local failure rates have been in other series of patients treated with radiation therapy alone but without excision of the primary tumor (CALLE et al. 1978, 1983; AMALRIC et al. 1982). Acceptable local control is obtained by substantially increasing the dose of radiation therapy, although cosmetic results are then sacrificed (AMALRIC et al. 1982; PIERQUIN et al. 1980). Tumor size itself has not been shown to be a significant risk factor for local recurrence after excisional biopsy and radiation therapy. In the JCRT series, local recurrence rates were similar for all tumors up to 5 cm in size (RECHT et al. 1985). Similarly, the NSABP B-06 trial reported that the local recurrence rate was 6.5% for T1 tumors and 9.6% for T2 tumors (FISHER et al. 1985).

The amount of breast tissue removed at the time of conservative surgery prior to radiation therapy remains controversial. Some institutions advocate a wide excision; for example, the Institut Curie advocates removal of approximately 2 cm of unaffected breast tissue (CALLE et al. 1978). Wide margins, however, do not appear necessary provided that adequate doses of radiation are given. At the Institut Gustave-Roussy, low boost doses are typically utilized, and the local recurrence rate seen in patients treated with quadrantectomy is 9% and 5% in patients treated with excisional biopsy (CLARKE et al. 1985). Thus, equivalent results can be achieved with either wider excisions and lower doses of radiation therapy, or with smaller gross excisions and higher doses of radiation therapy. This inverse relationship appears to hold for all infiltrating ductal type tumors.

Further controversy exists as to whether patients with microscopically involved margins can be treated with radiation therapy. The JCRT experience as well as that of the Institut Gustave-Roussy suggests that a boost radiation dose of at least 6000 cGy to the primary tumor site can accomplish local control, as long as the patient does not have an extensive intraductal component (EIC).

Investigators at the JCRT have studied the influence of pathologic features such as nuclear grade, size of the primary, clinical axillary status, lymphatic vessel invasion and blood vessel invasion on the subsequent risk of recurrence (SCHNITT et al. 1984; HARRIS et al. 1985a). The only feature shown to have a statistically significant impact on local recurrence rate was the presence of an EIC. An EIC is defined as the combination of prominent intraductal cancer within the infiltrating tumor and any amount of intraductal cancer present in grossly normal adjacent breast tissue. Alternatively, EIC is defined as a predominantly intraductal cancer with foci of invasion. As seen in Fig. 12.7, if an EIC is seen in either T1 or T2 tumors, the risk of local recurrence is significantly higher than in non-EIC tumors of similar size.

As seen in Table 12.1, a detailed study of 584 tumors divided into 1 cm increments showed no increase in local recurrence rates with larger tumor sizes. This was true whether the tumor was estrogen receptor (ER)-positive or ER-negative. However, with every 1 cm increment, a significant increase in local recurrence rates was demonstrated when the tumor had an EIC (EBERLEIN et al. 1990). We then studied the local recurrence rate in relation to the

Table 12.1. Local recurrence rate for each tumor (from Eberlein et al. 1990)

	Tumor size (cm)											
	0–1		1.1–2		2.1–3		3.1–4		4.1–5		Total	
	R/P	%	R/P	%	R/P	%	R/P	%	R/P	%	R/P	%
EIC –	8/70	11	10/155	6	11/124	9	2/49	4	0/20	0	31/418	7
EIC +	14/33	42	7/53	13	11/48	23	11/26	42	1/6	17	44/166	27
Total	22/103	21	17/208	8	22/172	13	13/75	17	1/26	4	75/584	13

R/P, number of recurrences/number of patients; EIC, extensive intraductal component

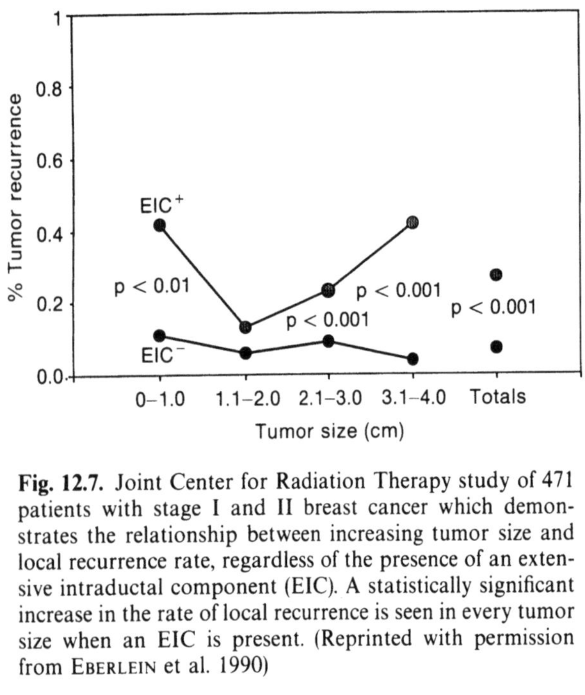

Fig. 12.7. Joint Center for Radiation Therapy study of 471 patients with stage I and II breast cancer which demonstrates the relationship between increasing tumor size and local recurrence rate, regardless of the presence of an extensive intraductal component (EIC). A statistically significant increase in the rate of local recurrence is seen in every tumor size when an EIC is present. (Reprinted with permission from Eberlein et al. 1990)

Table 12.2. Five-year actuarial rate of recurrence of the breast tumor in relation to the extent of breast resection and presence of extensive intraductal component (EIC) (from Vicini et al. 1991)

Tumor size		Extent of breast resection			*p* Value
		Smallest (%)	Intermediate (%)	Largest (%)	
EIC +	T1	29	22	10	0.07
	T2	36	26	9	0.04
EIC –	T1	9	2	0	0.02
	T2	6	2	3	n.s.

extent of breast resection (Vicini et al. 1991). As seen in Table 12.2, in an EIC-negative tumor, the extent of breast resection has much less significance in determining local recurrence rate than in EIC-positive tumors. The association of EIC with a high risk of local recurrence seems to be due to a greater residual tumor burden following simple gross excision. In patients who have undergone re-excision of the primary tumor site, patients with EIC-positive tumor in the initial specimen are more likely to have residual cancer on the re-excision specimen than patients with EIC-negative tumors (Brenner et al. 1985). Thirty-seven percent of patients with an EIC-positive tumor had substantial intraductal cancer in the re-excision as compared with only 7% of patients with EIC-negative tumors. The presence of an EIC did not predict for local recurrence in the Villejuif series, since a quadrantectomy or very wide excision was used (Clarke et al. 1985). Gross excisional biopsy with inked margins, therefore, is recommended for T0 and T1 lesions. If no EIC is seen, radiation therapy is utilized. If an EIC is identified, the patient may choose mastectomy or undergo wider excision with inked margins. If the margins are negative, radiation therapy is administered. If the margins are positive and an extensive amount of intraductal disease is seen in the re-excision, mastectomy is usually recommended (Fig. 12.8). Similarly, incisional biopsy is recommended for T2 lesions, with careful evaluation of the intraductal component (Fig. 12.9). If no EIC is seen, gross excision with inked margins is recommended followed by radiation therapy. If an EIC is present, a wider excision with inked margins is recommended. Again, if the margins are negative, radiation therapy is given; and if the margins are positive with substantial intraductal disease in the wide excision, mastectomy is usually recommended.

12.10 Technical Aspects of Conservative Breast Surgery

Careful evaluation of prebiopsy mammograms is the first step in evaluating a patient for conservative breast surgery. Evaluation of lesions that would

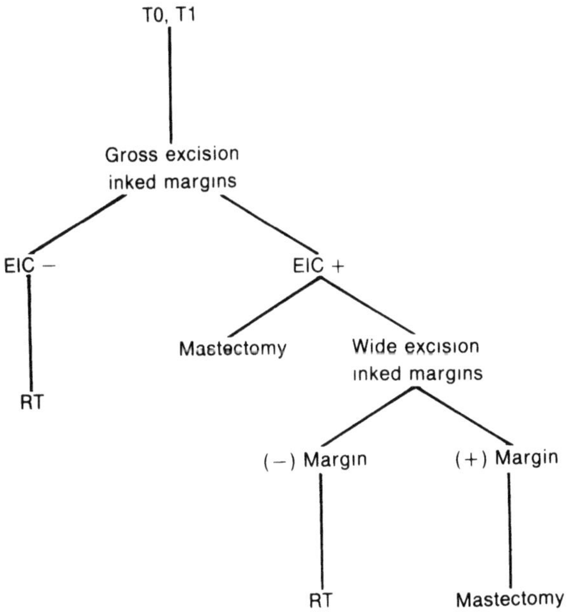

Fig. 12.8. Algorithm for treatment of T0 T1 breast cancer. (*RT*, radiation therapy; *EIC*, extensive intraductal component)

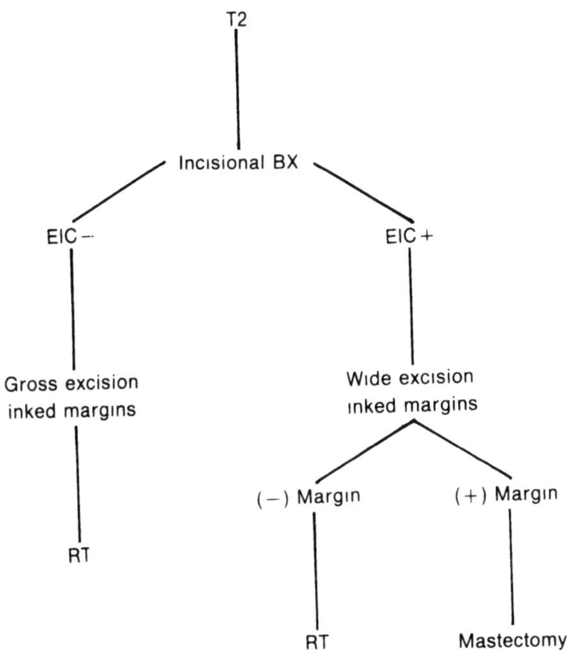

Fig. 12.9. Algorithm for treatment of T2 breast cancer. (*RT*, radiation therapy; *EIC*, extensive intraductal component; *BX*, biopsy)

contraindicate breast-conserving surgery due to their location or the overall extent of their mammographic abnormality is important. Following biopsy, evaluation is important to determine the exact histology of the tumor, the presence or absence of an EIC, and the location of the tumor with

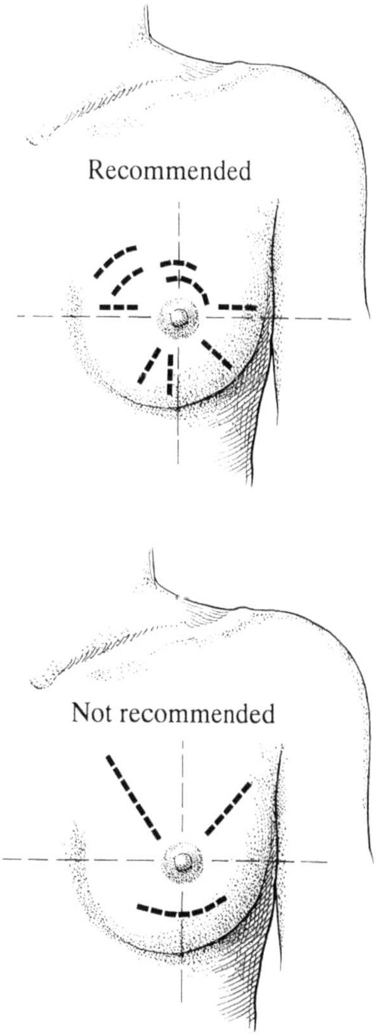

Fig. 12.10. Cosmesis is best maintained using circular incisions in the upper half of the breast with radial incisions in the lower half of the breast

respect to the margins. This information is necessary to plan the re-excision, if indicated. This planning may also be assisted by a postbiopsy mammogram with magnification views to evaluate residual calcifications or other mammographic defects. If necessary, these residual calcifications can be encompassed in the re-excision with a needle-directed approach. Ductal carcinoma in situ often tracks toward the nipple, and caution must be taken to be skeptical of frozen section reports if they are negative, since ductal carcinoma can be easily missed on frozen section.

General principles of breast-conserving surgery include keeping the incision in the lines of Langerhans and as central as possible in the breast (Fig. 12.10). Some surgeons prefer radial incisions inferior to the nipple, but these should generally be avoided superior to the nipple. Obviously, transverse or vertical incisions are to be avoided. In general, limiting the volume of the breast removed is a good policy, unless a wide excision is necessary due to an EIC. Limiting the skin excised will minimize the cosmetic deformity of the breast and will assist in avoiding a misshapen breast. Although important in any surgical procedure, good hemostasis is paramount in breast-conserving surgery. Excellent hemostasis can avoid the use of drains in the breast. Orientation of the excision in a tangential plane in the breast will often assist in the creation of flaps which can be brought together by gravity with a minimal number of sutures. In general, the fewer sutures deep in the breast, the better the cosmetic effect. Finally, separate breast and axillary incisions will avoid unnecessary radiation to a pathologically negative axilla.

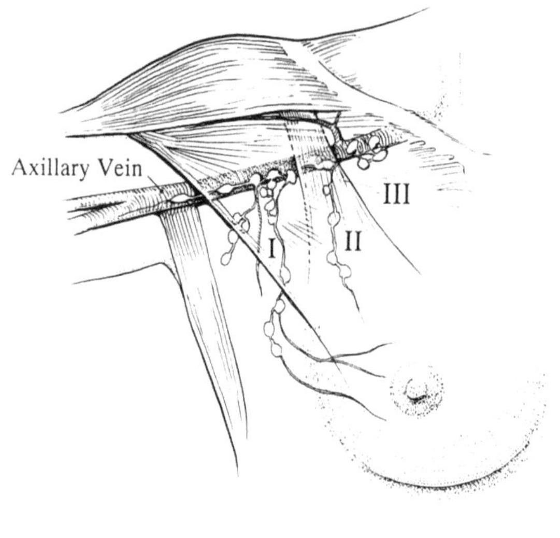

Fig. 12.11. Extent of axillary dissections. Level I sampling involves the nodes around the axillary tail of the breast. Level II removal requires the nodes up to the axillary vein, while Level III includes both the nodes above the axillary and beneath the pectoralis major

12.11 Axillary Lymph Node Dissection

Axillary lymph node dissection has become controversial. With recommendations to treat node-negative patients, some physicians advocate the elimination of axillary lymph node dissections. Thus, questions arise as to how to adequately stage the axilla, identify pathologically positive lymph nodes, and prevent axillary recurrence.

Axillary lymph node dissection serves several functions. Patients with pathologically positive axillary lymph nodes are at a much greater risk for distant relapse and are, therefore, considered for adjuvant systemic therapy of either chemotherapy or hormonal therapy. In patients with clinically suspicious axillary lymph nodes, dissection may be helpful not only to adequately stage the disease but also to remove gross and bulky disease, thereby facilitating radiotherapy with lower doses and less risk. Since axillary lymph node dissections can prevent tumor recurrence in the axilla, this surgery should be extensive enough to detect pathologically positive nodes as well as to provide a high level of local control. Axillary dissection may also minimize the risk of complication or cosmetic deformity.

Several studies have shown that in patients with pathologically negative level I or level II axillary lymph nodes, it is rare to have a pathologically positive level III lymph node (Rosen et al. 1983; Danforth et al. 1986). Level III lymph nodes, which are the apical nodes underneath the pectoralis minor muscle, can substantially add to the morbidity of an axillary dissection (Fig. 12.11). A study from the JCRT reported that as the level of lymph node dissection increases, the number of nodes obtained also increases (Table 12.3). The percentage of pathologically positive nodes does not substantially change, however, nor does the percentage of pathologically positive nodes from a clinically negative axilla change. Therefore, adequate staging of the axilla appears to be achieved with approximately ten nodes from a level II dissection (Rose et al. 1983; Fisher et al. 1981). Other studies have shown that, in the instance of histologically positive nodes, a limited axillary dissection was similar to a complete axillary dissection when more than five nodes were obtained. We therefore recommend a level I–II dissection that includes full visualization of the axillary lymph nodes without stripping the adventitia from the vein. We also advocate not to remove level III lymph nodes, since either stripping the axillary vein or removing the level III nodes can increase the likelihood of arm edema from 6% to 36% when axillary irradiation is given (Larson et al. 1984). When axillary irradiation is utilized without axillary lymph node dissection, the risk of arm edema is approximately 4%. Thus, the combination of axillary dissection and full axillary irradiation results in a significant risk of arm edema. Studies from the JCRT have demonstrated that radiation therapy or axillary lymph node dissection are very effective in preventing axillary lymph node recurrence. Thus, a level I–II

Table 12.3. Relationship of node positivity of type of axillary dissection

	Minimum		Moderate		Maximum	
	n	%	*n*	%	*n*	%
Number of patients	116		185		65	
Number of nodes (median)	6		9		11	
Node positive[a]	45/116	39	64/185	35	20/65	31
Node negative[b]	22/86	26	42/162	26	13/58	22

[a] Pathologically positive
[b] Pathologically negative

dissection provides accurate staging and protection against local recurrence with few complications. A level I lymph node dissection identifies most node-positive patients and coupled with radiation therapy, protects against local recurrence. However, a level I dissection may fail to assess the true extent of disease.

12.12 Conclusion

Randomized prospective trials of treatments for primary breast cancer show that conservative surgery and primary radiation therapy result in equivalent survival when compared with mastectomy. Discussion has been provided regarding patient selection, the criteria employed for electing conservative surgery, as well as the techniques for optimal cosmetic results. Gross excision of primary tumors is adequate when an EIC is not seen; however, when extensive intraductal disease is identified, wide excision is required. This type of tumor is generally associated with a relatively large tumor burden; therefore, if wide local excision reveals extensive disease with positive margins, then mastectomy is usually a better treatment option to prevent local recurrence. Otherwise, the patient is still a good candidate for primary radiation therapy. Finally, a level I–II axillary lymph node dissection, which identifies the axillary vein but does not strip the adventitia, provides adequate staging and prevention of axillary recurrence without significant increase in risk of complication or morbidity.

Future advances in the conservation management of primary breast cancer will identify those patients who are poor candidates for primary radiation therapy and will integrate primary radiation therapy with systemic adjuvant treatment. Further progress in the management of primary breast cancer will also be made through improved imaging techniques such as magnetic resonance imaging, superior identification of pathologic risk factors, and identification of more efficacious systemic therapies.

References

Aberizk WJ, Silver B, Henderson IC et al (1986) The results of radiation therapy for locally recurrent breast carcinoma after mastectomy. Cancer 58: 1214–1218

Amalric R, Santamarie F, Robert F et al (1982) Radiation therapy with or without primary limited surgery for operable breast cancer: a 20-year experience at the Marseilles Cancer Institute. Cancer 49: 30–34

Atkins H, Hayward JL, Klugman DL et al (1972) Treatment of early breast cancer: a report after ten years of clinical trial. BMJ 2: 423–429

Bartelink H, Van Dam F, Van Dongen J (1985) Psychological effects of breast conserving therapy in comparison with radical mastectomy. Int J Radiat Oncol Biol Phys 11: 381–385

Beadle GF, Come S, Henderson IC et al (1984a) The effect of adjuvant chemotherapy on the cosmetic results after primary radiation treatment for early stage breast cancer. Int J Radiat Oncol Biol Phys 10: 2131–2137

Beadle GF, Harris JR, Silver B et al (1984b) Cosmetic results following primary radiation therapy for early breast cancer. Cancer 54: 2911–2918

Beck TM, Hart NE, Woodard DA et al (1983) Local or regionally recurrent carcinoma of the breast: results of therapy in 121 patients. J Clin Oncol 1: 400–405

Bedwinek JM, Fineberg B, Lee J et al (1981) Analysis of failure following local treatment of isolated locoregional recurrence of breast cancer. Int J Radiat Oncol Biol Phys 7: 581–585

Blichert-Toft M, Andersen JA, Andersen KW et al (1988) A Danish randomized trial comparing breast-preserving therapy with mastectomy in mammary carcinoma. Acta Oncol 27: 671–677

Bonadonna G, Valagussa P, Zucali R et al (1983) Feasibility of adjuvant chemotherapy plus radiotherapy in operable breast cancer. In: Harris JR, Hellman S, Silen W (eds) Conservative management of breast cancer. Lippincott, Philadelphia, pp 321–328

Brenner MJ, Schnitt SJ, Connolly JL et al (1985) The use of re-excision in primary radiation therapy for stage I and II breast carcinoma. Int J Radiat Oncol Biol Phys 11(1): 151 (Abstract)

Calle R, Pilleron JP, Schlienger P et al (1978) Conservative management of operable breast cancer: ten years experience at the Foundation Curie. Cancer 42: 2045–2053
Calle R, Vilcoq JR, Pilleron P et al (1983) Conservative treatment of operable breast carcinoma by irradiation with or without limited surgery – ten-year results. In: Harris JR, Hellman S, Silen W (eds) Conservative management of breast cancer. Lippincott, Philadelphia, pp 3–10
Clarke DH, Le MG, Sarrazin D et al (1985) Analysis of locoregional relapses in patients with early breast cancers treated by excision and radiotherapy: Experience of the Institut Gustave-Roussy. Int J Radiat Oncol Biol Phys 11: 137–145
Clarke RM (1983) Alternatives to mastectomy – the Princess Margaret Hospital experience. In: Harris JR, Hellman S, Silen W (eds) Conservative management of breast cancer. Lippincott, Philadelphia, pp 35–46
Danforth DN, Findlay PA, McDonald HD et al (1986) Complete axillary lymph node dissection for stage I–II carcinoma of the breast. J Clin Oncol 4: 655–662
Donegan WL, Perez-Mesa CM, Watson FR (1966) A biostatistical study of locally recurrent breast carcinoma. Surg Gynecol Obstet 122: 529–540
Eberlein TJ, Connolly JL, Schnitt SJ et al (1990) Predictors of local recurrence following conservative breast surgery and radiation therapy: the influence of tumor size. Arch Surg 125: 771–777
Findlay P, Lippman M, Danforth D et al (1985) A randomized trial comparing mastectomy to radiotherapy in the treatment of stage I–II breast cancer: a preliminary report. Proc Am Soc Clin Oncol 4: C-230.
Fisher B, Wolmark N, Bauer M et al (1981) The accuracy of clinical nodal staging and of limited axillary dissection as a determinant of histologic nodal status in carcinoma of the breast. Surg Gynecol Obstet 152: 765–772
Fisher B, Bauer M, Margolese R et al (1985) Five-year results of a randomized clinical trial comparing total mastectomy and segmental mastectomy with or without radiation in the treatment of breast cancer. N Engl J Med 312: 665–673
Haagensen CD (1971) Diseases of the breast, 2nd edn. Saunders, Philadelphia
Harris JR, Recht A, Amalric R et al (1984) Time course and prognosis of local recurrence following primary radiation therapy for early breast cancer. J Clin Oncol 2: 37–41
Harris JR, Connolly JL, Schnitt SJ et al (1985a) The use of pathologic features in selecting the extent of surgical resection necessary for breast cancer patients treated with primary radiation treatment. Ann Surg 201: 164–169
Harris JR, Recht A, Schnitt S et al (1985b) Current status of conservative surgery and radiotherapy as primary local treatment for early carcinoma of the breast. Breast Cancer Res Treat 5: 245–255
Hayward JL (1977) The Guy's trial of treatments of 'early' breast cancer. World Surg 1: 314–216
Hayward JL (1983) The Guy's hospital trials on breast conservation. In Harris JR, Hellman S, Silen W (eds) Conservative management of breast cancer. Lippincott, Philadelphia, pp 77–90
Kurtz JM, Spitalier JM, Amarlic R (1983) Late breast recurrence after lumpectomy and irradiation. Int J Radiat Oncol Biol Phys 9: 1191–1194
Kurtz JM, Amalric R, Delouche G et al (1985) The second ten years: long-term risks of breast conservation. Int J Radiat Oncol Biol Phys 11(1): 184–185 (Abstract)
Larson D, Weinstein M, Goldberg I et al (1984) Arm edema is influenced by the extent of axillary surgery in patients treated with primary radiation therapy. Int J Radiat Oncol Biol Phys 10(2): 78 (Abstract)
Montague ED (1984) Conservative surgery and radiation therapy in the treatment of operable breast cancer. Cancer 53: 700–704
National Institutes of Health Consensus Conference (1991) Treatment of early stage breast cancer. JAMA 265: 391–395
Osborne MP, Ormiston N, Harmer CL et al (1984) Breast conservation in the treatment of early breast cancer. Cancer 53: 349–355
Pierquin B, Owen R, Maylin C et al (1980) Radical radiation therapy of breast cancer. Int J Radiat Oncol Phys 6: 17–24
Recht A, Silver B, Harris JR (1984) The patterns of failure within the treated breast following primary radiation therapy. Int J Radiat Oncol Biol Phys 10(2): 79 (Abstract)
Recht A, Silver B, Schnitt S et al (1985) Breast relapse following primary radiation therapy for early breast cancer. I. Classification, frequency, and salvage. Int J Radiat Oncol Biol Phys 11: 1271–1276
Rose CM, Botnick LE, Goodman RL et al (1983) The role of limited axillary dissection in the treatment of breast cancer by primary irradiation. In Harris JR, Hellman S, Silen W (eds) Conservative management of breast cancer. Lippincott, Philadelphia, pp 155–162
Rosen PP, Lesser ML, Kinne DW et al (1983) Discontinuous or "skip" metastases in breast carcinoma. Ann Surg 197: 276–283
Sarrazin D, Le M, Rouesse J et al (1984) Conservative treatment versus mastectomy in breast cancer tumors with macroscopic diameter of 20 millimeters or less: the experience of the Institut Gustave-Roussy. Cancer 53: 1209–1213
Schain W, Edwards B, Gorrell CR et al (1983) Psychosocial and physical outcomes of primary breast cancer therapy: mastectomy vs excisional biopsy and irradiation. Breast Cancer Res Treat 3: 377–382
Schnitt SJ, Connolly JL, Harris JR et al (1984) Pathologic predictors of early local recurrence in stage I and II breast cancer treated by primary radiation therapy. Cancer 53: 1049–1057
Smith BL, Bertagnolli MM, Klein BB et al (1992) Evaluation of the contralateral breast: the role of biopsy at the time of treatment of primary breast cancer. Ann Surg 216(1): 17–21
Svensson GK, Kase KR, Chin LM et al (1981) Dose to the opposite breast as a result of primary radiation therapy for carcinoma of the breast. Int J Radiat Oncol Biol Phys 7: 1209 (Abstract)
Toonkel LM, Fix I, Jacobson LH et al (1983) The significance of local recurrence of carcinoma of the breast. Int J Radiat Oncol Biol Phys 9: 33–39
Valagussa P, Bonadonna G, Veronesi U (1985) Patterns of relapse and survival following radical mastectomy: analysis of 716 consecutive patients. Cancer 56: 1269–1273
Veronesi U (1985) Randomized trials comparing conservative techniques with conventional surgery: an overview. In: Tobias JS, Peckham MJ (eds) Primary management of breast cancer: alternatives to mastectomy. Edward Arnold, London, pp 131–152
Veronesi U, Saccozzi R, Del Vecchio M et al (1981) Comparing radical mastectomy with quadrantectomy, axillary dissection, and radiotherapy in patients with small cancers of the breast. N Engl J Med 305: 6–11
Vicini FA, Eberlein TJ, Connolly JL et al (1991) The optimal extent of resection for patients with stages I or II breast cancer treated with consecutive surgery and radiotherapy. Ann Surg 214(3): 200–205

13 What Is the Role of Adjuvant Chemotherapy in Postmenopausal Women with Operable Breast Cancer?

JAMES N. INGLE

CONTENTS

13.1	Introduction	129
13.2	Postmenopausal Women with Resected Node-Positive Breast Cancer	129
13.3	The Overview or Meta-analysis of Adjuvant Trials	130
13.3.1	Overview of Tamoxifen in Women Aged 50 Years and Over	130
13.3.2	Overview of Polychemotherapy in Women Aged 50 Years and Over	131
13.4	Clinical Trials of Adjuvant Therapies	134
13.4.1	The Relative Efficacy of Tamoxifen Versus Polychemotherapy in Postmenopausal Women with Positive Nodes	134
13.4.2	Evaluation of Adding Chemotherapy to Tamoxifen	136
13.5	Chemohormonal Therapy: Findings from the Overview	138
13.6	Use of Chemotherapy in Selected Subsets	139
13.6.1	Evaluation in Hormone Receptor-Negative Postmenopausal Women with Positive Nodes	139
13.6.2	Evaluation in Postmenopausal Women with Negative Nodes	140
13.7	Alternative Adjuvant Therapy in Postmenopausal Women: Combination Hormonal Therapy	140
13.8	Conclusions	140
	References	141

13.1 Introduction

The role of adjuvant chemotherapy in postmenopausal women with resected primary breast cancer is still being elucidated. Clinical oncologists have gone through several distinct phases regarding the value of this modality. Strong enthusiasm for its use was ushered in during the mid-1970s, largely due to early results from the first Milan cyclophosphamide, methotrexate, and 5-fluorouracil (CMF) trial that showed a statistically significant advantage in terms of treatment failure for women treated with CMF over control (BONADONNA et al. 1976). When patients were evaluated according to menopausal status, this advantage was found to be present for both premenopausal and postmenopausal women. An accompanying editorial hailed this treatment as a major advance and advocated its use in women who could not participate in a research program (HOLLAND 1976). However, enthusiasm largely dissipated when subsequent updates of the Milan trial revealed a lack of significant advantage for CMF over control in postmenopausal women (BONADONNA et al. 1977, 1978).

In 1980, the National Institutes of Health (NIH) Consensus Development Conference Panel noted that the preliminary nature of information on adjuvant chemotherapy in postmenopausal women precluded a definitive statement as to its role. It was advocated that clinical investigations continue and that they include concurrent controls receiving only surgical treatment (NIH CONSENSUS DEVELOPMENT PANEL 1980). Since this consensus conference, a great deal of work has been accomplished. We are in a phase of renewed interest in adjuvant chemotherapy for postmenopausal women. Information from clinical trials and the recently published overview will be considered.

13.2 Postmenopausal Women with Resected Node-Positive Breast Cancer

Postmenopausal women with axillary nodal metastasis are at substantial risk for disease recurrence following definitive local regional treatment. It was concluded at the NIH Consensus Development Conference in 1985 that tamoxifen was indicated as standard adjuvant treatment in women whose tumors were estrogen receptor (ER) positive (NCI CONSENSUS CONFERENCE 1985). This position was substantially influenced by presentations given by Richard Peto prior to the conference (and subsequently published; EARLY BREAST CANCER

JAMES N. INGLE, M.D., Consultant, Division of Medical Oncology, Mayo Clinic, Betty J. Foust, M.D., and Parents' Professor of Oncology, Mayo Medical School, 200 1st Street SW, Rochester, MN 55905, USA

Trialists' Collaborative Group 1988) on an overview that showed a 20% reduction in annual odds of death produced by tamoxifen. Whereas the 1985 Consensus Development Conference concluded that combination chemotherapy was of established value in premenopausal women with positive nodes, no such value could be established for postmenopausal women.

Tamoxifen is well-established for the management of postmenopausal women with ER-positive tumors. It is relatively nontoxic, easy to administer, and is applicable to the majority of postmenopausal women. In one large experience, the proportion of women with ER-positive tumors increased from slightly more than 60% at age 50, to more than 80% at age 80, and the median ER value increased from about 20 fmol/mg cytosol protein to over 120 fmol, respectively (Jordan et al. 1988). Although questions remain, such as to the optimal duration of therapy and the use in women with ER-negative tumors, tamoxifen has an established efficacy that must be considered when addressing the question of the role of chemotherapy.

13.3 The Overview or Meta-analysis of Adjuvant Trials

Specific clinical trials can be identified that have had a profound impact on clinical practice and future directions of clinical research in treating early breast cancer with adjuvant chemotherapy. However, it is well-known that considering selected individual trials involves problems of selection and publication bias, and many trials do not have sample sizes adequate to identify moderate differences in efficacy between therapeutic approaches. Therefore, along with reviewing individual trials, it is important to look at overviews of trials in which these problems are eliminated.

The Early Breast Cancer Trialists' Collaborative Group (EBCTCG) has published three reports within the past several years on the role of adjuvant therapies in treating early breast cancer (EBCTCG 1988, 1990, 1992). Several pertinent features of the methodology used are of note. Each randomized trial is considered separately and the number of observed (O) events (i.e., recurrence, death) is compared with the number of events expected (E) to occur if the treatment arms were equivalent. Except for random variability, the difference between observed and expected (O − E) should be close to zero if the treatments are equivalent. Following a determination of O − E and a measure of variability (variance, V) for each trial, the overview of multiple trials adds these values to examine the overall effect. Thus, patients from one trial are not added to patients from other trials; rather, the differences of multiple individual trials are considered together in the overview. In addition, the values for O − E and V can be used to estimate the ratio of the annual odds of an event, e.g., disease recurrence or death. For example, an odds ratio of 0.8 comparing a given treatment with control indicates a 20% reduction in the annual odds of the event being considered. In the following discussion of results from the most recent overview (EBCTCG 1992), the reductions are indicated by percent 1 +/− percent 2. Percent 1 is the estimated reduction and percent 2 is the standard deviation.

The most recent overview presents analyses of both direct and indirect randomized comparisons (EBCTCG 1992). In brief, indirect comparisons do not directly compare treatment groups of interest from separate studies. Rather, in an indirect comparison, each treatment is first compared with its own control and then the results of the different trials are compared with each other. The authors of the overview (EBCTCG 1992) clearly state that "the weight that can be given to such indirect randomized comparisons (or, indeed, to extrapolation of any trial results to other circumstances) is a matter of judgement on which opinion may differ substantially, and on which the present report takes no definite stand." A somewhat more critical perspective recently concluded that an overview should be viewed as a valuable objective descriptive technique that can provide qualitative conclusions about broad treatment policies, but whose quantitative results have to be interpreted cautiously (Thompson and Pocock 1991). This cautionary note appears appropriate for reviewing a work of such substantial importance as the overview on early breast cancer (EBCTCG 1992).

With this caution in mind, we will review the 1992 EBCTCG overview – which included 133 randomized trials involving almost 75000 women with data spanning 10 years – to examine the role of chemotherapy in postmenopausal women.

13.3.1 Overview of Tamoxifen in Women Aged 50 Years and Over

Table 13.1 shows the overview data assessing the impact of tamoxifen in women over the age of 50.

Table 13.1. Overall effects of tamoxifen in women aged 50 years or over (from EARLY BREAST CANCER TRIALISTS' COLLABORATIVE GROUP 1992)

	Number randomized	Reduction in average annual odds			
		Disease recurrence or death		Death from any cause	
	n	%	SD	%	SD
All trials					
TAM vs no TAM	21 280	29	(2)	20	(2)
Indirect comparisons					
I. By accompanying treatment					
a. TAM alone vs nothing	13 145	30	(2)	19	(3)
b. TAM + chemo vs same chemo alone	8 135	28	(3)	20	(4)
II. By nodal status[a]					
a. Node-negative	9 473	28	(4)	16	(5)
b. Node-positive	11 807	33	(2)	22	(3)
III. By ER status					
a. ER poor (or < 10 fm/mg)	3 311	16	(5)	16	(6)
b. ER-positive (or > 10 fm/mg)	10 845	36	(3)	23	(4)
c. ER unknown	7 153	26	(3)	17	(4)

TAM, tamoxifen; SD, standard deviation; chemo, chemotherapy; ER, estrogen receptor

[a] Node-negative is defined here as nodes diagnosed negative on sample or dissection. All other women were defined as node-positive.

Substantial and statistically significant reductions are produced in both the annual odds of recurrence (29% ± 2%) and death (20% ± 2%). This benefit for tamoxifen was seen when treatment was considered with tamoxifen alone or when tamoxifen was added to chemotherapy. When examined by nodal status, benefit was seen in both node-negative and node-positive subsets. When examined by ER status, results were highly positive, as expected, in ER-positive patients. It is interesting to note that value was also shown for tamoxifen in the ER-negative subset with reduction in annual odds of recurrence (16% ± 5%; $1p = 0.001$) and death (16% ± 6%).

13.3.2 Overview of Polychemotherapy in Women Aged 50 Years and Over

Tables 13.2 and 13.3 show the overall effects of polychemotherapy from the recent EBCTCG overview (EBCTCG 1992). With respect to annual odds of disease recurrence, it can be seen that in the age groups "50–59, post" and "60–69, any" substantial reductions were identified (29% ± 5% and 20% ± 5%, respectively). Table 13.3 shows graphically that there is a reduction in mortality associated with the use of polychemotherapy, albeit less than in premenopausal women. Considering women at least 50 years of age, the overview found a significant reduction in the annual odds of death (12% ± 4%; $p < 0.002$). The identification of the positive impact of polychemotherapy in women aged 50 years and over was considered evidence of a "quantitative" (i.e., same direction of effect, but different magnitude) rather than "qualitative" (i.e., opposite direction of effect) difference in effect given the relatively greater effect in younger women.

Table 13.4 provides a further breakdown of the chemotherapy data in women of 50 years of age and over. Line IIa shows the impact of prolonged polychemotherapy alone versus no treatment with reductions in risk of recurrence (24% ± 4%) and death (14% ± 5%). These data contrast with the most influential single trial evaluating polychemotherapy from Milan that compared CMF with observation in 197 postmenopausal women. Fourteen-year results demonstrated no significant benefit for chemotherapy in either relapse-free or overall survival, with survival curves essentially superimposable (BONADONNA and VALAGUSSA 1989). Advocates of the overview analysis appropriately point out that trials such as the very influential Milan trial are too small from the standpoint of sample size to detect moderate differences in outcome.

Table 13.2. Recurrence in polychemotherapy trials (adapted from EARLY BREAST CANCER TRIALISTS' COLLABORATIVE GROUP 1992)

Age (years)[a]	Menopausal status[b]	Events/patients		Chemotherapy events[a]		Annual odds of event		
		Chemotherapy group	Control group[b]	O − E	Variance of O − E	Ratio (and confidence limits), chemotherapy:control[c]	Reduction	
							%	SD
< 50	pre	655/1632	758/1506	−134.4	296.2		36	5
< 50	post	46/101	66/124	−8.0	17.6		37	19
50–59	pre	231/438	276/473	−30.2	104.3		25	9
50–59	post	574/1563	691/1565	−88.3	257.3		29	5
60–69	any	685/1876	812/1898	−69.5	309.3		20	5
70 +	any	53/130	54/144	3.7	18.7			
	Total	2244/5740 (39.1%)	2657/5710 (46.5%)	− 326.7	1003.4		28	3

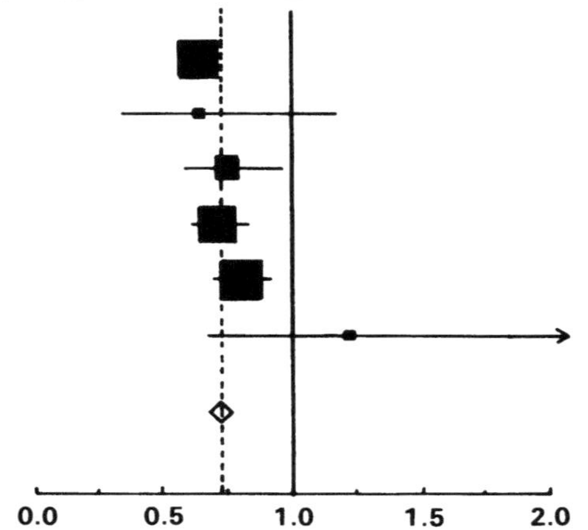

Chemotherapy better Chemotherapy worse
Treatment effect $2p < 0.00001$

O − E, observed minus expected
[a] Test for age trend = 3.4 SD; $2p = 0.0006$
[b] Test for menopausal trend = 0.8 SD; not significant. Premenopausal here includes pre- and perimenopausal patients. Patients of unknown menopausal status were arbitrarily classified as premenopausal if age less than 50 years.
[c] Black squares, 99%. Confidence limits, white triangles, 95% confidence limits

Table 13.3. Mortality in polychemotherapy trials (adapted from EARLY BREAST CANCER TRIALISTS' COLLABORATIVE GROUP 1992)

Age (years)[a]	Menopausal status[b]	Deaths/patients: Chemotherapy group	Deaths/patients: Control group[c]	Chemotherapy deaths: O − E	Chemotherapy deaths: Variance of O − E	Annual odds of death: Ratio (and confidence limits) chemotherapy:control[c]	Reduction %	Reduction SD
< 50	pre	503/1632	562/1506	−70.8	240.7		25	6
< 50	post	41/101	48/124	−2.7	14.7			
50–59	pre	183/438	226/473	−23.2	90.4		23	9
50–59	post	443/1563	476/1565	−29.1	203.3		13	7
60–69	any	516/1876	585/1898	−25.3	241.1		10	6
70 +	any	46/130	46/144	3.8	16.9			
	Total	1732/5740 (30.2%)	1943/5710 (46.5%)	−147.4	807.1		17	3

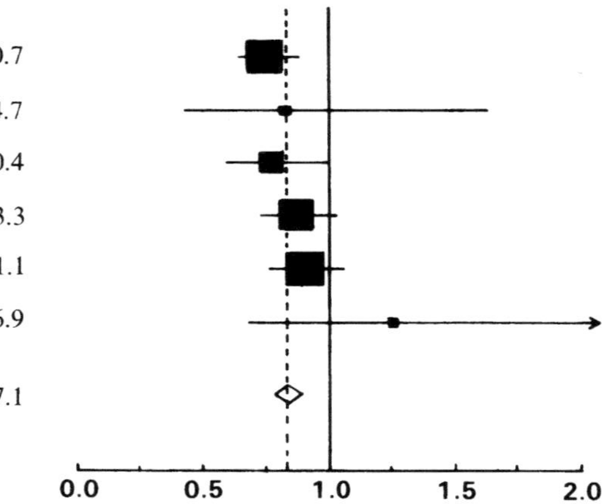

Chemotherapy better   Chemotherapy worse
Treatment effect $2p < 0.00001$

O − E, observed minus
[a] Test for age trend = 2.5 SD; $2p = 0.01$
[b] Test for menopausal, trend = 1.6 SD; not significant. Premenopausal here includes pre- and perimenopausal patients. Patients of unknown menopausal status were arbitrarily classified as premenopausal if age less than 50 years.
[c] Black squares, 99% confidence limits; white triangles, 95% confidence limits.

Table 13.4. Overall effects of chemotherapy in women aged 50 years and over (from EARLY BREAST CANCER TRIALISTS' COLLABORATIVE GROUP 1992)

	Number randomized	Reduction in average annual odds			
		Disease recurrence or death		Death from any cause	
	(n)	%	SD	%	SD
All trials					
Chemo vs No chemo	12 300	17	3	9	3
Indirect Comparisons					
I. Prolonged polychemotherapy vs no chemo	7 666	24	3	13	4
II. Breakdown according to concurrent TAM					
a. Prolonged polychemo vs no adjuvant	3 746	22	4	14	5
b. Prolonged polychemo + TAM vs TAM alone	3 932	26	5	10	7
III. Breakdown according to nodal status[a]					
a. Node-negative	1 361	27	9[b]	23	11[b]
b. Node-positive	6 305	23	4	11	4

TAM, tamoxifen; SD, standard deviation; chemo, chemotherapy

[a] Node-negative is defined here as nodes diagnosed negative by sample or dissection. All other women were defined as node positive.

[b] Considered statistically unstable

13.4 Clinical Trials of Adjuvant Therapies

13.4.1 The Relative Efficacy of Tamoxifen Versus Polychemotherapy in Postmenopausal Women with Positive Nodes

The benefit of polychemotherapy per se appears to be less than that for tamoxifen alone (Table 13.1) (EBCTCG 1992). In this regard, trials that directly compare tamoxifen alone with chemotherapy alone are of particular interest. Table 13.5 outlines major trials that provide this direct comparison. A German trial, the GABG Trial 1, randomized "low risk" patients, defined as having one to three involved axillary nodes and hormone receptor positive cancers, to either tamoxifen alone (30 mg/day for 2 years) or six cycles of CMF (C, 500 mg/m^2; M, 40 mg/m^2; F, 600 mg/m^2; all given intravenously on days 1 and 8 every 4 weeks) (JONAT et al. 1989). They analyzed the results in 157 women aged 50 years and over and found patients treated with tamoxifen did significantly better than those treated with CMF in disease-free survival (DFS) ($p = 0.003$), despite the fact that only about one-quarter of the patients relapsed. Survival data were still very early in that only 6% of the tamoxifen patients and 9% of the CMF patients had died, although a slight but not significant ($p = 0.5$) separation in curves was noted in favor of tamoxifen.

A multicenter trial from Italy (GROCTA) contained three arms, two of which provide data comparing tamoxifen alone with chemotherapy alone (BOCCARDO et al. 1990). The tamoxifen arm was remarkable for the duration of therapy, i.e., 10 mg daily for 5 years, which is consistent with current clinical practice. The chemotherapy employed involved six cycles of CMF (C, 500 mg/m^2; M, 40 mg/m^2; F, 600 mg/m^2; given intravenously every 3 weeks) followed by four courses of epirubicin (75 mg/m^2 intravenously every 3 weeks). Eligibility criteria included axillary node metastasis, examination of ten or more nodes, an ER value of at least 10 fmol/mg protein, and age between 35 and 65 years. An analysis of only postmenopausal women involved 89 patients treated with tamoxifen alone and 84 patients treated with chemotherapy alone. DFS and overall survival were significantly better for patients treated with tamoxifen. However, the survival analysis must be considered early, as only 10 of 89 (11%) of the tamoxifen patients and 22 of 84 (26%) chemotherapy patients had died.

A third trial of substantial importance for considering the relative value of tamoxifen versus chemotherapy is that of the Southwest Oncology Group (SWOG) 7827, which has been published in abstract form only (RIVKIN et al. 1990). This trial involved 894 eligible postmenopausal women with positive nodes known to be ER-positive random-

Table 13.5. Major clinical trials evaluating hormonal and chemotherapy in postmenopausal women with node-positive breast cancer

Trial	Reference	Arms of protocol	Number of patients	Comments	Comparison of arms	Results (*p*-values) DFS	OS
GABG 1	JONAT et al. (1989)	"Low Risk" (1–3 + nodes)					
		1. T (30 mg/day, 2 years)	89	Age ≥ 50 years	1 > 2	0.003	0.5
		2. CMF (6 cycles)	68	Accrual 1981–1988			
GROCTA	BOCCARDO et al. (1990)	1. T (10 mg tid, 5 years)	89	Postmenopausal subset	1 > 2	0.000	0.008
		2. CMF × 6, E × 4	84		1 vs 3	0.42	0.8
		3. Both 1 and 2	94	Median follow-up: 40 months; Accrual 1983–1987	3 > 2	0.000	0.003
SWOG 7827	RIVIKIN et al. (1990)	1. T (10 mg bid, 1 year)	894 eligible	Postmenopausal		5-year survival (%)	
		2. CMFVP (1 year)		Accrual 1979–1989		1. 77	
		3. Both 1 and 2				2. 78	
						3. 73	
Ludwig III	GOLDHIRSCH et al. (1989)	1. Observation	156	Postmenopausal	2 > 1	0.02	0.81
		2. T (20 mg/day) + P (7.5 mg/day) for 12 months	153	Median follow-up: 7 years	3 > 1	< 0.01	0.04
		3. CMFPT (12 months)	154	Accrual 1978–1981	3 > 2	< 0.01	0.08
NSABP B-16	FISHER, et al. (1990a)	1. T (10 mg bid, 5 years)	376	Age ≥ 50 years	2 > 1	0.0004	0.04
		2. AC × 4 (q21 days) + T (5 years)	377	Accrual 1984–1989	3 > 1	0.0002	0.3
		3. PmF × 17 (q6 weeks) + T (5 years)	73		4 > 1	0.07	0.3
		4. PmF × 17 (q6 weeks) + A × 10 (q3 weeks) + T (5 years)	298				
DBCG 82C	MOURIDSEN et al. (1988)	1. RT + T (30 mg/day, 1 year)	457	Postmenopausal		4-year actual survival (%)	
		2. T (30 mg/day, 1 year)	458	Accrual 1982–		1. 71	
		3. CMF× 9 + T (30 mg/day, 1 year)	432	(still accruing at time of report)		2. 68	
						3. 66	
Case Western Reserve	PEARSON et al. (1989)	1. T (20 mg bid, 3 years)	48	Postmenopausal	2 > 1	0.04	0.11
		2. CMFVP (1 year) + T (20 mg bid, 3 years)	46	Median follow-up: 55 months			

T; tamoxifen; C, cyclophosphamide; M, methotrexate, F, 5-fluorouracil; E, epirubicin; V, vincristine; P, prednisone; A, Adriamycin (doxorubicin); Pm, L-phenylalanine mustard; RT, radiation therapy; >, superior to; DFS, disease-free survival; OS, overall survival.

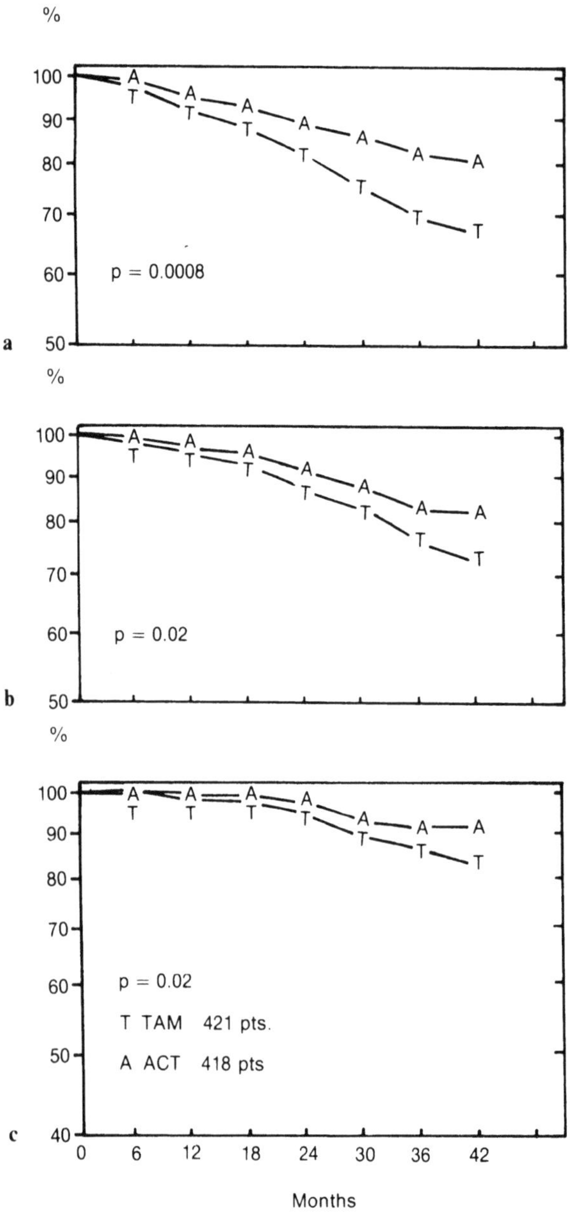

Fig. 13.1. Results from NSABP B-16. (*TAM*, tamoxifen; *ACT*, Adriamycin, cyclophosphamide, tamoxifen; from FISHER et al. 1990c) **a** Disease-free survival of all patients; **b** distant Disease-free survival of all patients; **c** survival of all patients

shown in Fig. 13.1 (FISHER et al. 1990c) reveals a continued statistically significant advantage for AC plus tamoxifen over tamoxifen alone (p values: 0.0008, 0.02, and 0.02, respectively). Concerns relating to this study include the relatively short follow-up of the patients, the inclusion of women with negative ER (15% of tamoxifen-alone patients and 20% of AC plus tamoxifen patients had an ER value of 0–9 fmol) and the inclusion of some premenopausal women due to using age requirement, rather than actual menopausal status. Regarding the last point, this can involve a substantial proportion of patients, as illustrated in an adjuvant trial conducted by the North Central Cancer Treatment Group (NCCTG) in which 19% of the 400 premenopausal women were 50 years of age or older (INGLE et al. 1989).

Arms one and three of the GROCTA Trial (BOCCARDO et al. 1990) (Table 13.5) address the value of adding chemotherapy to tamoxifen. As previously discussed, tamoxifen alone (10 mg 3 times daily for 5 years) was superior to chemotherapy (six cycles of CMF followed by four cycles of epirubicin). In comparing the combined approach using chemotherapy plus tamoxifen versus tamoxifen alone, there was a slight separation in the DFS curves favoring the former; however, this did not achieve statistical significance and there was no difference in overall survival. A concern must be raised regarding the maturity of this trial as only 21 of 89 patients (24%) on the tamoxifen arm experienced an event and only 10 (11%) have died compared with 20 of 94 (21%) and 11 (12%), respectively, on the chemotherapy plus tamoxifen arm. Further maturation of the data is necessary to draw final conclusions.

The Danish Breast Cancer Cooperative Group (DBCG) reported preliminary results of a trial (DBCG 82C) involving postmenopausal women less than 70 years of age; the trial was still open for patient entry when the report was published in 1988 (MOURIDSEN et al. 1988). Patients were eligible if axillary nodes were positive for tumor, if tumor size was greater than 5 cm in diameter, or if the tumor invaded skin or deep fascia. The three arms of the study were radiation therapy (RT) plus tamoxifen (30 mg per day for 1 year), tamoxifen alone, or tamoxifen plus CMF (C, 600 mg/m^2; M, 40 mg/m^2; F, 600 mg/m^2; administered intravenously every 4 weeks) for nine cycles. At 2 years, median time of observation involving 1347 patients, life-table analysis revealed relapse-free survival at 4 years to be 60% for the RT plus tamoxifen group, 49% for the tamoxifen alone group, and 56% for the tamoxifen plus CMF group ($p = 0.03$). The survival rates were 71%, 68%, and 66%, respectively. Further maturation of the completed trial is necessary.

The Case Western Reserve Group reported a small trial involving 94 postmenopausal patients with axillary nodal metastasis and an ER value of at least 3 fmol/mg cytosol protein (PEARSON et al. 1989). Patients were randomized to tamoxifen alone (20 mg twice daily for 3 years) or tamoxifen plus 1 year of CMFVP. At the time of their report, median follow-up was 55 months. Disease recurrence and death had been observed in 42% and 31%, respectively, of 48 patients on tamoxifen alone; and 24% and 15%, respectively, in 46 patients on the chemohormonal regimen. DFS was significantly better with CMFVP plus tamoxifen (log-rank $p = 0.04$, multivariate analysis $p = 0.03$). Overall survival favored CMFVP plus tamoxifen, but did not achieve statistical significance ($p = 0.11$). Concerns regarding this trial include the small sample size and the inclusion of patients with ER values in the range of 3–9 fmol.

Based on the review of these major trials, conflicting findings are evident on the value of adding chemotherapy to tamoxifen in postmenopausal women with ER-positive disease. Several trials indicate an advantage that is not corroborated by others. There does not appear to be adverse interaction between concurrent tamoxifen and chemotherapy. This is consistent with the findings of Brünner et al. that, in contrast to in vitro conditions, the growth-inhibitory effect of tamoxifen on MCF-7 cells grown in vivo (in nude mice) is not mediated through a perturbation of the cell cycle (Brünner et al. 1989).

13.5 Chemohormonal Therapy: Findings from the Overview

Using the information from available major studies, we can review the results of the recent overview on the value of adding chemotherapy to tamoxifen in postmenopausal women (EBCTCG 1992). Table 13.6 presents indirectly estimated effects of combining polychemotherapy with tamoxifen in women aged at least 50 years based on the individual results for tamoxifen and for chemotherapy. Several features of this table are of note. Line IIb indicates a substantial benefit of adding chemotherapy to tamoxifen, at least in terms of reduction in annual odds of recurrence, i.e., 26% ± 5%. All three of the indirect estimations of value of adding chemotherapy and tamoxifen indicate substantially higher benefits than with either alone.

The authors of the overview presented estimates of proportional reduction in annual mortality and absolute reduction in 10-year mortality for tamoxifen alone, polychemotherapy alone, and for the combination in women 50 years of age and older (Table 13.7) (EBCTCG 1992). From this table one would conclude that there is a 50% improvement in efficacy by adding polychemotherapy to tamoxifen, i.e., the proportional reduction in annual mor-

Table 13.6. Indirect estimations of the effects of concurrent prolonged polychemotherapy and about 2 years of tamoxifen in women aged 50 years and over (from Early Breast Cancer Trialists, Collaborative Group 1992)

Type of adjuvant therapy compared	Number aged ≥ 50 years	Typical reduction in annual odds			
		Recurrence or prior death		Death from any cause	
		%	SD	%	SD
I. Effects of adding TAM					
a. TAM alone vs no adjuvant therapy	13 114	30	2	19	3
b. Chemo + TAM vs Chemo alone	8 148	28	3	20	4
c. TAM vs same but without TAM (overview of Ia and Ib)	21 262	29	2	20	2
II. Effects of adding chemo					
a. Chemo alone vs no adjuvant therapy	3 745	22	4	14	5
b. Chemo + TAM vs TAM alone	3 932	26	5	10	7
c. Chemo vs same but without chemo (overview of IIa and IIb)	7 677	23	3	12	4
III. Indirectly estimated effects of chemo + TAM vs no adjuvant therapy					
a. Adding chemo to TAM (IA + IIb)	–	48	4	27	6
b. Adding TAM to chemo (Ib + IIa)	–	44	4	31	5
c. Ignoring any interactions (Ic + IIc)	–	45	3	30	4

TAM, tamoxifen; SD, standard deviation; chemo, polychemotherapy.

ized to one of three arms (Table 13.5). Two of the arms related to tamoxifen or chemotherapy alone; the tamoxifen regimen consisted of 10 mg twice daily for 1 year and the chemotherapy alone arm consisted of CMF plus vincristine and prednisone (CMFVP) for 1 year. The 5-year survivals were 77% and 78%, respectively, and the death hazard ratio (tamoxifen/CMFVP) was 0.98 (95% confidence interval, 0.69–1.39). Thus, even when using a suboptimal duration of tamoxifen, there was no indication that chemotherapy was superior to this agent.

The overview and individual trial data provide a firm basis for considering tamoxifen as the established adjuvant therapy in hormone receptor-positive women with node-positive disease. There is no justification for choosing chemotherapy alone over tamoxifen in such women and the primary question is whether combination chemotherapy added to tamoxifen (chemohormonal therapy) is superior to tamoxifen alone.

13.4.2 Evaluation of Adding Chemotherapy to Tamoxifen

Several important clinical trials exist that directly compare chemotherapy plus tamoxifen with tamoxifen alone. Even though all but one of these trials consisted of three arms, focus will be only on the arms providing direct comparisons of chemohormonal therapy versus tamoxifen.

One of the oldest trials is that of Ludwig III, in which postmenopausal women 65 years of age and younger with axillary nodal metastasis were randomized to observation, tamoxifen 20 mg per day plus prednisone 7.5 mg/day for 12 months, or CMF (C, 100 mg/m^2 orally on days 1–14; M, 40 mg/m^2 and F, 600 mg/m^2 intravenously on days 1 and 8; all given in 28-day cycles) for 12 cycles along with tamoxifen and prednisone as in the endocrine therapy alone arm (Ludwig Breast Cancer Study Group 1984). ER positivity was defined as at least 10 fmol/mg cytosol protein, but receptor results were available for only 49% of the patients. ER-positive and ER-negative patients comprised 34% and 21% of the observation patients, 29% and 20% of the hormonal therapy patients, and 38% and 12% of the chemohormonal patients, respectively. The recent 9-year, median follow-up time results showed DFS rates of 19% for observation, 31% for the hormonal therapy group, and 41% for the chemohormonal group (Goldhirsch et al. 1990, 1991). The chemohormonal approach was significantly superior to the hormonal therapy alone. The overall survival rates were 38%, 41%, and 51%, respectively. Whereas hormonal therapy alone with tamoxifen plus prednisone for 1 year did not produce a significant survival advantage over observation, there was a significant advantage for chemohormonal therapy alone over hormonal therapy alone. When examined by ER status, the advantage for the chemohormonal therapy over hormonal therapy alone was statistically significant only in the ER-negative subsets (Goldhirsch et al. 1991). The short duration of tamoxifen, the inclusion of ER-negative patients, and a substantial proportion of patients (about one-half) without receptor data can be viewed as deficiencies of this trial when considering the value of chemohormonal therapy vis-à-vis tamoxifen in ER-positive women.

Two arms of SWOG 7827 (Rivkin et al. 1990) address the value of adding chemotherapy to tamoxifen. This trial involved postmenopausal women with ER-positive tumors, and arms one and three (Table 13.5) addressed the value of tamoxifen alone for 1 year versus the same tamoxifen plus 1 year of CMFVP. The 5-year survival rates were 77% and 73%, respectively, with a death hazard ratio (tamoxifen/CMFVP plus tamoxifen) of 0.77 (95% confidence interval, 0.55–1.08). Thus, again, even when using the suboptimal duration of tamoxifen, there was no indication that the chemohormonal therapy was superior.

A very important trial addressing the value of adding chemotherapy to tamoxifen is the National Surgical Adjuvant Breast and Bowel Project (NSABP) trial B-16 (Fisher et al. 1990a). This trial involved women of at least 50 years of age with node-positive breast cancer who were considered "responsive to tamoxifen," defined as aged 50–59 years with progesterone receptor values of at least 10 fmol/mg cytosol protein or as aged at least 60 years regardless of receptor status. There were four arms to this trial (Table 13.5), but the two of greatest interest are arms one and two that involve tamoxifen alone at a dose of 10 mg twice daily for 5 years or this same tamoxifen regime plus doxorubicin (Adriamycin, A) and cyclophosphamide (AC; A, 60 mg/m^2 and C, 600 mg/m^2, both intravenously every 3 weeks) for four cycles. Actuarial life-table analyses were utilized to estimate outcome at 3 years. The chemohormonal approach was significantly better than tamoxifen alone in terms of DFS ($p = 0.0004$), distant DFS (p, 2-sided, $= 0.04$), and overall survival ($p = 0.04$). An update of these data

Table 13.7. Proportional and absolute reductions in mortality in women 50 years of age and over (from EARLY BREAST CANCER TRIALISTS' COLLABORATIVE GROUP 1992)

	Proportional reduction in annual mortality		Absolute reduction in 10-year mortality	
	%	SD	%	SD
Polychemotherapy alone[a]	12	4	5	2
Tamoxifen alone[b]	20	2	8	1
Polychemotherapy plus tamoxifen	30	5	12	2

[a] For example, more than 6 months of cyclophosphamide, methotrexate, 5-fluorouracil.
[b] Median of 2 years.

tality increases from 20% to 30% and the absolute reduction in 10-year mortality increases from 8% to 12%. Of substantial concern is that this will be interpreted as proving that chemohormonal therapy is the superior approach. The availability of the overview and the indicated benefit for adding chemotherapy does not obviate the need for determining merit through direct randomized trials. The conflicting findings and the shortcomings of the available studies, as previously discussed, must be kept clearly in mind when considering the findings of the overview. Additional research is needed to evaluate the role of chemotherapy in addition to tamoxifen in postmenopausal women with hormone receptor-positive and node-positive breast cancer. A Breast Intergroup Trial is currently active comparing tamoxifen alone (20 mg/day for 5 years) versus CAF (C, 100 mg/m^2 orally on days 1–14; A, 30 mg/m^2 and F, 500 mg/m^2 both administered intravenously on days 1 and 8 every 28 days) for six cycles along with tamoxifen given either concurrently or sequentially. This trial (INT 0100) is coordinated by SWOG with participation by NCCTG, the Eastern Cooperative Oncology Group (ECOG), and Cancer and Leukemia Group B. There is strong support from a national standpoint to determine the value of adding chemotherapy to tamoxifen in postmenopausal women with ER-positive breast cancer.

13.6 Use of Chemotherapy in Selected Subsets

13.6.1 Evaluation in Hormone Receptor-Negative Postmenopausal Women with Positive Nodes

The NIH Consensus Development Conference concluded in 1985 that "for postmenopausal women with positive nodes and negative hormonal receptor levels, chemotherapy may be considered but cannot be recommended as standard practice" (NCI CONSENSUS CONFERENCE 1985). At present, there are no clinical trials that show a survival advantage for systemic therapy in this setting. Of interest is that a trial of the ECOG demonstrated that adjuvant chemotherapy with CMFP plus tamoxifen provided a relapse-free survival advantage over observation in ER-negative patients ($p < 0.001$, in multivariate analysis), but not in ER-positive patients (TAYLOR et al. 1989). However, the sample size was small in the ER-negative subset, with only 31 patients on CMFP plus tamoxifen and 35 on observation, and there was no survival advantage. The overview suggested some advantage for tamoxifen even in ER-negative women aged at least 50 years (Table 13.1), but the value of tamoxifen alone or combined with chemotherapy in such patients remains to be established.

Although there is a paucity of data in hormone receptor-negative node-positive postmenopausal women, some enthusiasm can be generated for the use of chemotherapy in such patients. Bonadonna et al. point out that there is evidence for a beneficial effect of adjuvant chemotherapy in postmenopausal patients based on several recent reports (BONADONNA et al. 1991). They note that in two recently published trials from Milan (MOLITERNI et al. 1991; BUZZONI et al. 1991) a difference in outcome between premenopausal and postmenopausal women was not observed, which they concluded was probably due to the administration of full dose chemotherapy in the postmenopausal women. Neither of these trials had a no-treatment control arm. A Mayo Clinic/NCCTG trial did have an observation control arm and found a relapse-free survival advantage for both chemotherapy (CFP) alone and combined with tamoxifen (INGLE et al. 1990). However, only 31% of patients in this trial were known to be ER-negative and as yet there is no survival advantage in this subset. Of particular interest with respect to the question of chemotherapy in ER-negative women are data from trials in node-negative women given below.

13.6.2 Evaluation in Postmenopausal Women with Negative Nodes

In June 1990, the NIH held a consensus development conference on early stage breast cancer at which the major trials addressing the value of chemotherapy in node-negative patients were considered. Several trials are particularly noteworthy and have unquestionably influenced clinical practice. The NSABP B-13 trial compared observation with 12 monthly cycles of adjuvant chemotherapy with methotrexate, 5-fluorouracil, and leucovorin in women with resected node-negative breast cancer with an ER value of less than 10 fmol/mg cytosol protein (Fisher et al. 1990b). In patients 50 years of age or older there was an advantage to adjuvant therapy both in terms of DFS ($p = 0.0006$) and overall survival ($p = 0.004$). Further maturation of this trial and publication in full manuscript form will be of great interest.

The ECOG reported a trial in women with node-negative breast cancer considered to be at high risk for recurrence based on an ER-negative status or tumor size of at least 3 cm in diameter (Mansour et al. 1989). Patients were randomized to observation or six cycles of CMFP (C, 100 mg/m^2 orally on days 1–14, M, 40 mg/m^2 on days 1 and 8; F, 600 mg/m^2 on days 1 and 8; P, 40 mg/m^2 orally on days 1–14; planned cycle length was 28 days). With a median follow-up time of 4.5 years and considering all 425 eligible patients, the DFS was significantly better in the treated group than the control (5-year DFS, 83% and 61%, respectively; log-rank, $p < 0.0001$) (Tormey et al. 1990). Analysis according to menopausal status revealed benefit in both premenopausal and postmenopausal subsets. Considering 159 postmenopausal women, 5-year DFS was 79% for the treated group and 60% for the control group ($p = 0.03$). Considering just the 115 postmenopausal women who were ER-negative, 5-year DFS was 80% for the treated group and 67% for the control group, but this difference was not statistically significant ($p = 0.20$). There were only 44 postmenopausal patients who were ER-positive, but there was an advantage for CMFP in terms of DFS ($p = 0.05$) and survival ($p = 0.09$). One must be cautious in multiple subset analyses, particularly with such small numbers.

Table 13.4 displays the findings from the overview evaluating chemotherapy in node-negative women of 50 years of age and older (EBCTG 1992). It can be seen that there was a substantial reduction in odds of disease recurrence or death, but the number of patients analyzed was relatively small and the findings were considered statistically unstable. Data from NSABP B-13 noted above provides compelling evidence for the value of combination chemotherapy in ER-negative node-negative postmenopausal women. In ER-positive, node-negative women, however, the value of adding chemotherapy to tamoxifen needs to be determined.

13.7 Alternative Adjuvant Therapy in Postmenopausal Women: Combination Hormonal Therapy

Research is ongoing which examines another means of improving the efficacy of adjuvant therapy in postmenopausal women with resected ER-positive breast cancer. This involves a study of combination hormonal therapy utilizing tamoxifen plus fluoxymesterone. The basis for interest in this approach comes from a randomized trial in postmenopausal women with metastatic disease in which women were randomized to tamoxifen alone or combined with fluoxymesterone (Ingle et al. 1991). Among women with an ER value of 10 fmol or greater, there was a statistically significant advantage for the combination in terms of response rate and time of disease progression. Of particular note was that in women 65 years of age or older, there was a survival advantage (Cox model, $p = 0.06$) for those treated with tamoxifen plus fluoxymesterone. This regimen is currently being compared with tamoxifen alone in the adjuvant setting in a NCCTG trial in postmenopausal women of any age with negative nodes and women aged 65 years or older with positive nodes. This trial is important because a purely hormonal approach may be more appropriate and acceptable to many postmenopausal women, especially those who are elderly, than one involving chemotherapy.

13.8 Conclusions

Systemic adjuvant therapy with tamoxifen has been established to be of value in postmenopausal women with resected node-positive hormone receptor-positive disease. The value of adding combination chemotherapy to tamoxifen remains to be established despite the findings of the overview and the availability of data suggesting an advantage. An analogous situation exists for women who are node-negative and receptor-positive. In ER-negative women, chemotherapy appears more encouraging in node-negative than node-positive patients, but there is a paucity of data for the latter subgroup. Further work is needed to determine the value of chemotherapy plus tamoxifen adjuvant therapy in postmenopausal hormone receptor-negative women. It is essential that the oncology community be strongly committed to clinical trials directed at resolving these important issues. Although further investigations are needed, it is likely that chemotherapy will be playing a larger role in the future in adjuvant therapy of postmenopausal women with resected breast cancer. The findings of the recent overview were more positive than expected in terms of benefit of adjuvant chemotherapy in postmenopausal women. This should provide a positive stimulus for further research efforts.

References

Boccardo F, Rubagotti A, Bruzzi P et al (1990) Chemotherapy versus tamoxifen versus chemotherapy plus tamoxifen in node-positive, estrogen receptor-positive breast cancer patients: results of a multicentric Italian study. J Clin Oncol 8: 1310–1320

Bonadonna G, Valagussa P (1989) Systemic therapy in resectable breast cancer. Hematol Oncol Clin N Am 3: 727–742

Bonadonna G, Brusamolino E, Valagussa P et al (1976) Combination chemotherapy as an adjuvant treatment in operable breast cancer. N Engl J Med 294: 405–410

Bonadonna G, Rossi A, Valagussa P et al (1977) The CMF program for operable breast cancer with positive axillary nodes. Cancer 39: 2904–2915

Bonadonna G, Valagussa P, Rossi A et al (1978) Are surgical adjuvant trials altering the course of breast cancer? Semin Oncol 5: 450–464

Bonadonna G, Valagussa P, Brambilla C et al (1991) Adjuvant and neoadjuvant treatment of breast cancer with chemotherapy and/or endocrine therapy. Semin Oncol 18: 515–524

Brünner N, Bronzert D, Vindelov LL et al (1989) Effect on growth and cell cycle kinetics of estradiol and tamoxifen on MCF-7 human breast cancer cells grown in vitro and in nude mice. Cancer Res 49: 1515–1520

Buzzoni R, Bonadonna G, Valagussa P et al (1991) Adjuvant chemotherapy with doxorubicin plus cyclophosphamide, methotrexate, and fluorouracil in the treatment of resectable breast cancer with more than three positive axillary nodes. J Clin Oncol 9: 2134–2140

Early Breast Cancer Trialists' Collaborative Group (1988) Effects of adjuvant tamoxifen and of cytoxic therapy on mortality in early breast cancer: an overview of 61 randomized trials among 28 896 women. N Engl J Med 319: 1681–1692

Early Breast Cancer Trialists' Collaborative Group (1990) Treatment of early breast cancer, vol I. Worldwide evidence 1985–1990. A systematic overview of all available randomized trials of adjuvant endocrine and cytotoxic therapy. Oxford University Press, Oxford

Early Breast Cancer Trialists' Collaborative Group (1992) Systemic treatment of early breast cancer by hormonal, cytotoxic or immune therapy: 133 randomized trials involving 31 000 recurrences and 24 000 deaths among 75 000 women. Lancet 339: 1–15, 71–85

Fisher B, Redmond C, Legault-Poisson S et al (1990a) Postoperative chemotherapy and tamoxifen compared with tamoxifen alone in the treatment of positive-node breast cancer patients aged 50 years and older with tumors responsive to tamoxifen: results from the National Surgical Adjuvant Breast and Bowel Project B-16. J Clin Oncol 8: 1005–1018

Fisher B, Redmond C et al (1990b) NSABP B-13: methotrexate + 5-FU in women with estrogen receptor negative, node negative breast cancer. In: Treatment of early stage breast cancer: program and abstracts. NIH Consensus Development Conference, June 18–21, 1990. National Institutes of Health, Bethesda, Maryland, p 63

Fisher B, Redmond C, Brown A (1990c) Reply to letter to editor. J Clin Oncol 8: 1925–1926

Goldhirsch A, Castiglione M, Gelber RD (1990) Adjuvant chemoendocrine therapy in postmenopausal women with breast cancer and axillary-node metastases. Lancet 335: 1099–1100

Goldhirsch A, Gelber RD (1989) Adjuvant Chemo-endocrine therapy or endocrine therapy alone for postmenopausal patients: Ludwig studies III and IV Recent Results Cancer Res 115: 153–162

Goldhirsch A, Gelber RD, Castiglione M et al (1991) Adjuvant therapy of breast cancer. Eur J Cancer 27: 389–399

Holland JF (1976) Major advance in breast-cancer therapy. N Engl J Med 294: 440–441

Ingle JN, Everson LK, Wieand HS et al (1989) Randomized trial to evaluate the addition of tamoxifen to cyclophosphamide, 5-fluorouracil, prednisone adjuvant therapy in premenopausal women with node-positive breast cancer. Cancer 63: 1257–1264

Ingle JN, Krook JE, Schaid DJ et al (1990) Randomized trial in postmenopausal women with node-positive breast cancer: observation versus adjuvant therapy with cyclophosphamide, 5-fluorouracil, prednisone with or without tamoxifen. Results with seven year median follow-up. In: Salmon SE (ed) Adjuvant therapy of cancer VI. Saunders, Philadelphia, pp 216–225

Ingle JN, Twito DI, Schaid DJ et al (1991) Combination hormonal therapy with tamoxifen plus fluoxymesterone versus tamoxifen alone in postmenopausal women with metastatic breast cancer: an updated analysis. Cancer 67: 886–891

Jonat W, Kaufmann M, Abel U (1989) Chemo- or endocrine adjuvant therapy alone or combined in postmenopausal patients (GABG Trial I). Recent Results Cancer Res 115: 163–169

Jordan VC, Wolf MF, Mirecki DM et al (1988) Hormone receptor assays: clinical usefulness in the management of carcinoma of the breast. In: Batsakis J, Savory J (eds) Critical reviews in clinical laboratory sciences, vol 26. CRC Press, Boca Raton, Florida, p 97–152

Ludwig Breast Cancer Study Group (1984) Randomised

trial of chemo-endocrine therapy, endocrine therapy, and mastectomy alone in postmenopausal patients with operable breast cancer and axillary node metastasis. Lancet i: 1256–1260

Mansour EG, Gray R, Shatila AH et al (1989) Efficacy of adjuvant chemotherapy in high-risk node-negative breast cancer: an intergroup study. N Engl J Med 320: 485–490

Moliterni A, Bonadonna G, Valagussa P et al (1991) Cyclophosphamide, methotrexate, and fluorouracil with and without doxorubicin in the adjuvant treatment of resectable breast cancer with one to three positive axillary nodes. J Clin Oncol 9: 1124–1130

Mouridsen HT, Rose C, Overgaard M et al (1988) Adjuvant treatment of postmenopausal patients with high risk primary breast cancer: results from the Danish adjuvant trials DBCG 77C and DBCG 82C. Acta Oncologica 27: 699–705

NCI Consensus Conference (1985) Adjuvant chemotherapy for breast cancer. JAMA 254: 3461–3463

NIH Consensus Development Panel (1980) NIH consensus development statement. Adjuvant chemotherapy of breast cancer. N Engl J Med 303: 831–832

Pearson OH, Hubay CA, Gordon NH et al (1989) Endocrine versus endocrine plus five-drug chemotherapy in postmenopausal women with stage II estrogen receptor-positive breast cancer. Cancer 64: 1819–1823

Rivkin S, Green S, Metch B et al (1990) Adjuvant combination chemotherapy (CMFVP) vs tamoxifen (TAM) vs CMFVP + Tam for postmenopausal women with ER + operable breast cancer and positive axillary lymph nodes: an intergroup study. Proc Am Soc Clin Oncol 9: 24

Taylor IV SG, Knuiman MW, Sleeper LA et al (1989) Six-year results of the Eastern Cooperative Oncology Group trial of observation versus CMFP versus CMFPT in postmenopausal patients with node-positive breast cancer. J Clin Oncol 7: 879–889

Thompson SG, Pocock SJ (1991) Can meta-analyses be trusted? Lancet 338: 1127–1130

Tormey DC, Eudey L, Mansour EG et al (1990) INT-0011: CMFP versus observation in high-risk node negative breast cancer patients. In: Treatment of early stage breast cancer: program and abstracts, NIH Consensus Development Conference, June 18–21, 1990. National Institutes of Health, Bethesda, Maryland, pp 61–62

14 How Should We Treat Ductal Carcinoma In Situ?

Abram Recht

CONTENTS

14.1 Introduction . . . 143
14.2 Epidemiology . . . 143
14.3 Clinical and Radiologic Presentation . . . 144
14.4 Pathologic and Biologic Characteristics of Potential Clinical Significance . . . 144
14.5 Distribution of Tumor in the Breast . . . 146
14.6 Incidence of Occult Invasion . . . 146
14.7 Axillary Node Involvement . . . 147
14.8 Review of the Results of Treatment . . . 147
14.8.1 Mastectomy . . . 147
14.8.2 Conservative Surgery Alone . . . 147
14.8.3 Conservative Surgery and Radiotherapy . . . 149
14.9 Tamoxifen as Adjuvant Therapy and as Prophylactic Therapy Against Developing Contralateral Breast Cancers . . . 150
14.10 Management Recommendations . . . 150
14.10.1 Pretreatment Evaluation . . . 150
14.10.2 Selection of Treatment Options . . . 151
14.10.3 Surgical Techniques . . . 151
14.10.4 Radiotherapy Techniques . . . 152
14.10.5 Follow-Up and Management of Breast Recurrence . . . 152
14.11 Conclusion . . . 152
References . . . 152

14.1 Introduction

The management of patients with ductal carcinoma in situ (DCIS) is among the most controversial topics in the field of breast cancer. In the past, DCIS was an uncommon lesion that usually presented as a palpable mass. With the advent of screening mammography the incidence of DCIS has increased markedly. The success of breast-conserving treatment for invasive carcinomas (National Institutes of Health 1991) has also led to increased interest in avoiding mastectomy in patients with noninvasive cancers. However, the traditional therapy of DCIS has been mastectomy. Therefore, little information is available on the results of treatment with conservative surgery, either alone or in combination with radiotherapy.

This chapter will discuss the epidemiological, clinical, radiological, pathological, and biologic characteristics of DCIS and the results of past treatment efforts. A detailed description of the histopathology of DCIS may be found elsewhere (Schnitt et al. 1988; Schnitt 1991). The special aspects of the pathology and treatment of Paget's disease of the nipple will not be discussed here; see Osteen (1991) for details on that topic. The management of patients with lobular carcinoma in situ (LCIS), which may be increasing in incidence, is also dealt with elsewhere (Fryberg et al. 1987; Kinne 1991; Recht et al. 1989).

14.2 Epidemiology

In the past, DCIS comprised approximately 1%–5% of all breast cancer cases (Rosen et al. 1980; Rosner et al. 1980). However, widespread adoption of screening mammography has made this a far more common diagnosis. In the Breast Cancer Detection Demonstration Project, 31% of cancers detected only by screening mammography were noninvasive (Baker 1982). The relative rate of discovery of in situ breast cancers nearly tripled in the San Francisco–Oakland metropolitan region between the 1974–1982 base period and 1986, constituting 11% of all breast cancer cases (Austin et al. 1989). Among white women in the Detroit area, the incidence of DCIS in 1973–1974 was 1.5 per 100000 women; in 1987–1988, the incidence had increased nearly sixfold to 8.66 per 100000 women (Lemanne et al. 1991).

Very little information has been published concerning the risk factors for the development of DCIS specifically (as opposed to other types of breast cancer). A survey performed by the American College of Surgeons in patients treated before

Abram Recht M. D., Associate Professor; Joint Center for Radiation Therapy, Department of Radiation Oncology Harvard Medical School, 330 Brookline Avenue, Boston, MA 02215, USA

1972 showed that the ratio of noninvasive carcinomas (including LCIS) in white patients compared to black patients was 11.7:1, which was similar to the ratio of 12.3:1 for invasive carcinomas (ROSNER et al. 1980). None of the trials of screening mammography have yet reported data for DCIS separately from other cancers with regards to such important factors as age-specific incidence or relationship to family history, socioeconomic status, and race.

14.3 Clinical and Radiologic Presentation

These lesions present in a variety of ways, such as an incidental finding on a biopsy done for other reasons or as a small nonpalpable focus on a mammogram; they also may present as a palpable but localized mass or as diffuse involvement of one or more quadrants of the breast. Nipple discharge is sometimes the sole finding. Currently most patients with DCIS in Europe and North America present with nonpalpable lesions discovered by mammography.

Clustered microcalcifications are the most common finding on mammograms, but this can also occur in invasive or benign lesions. The comedo histologic subtype tends to produce casting or branched and linear calcifications, whereas noncomedo histologic subtypes produce granular calcifications or masses (BRANDON et al. 1990). Lesions with multiple or mixed histologic subtypes of DCIS tend to have radiologic features of both comedo and noncomedo types.

The relationship between the manner of presentation of the lesion and the risk of recurrence with any particular form of treatment is uncertain. Patients with palpable tumors have been reported to have a higher risk of local failure after treatment with either mastectomy or breast-conserving surgery (with or without radiotherapy) than patients presenting with only mammographic findings (CIATTO et al. 1990). In the few other reports that analyze results according to the method of presentation (e.g., SOLIN et al. 1991), no difference in outcome has been noted.

14.4 Pathologic and Biologic Characteristics of Potential Clinical Significance

Out of several histologic subtypes of DCIS the most common are the comedo, cribiform, solid, papillary, and micropapillary (SCHNITT et al. 1988; SCHNITT 1991). These are readily recognizable, for the most part, although more than one subtype may be found in a single lesion. It may be difficult at times to distinguish DCIS from atypical ductal hyperplasia or DCIS with focal areas of invasion. DCIS may also extend into lobules (and LCIS into extralobular ducts), thus occasionally leading to confusion between the two entities. Some lesions have cytologic features intermediate between DCIS and LCIS; their behavior is not well-described. DCIS and LCIS may coexist, in which case the patient's subsequent course appears similar to when only DCIS is found (KINNE et al. 1989).

These different histologic subtypes may have different likelihoods of progression to invasive disease or of local control with breast-conserving treatment, but at present such differences are poorly understood. Most clinical series do not distinguish between histologic subtypes in reporting outcome. Two studies of patients following biopsy of an unrecognized cribiform or papillary DCIS have shown a substantial rate of progression to invasive disease near the biopsy site (27%–28%), but only after average intervals of 6 years and 9.7 years, respectively (range, 1–24 years) (PAGE et al. 1982; ROSEN et al. 1980). In contrast, in a series of nonpalpable lesions treated with planned wide excision, patients with comedo-type DCIS had a substantially higher recurrence rate than patients with other subtypes (LAGIOS et al. 1989; LAGIOS 1990).

One recent study of 26 patients with comedo-type DCIS has suggested that a significant proportion of such tumors may contain areas of hypoxic tumor cells (MAYR et al. 1991). The average diameter of breast ducts containing DCIS was 349 μm, compared to 90 μm for uninvolved ducts. Necrotic tumor was found in 94% of ducts with diameters greater than 360 μm, compared with in only 34% of ducts with diameters smaller than 360 μm. Since hypoxic cells are generally less sensitive to the effects of radiotherapy than well-oxygenated cells, this finding has potential implications for the extent of surgery required to manage patients with comedo DCIS.

Several investigators have examined the expression of the *neu*, or c-erbB-2, oncogene in these lesions. The first investigation of this oncogene was conducted by workers at the Netherlands Cancer Institute (VAN DE VIJVER et al. 1988a). Their largest reported series showed that overexpression of the *neu* oncogene protein occurred very frequently in comedo DCIS (41 of 53 cases, or 77%), occasionally in invasive ductal carcinoma (14% of 189 specimens), but only rarely in small cell papillary or cribiform types of DCIS (0 of 50 cases) (VAN DE VIJVER et al. 1988b). Others report similar findings regarding a higher level of oncogene activity in noninvasive ductal tumors than in invasive ductal tumors, and a higher level of activity in comedo subtypes than in noncomedo subtypes (ALLRED et al. 1990; BARTKOVA et al. 1990; BENZ et al. 1991; LODATO et al. 1990).

However, the relationship of *neu* oncogene expression to the subsequent behavior of these lesions has not been established. In one series of patients treated with excision alone, the local recurrence rate was 10% (4 of 42 cases) when the cell membrane stained positively for the erbB-2 protein and 7% (3 of 43) when no staining was found (LOCKER et al. 1991). Other groups have not yet reported the clinical outcome of their patients.

The thymidine labelling index, a measure of proliferative activity, is higher for comedo DCIS than for cribiform or papillary DCIS or LCIS (MEYER 1986). A recent report documented a significant correlation between the presences of a high thymidine labelling index, a positive immunohistochemical staining for the erbB-2 protein, a comedo histologic subtype, and a large nuclear size (BARNES et al. 1991). However, in the majority of cases included in these two studies, measurements were performed on areas of DCIS found in conjunction with invasive breast cancer, and hence these findings may not reflect the true situation for cases of DCIS without invasion. In a study of 68 patients without evidence of invasion, tumors with a high S-phase fraction, measured by DNA flow cytometry, were more likely to be positive for erbB-2 and to exhibit a comedo pattern than were tumors with a lower S-phase fraction; however, the differences were not statistically significant (GOLDSCHMIDT et al. 1990).

One study of lesions detected by screening mammography suggested that ploidy may be a useful predictor of recurrence in patients treated with excision alone (COOKE 1988). Five of 15 aneuploid tumors recurred locally, compared to none of the 13 diploid tumors; follow-up was over 5 years. However, the relationship of ploidy to histologic subtype was not reported. A recent study of 84 patients from Trondheim, Norway suggested that patients with noncomedo diploid tumors had a substantially lower risk of recurrence after treatment by mastectomy or local excision (1 of 31 patients, or 3%) than did patients whose tumors were either of comedo type or aneuploid (9 of 38, or 24%) (AASMUNDSTAD and HAUGEN 1990). However, the overall incidence of recurrence among the 59 patients treated with mastectomy was 15%. This incidence is substantially higher than any previously reported mastectomy series (Table 14.1),

Table 14.1. Results of treatment with total mastectomy

Country or institution	Dates	Follows-up (months) Median	Range	Proportion nonpalpable	Distant or Local recurrence		Reference
				(%)	(%)	*n*	
Italy	1968–89	?	?	?	1	3/120	CIATTO et al. (1990)
MSKCC	1949–67	?	?	?	3	6/181	FARROW (1970)
Am Coll Surg	?–1972	?	?	?	8	14/181	BEDWANI et al. (1981) ROSNER et al. (1980)
MSKCC	1960–69	?	?	5	3	3/108	ASHIKARI et al. (1971)
Van Nuys CA	1979–90	?	?	?	1	1/97	SILVERSTEIN et al. (1991a)
MSKCC	1970–76	138	60–209	?	1	1/82	KINNE et al. (1989)
MSKCC	1965–75	?	?–132	42	0	0/74	ASHIKARI et al. (1977)
Oregon	1960–72	Minimum 120		?	9	6/68	SUNSHINE et al. (1985)
MD Anderson	1950–70	?	?	?	2	1/63	WESTBROOK and GALLAGHER (1975)
San Francisco	1972–80	?	?	?	2	1/48	LAGIOS et al. (1982)
BWH, Boston	1960 81	?	?	7	0	0/44	VON RUEDEN and WILSON (1984)
MSKCC	1953–72	?	?–120 +	13	3	1/37	WANEBO et al. (1974)
Virginia	1952–75	?	12–180	12	0	0/30	BROWN et al. (1976)
NSABP B-06	1976–84	?	50–141	?	5	1/28	FISHER et al. (1991)
Linkoping, Sweden	1978–84	77	48–106	79	0	0/28	ARNESSON et al. (1989)

?, no data

thus raising serious questions about the technical adequacy of surgery and/or the pathologic evaluation of specimens. The authors do not state whether patients treated with subcutaneous mastectomy were included in this series, which might be one possible explanation for their results (see Sect. 14.8.1).

Other biologic features of these tumors have been less well-studied. Estrogen and progesterone receptor proteins are known to be present in some cases of DCIS, but correlation with subsequent clinical outcome is unknown. (These assays are often not performed on the smaller lesions.) Chromosomal abnormalities were reported to occur in seven of eight cases of DCIS studied, but the clinical significance of this is again not known (NIELSEN et al. 1989).

Thus, as yet there is too little information to base the management of patients with DCIS on the histology or other biologic properties of the lesion. However, this is an area of intense interest and clinical correlations may be forthcoming in the next several years.

14.5 Distribution of Tumor in the Breast

Factors likely to be important in selecting patients for breast-conserving treatment include the distribution of tumor in the breast in relation to the index lesion, the incidence of true multicentric disease (i.e., tumors of independent origin in other quadrants of the breast), and whether the mammographic findings reflect the full extent of the tumor. Recent studies by Dr. Rolland Holland and his colleagues (Nijmegen, the Netherlands) have shown that the extent of the lesion pathologically is usually closely delineated by the extent of mammographic calcifications for the large-cell (comedo) subtype of DCIS (HOLLAND et al. 1990). Using a painstaking radiologic-pathologic correlation technique in which the distribution of tumor in the breast was carefully mapped, they found that only 8 of 50 cases (16%) had pathologic extension of tumor more than 2 cm beyond the boundaries of the radiologic abnormality. In contrast, the small-cell and well-differentiated subtypes may not produce any calcifications either radiologically or histologically. Even when they do, the pathologic extent of the lesion may be substantially underestimated. A discrepancy of greater than 2 cm in size between the pathologic and radiologic boundaries of the lesion was found in 15 of 32 cases (47%) of these noncomedo histologic subtypes (HOLLAND et al. 1990).

It is unclear whether so-called multicentric foci of tumor identified by past investigators (GUMP et al. 1987; LAGIOS et al. 1989; SCHWARTZ et al. 1980, 1989) were truly independently arising neoplasms or resulted from contiguous spread of tumor through the ducts. In fact, it seem likely that nearly all such cases represented clinically unappreciated spread from a single lesion. Holland found true multicentric disease (unconnected lesions) in only 1 of 82 cases (HOLLAND et al. 1990). In one study, multicentricity was much more frequent when the index lesion was more than 2.5 cm in size (13 of 25 cases, or 52%) than when the index lesion size was less than this (4 of 29 cases, 14%) (LAGIOS et al. 1989). The theoretical likelihood of developing multiple independent tumors in the breast should not depend on the size of the index lesion. Therefore, these results support Holland's conclusions.

Thus, it is rare that two or more independent ipsilateral tumors exist simultaneously in a patient with DCIS. Treatment efforts therefore can concentrate on controlling the index lesion. The extent of the tumor is usually defined accurately by the mammographic findings for comedo-type DCIS, but not for other histologic subtypes. However, the potential implications of these findings for breast-conserving management of patients are as yet unconfirmed by clinical experience.

14.6 Incidence of Occult Invasion

Another important factor to consider in making treatment decisions for patients with DCIS is the incidence of unsuspected invasive carcinoma following adequate excision and pathologic evaluation of the primary tumor. Unfortunately, the incidence of occult invasion in mastectomy specimens, either near the primary tumor or in other parts of the breast, has been examined only rarely in relation to other factors such as tumor size, presentation, or histologic type.

In one series, patients with lesions greater than 2.5 cm in size were more likely to have occult invasion (16 of 55 cases, or 29%) than were patients with smaller tumors (1 of 60 cases, or 2%) (LAGIOS et al. 1989). Of note, all four invasive tumors among the 90 patients with lesions 4.5 cm or smaller were found following inadequate initial excision. In another series, only 1 of 21 cases (5%) of lesions detected only on mammography had occult invasion, compared with 6 of 41 lesions (15%) of those presenting with a mass (FENTIMAN et al. 1986). No occult invasion was found at mastectomy performed for 20 mammographically detected lesions (SCHWARTZ et al. 1989) or for 30 cases of pure DCIS (RINGBERG et al. 1991) in two other series.

Other problems also make these reports difficult to interpret. The completeness of the initial biopsy varied from series to series, which probably affected the likelihood of finding residual invasive cancer at the time of mastectomy. Also, the thoroughness of sampling of the primary tumor and the remainder of the breast differed substantially among different institutions.

In summary, in patients with small lesions that are adequately excised and pathologically examined the risk of occult invasion appears to be very small. Hence, spread of tumor outside the breast by the time of diagnosis is unlikely.

14.7 Axillary Node Involvement

The incidence of axillary node metastases is 0%–1% when no evidence of invasion can be seen on routine light-microscopic examination (ASHIKARI et al. 1971; FENTIMAN et al. 1986; GUMP et al. 1987; KINNE et al. 1989; LAGIOS et al. 1982; SILVERSTEIN et al. 1991c; WESTBROOK and GALLAGHER 1975). Although it seems likely that nodal metastases occurred mainly in the patients with larger palpable tumors, this risk has not been reported in relation to the features of the primary tumor.

14.8 Review of the Results of Treatment

14.8.1 Mastectomy

The results of treating patients with DCIS with mastectomy are summarized in Table 14.1. A number of points regarding these series should be stressed. Most series included fewer than 100 patients, with limited or unstated length of follow-up. Since some lesions may be slow-growing, the ultimate recurrence rates may actually be somewhat higher than reported. For example, in one report DCIS was found on the chest wall of a patient 11 years after mastectomy for papillary DCIS; whether the new lesion was histologically similar to the initial one was not stated (GRAHAM et al. 1991). Patients in these series were also treated predominantly or exclusively before the routine use of mammography, and hence most presented with palpable masses. Locoregional and distant failures occurred in a few percent of patients in many series (range, 0%–14.5%), even in single-institution studies with careful pathologic review to exclude occult invasion. While some metastases may have been due to prior or later contralateral invasive breast carcinomas, clearly not all of them were. None of these series examined the clinicopathologic correlates of outcome in detail. Taken together, these series indicate that mastectomy prevents locoregional or distant failure for nearly, but certainly not all, patients.

The risk of local or distant recurrence would seem likely to be greatest for patients with large palpable lesions, since focal invasion might easily be missed when sampling a large surgical specimen. However, only one series has reported that lesion size may be a possible correlate of failure. In Italy, a collaborative study was performed involving 350 patients from 11 institutions (CIATTO et al. 1990). The average follow-up for the entire group was 66 months (range, 6–252 months). Among the 210 patients treated by mastectomy, three suffered recurrence in the mastectomy scar (two lesions were invasive and one was noninvasive). All three recurrences were among the approximately 50% of evaluable patients (exact number not given) who presented with a palpable mass. One of these patients subsequently died due to her recurrence.

The influence of histologic subtype on recurrence rates is not known. In one series, there was one recurrence among 47 patients with comedocarcinomas, compared to no recurrences among 50 patients with other lesions (SILVERSTEIN et al. 1991a).

One particular surgical procedure, subcutaneous mastectomy, warrants particular mention. This operation is known to leave behind substantial amounts of residual breast tissue, including tissue posterior to the nipple–areola complex (GOLDWYN 1977). One group reported a 9% incidence of local recurrence (3 of 34 cases) within 3 years of treatment of DCIS; one of these recurrences was invasive (ABBES et al. 1988). Therefore, subcutaneous mastectomy should not be used to treat patients with DCIS.

14.8.2 Conservative Surgery Alone

The results of treatment with excision alone (for lesions recognized to be malignant) are summarized in Table 14.2. The length of follow-up and number of patients in these series were limited. Results varied substantially, probably due to differences in surgical technique, completeness of pathologic evaluation of margins, and tumor-related factors that are only partially reported. Two of these studies illustrate the range of possible results with the use of conservative surgery alone, and how these results may depend on clinical and histologic factors.

A study conducted at Children's and Adults' Hospital of San Francisco included 79 patients with mammographically detected tumors less than 2.5 cm in size (median, 0.6 cm) (LAGIOS et al. 1982, 1989; LAGIOS 1990). Margins were carefully assessed by a painstaking pathologic–radiologic correlative technique. With a mean follow-up of 68 months, ten tumors (13%) recurred, most in the vicinity of the excision site (LAGIOS 1990). One-half of the recurrences were invasive. All patients were free of disease following salvage mastectomy or re-excision.

A much higher rate of breast recurrence was reported for a subset of patients entered on the National Surgical Adjuvant Breast and Bowel Project (NSABP) B-06 trial who were later classified as having DCIS (FISHER et al. 1986, 1991). The average pathologic size of these tumors was 2.2 cm, and only one case was nonpalpable. "Negative margins" were also defined by less rigorous methods than in Lagios's study. At average follow-up of 85 months, 43% of patients (9 of 21) recurred locally. All recurrences were near the tumor bed.

As noted earlier, the histologic subtype of DCIS may affect the risk of recurrence after treatment by conservative surgery alone. In Lagios's study, the incidence of local recurrence for patients with comedo DCIS was 23% (7 of 31 cases), 40% (2 of 5 cases) for patients with cribiform or papillary tumors of high nuclear grade with necrosis, and 10% (1 of 10 cases) for cribiform tumors of intermediate nuclear grade. No failures were found among 33 patients with micropapillary or cribiform lesions with low nuclear grade (LAGIOS 1990). However, as noted above, these lesions have different rates of proliferation and hence the time to recurrence also may be different, although this was not so in one study (GRAHAM et al. 1991). Further follow-up of other series will be needed to confirm Lagios's results.

Table 14.2. Results of treatment with excision alone

Country or institution	Dates	Follow-up (months)		Nonpalpable	Breast recurrence		Salvage	Reference
		Median	Range	(%)	(%)	n	n	
Italy	1968–89	?	?	?	6	6/103	4/6	CIATTO et al. (1990)
San Franciso	1975–?	?	?	100	13	10/79	10/10	LAGIOS (1990)
France	1970–81	?	?	?	42	of 74[a]	?	ASSELAIN et al. (1990)
Am Coll surg	?–1972	?	?	?	2	1/46	?	BEDWANI et al. (1981) ROSNER et al. (1980)
Linkoping, Sweden	1978–84	60	25–100	89	13	5/38	?	ARNESSON et al. (1989)
Royal Marsden/ St George's	1969–88	?	24–198	?	38	14/37	13/14	GRAHAM et al. (1991)
Royal Marsden	1972–82	?	?	?	63	22/35	20/22	PRICE et al. (1988)
Vancouver	1974–88	?	3–154	?	13	4/30	?	BAIRD et al. (1990)
MSKCC	1949–67	?	?	?	20	5/25	?	FARROW (1970)
NSABP B-06	1976–84	?	50–141	?	43	5/21	7/9	FISHER et al. (1991)
Milan	1973–82	?	?	?	36	7/19	5/7	SALVADORI 1988
MGH	1944–81	100	78–?	?	29	5/13	1/5	GALLAGHER et al. (1989)

?, no data
[a]Actuarial 10-year rate

The optimum extent of surgical resection for patients treated with excision alone is unclear. In one series, 4 of 38 patients (11%) treated with wide excision suffered local recurrence, compared with 2 of 65 patients (3%) treated with quadrantectomy (CIATTO et al. 1990). In a Swedish study employing a wide sector resection, three of eight patients suffered recurrence locally when the tumor extended to within 5 mm of the histologic resection margin; 2 of 33 patients suffered recurrence when the microscopic margin was greater than 5 mm (ARNESSON et al. 1989). It is of note that they found no relation between the size of the lesion and the risk of recurrence. However, the possible improvement in local tumor control achieved by very wide excision must be balanced against the adverse cosmetic results of more extensive surgery. Deforming surgery, such as quadrantectomy, may not be necessary, particularly if radiotherapy will be used.

Thus, the correlates of local recurrence following treatment with conservative surgery alone are poorly understood. However, acceptably low failure rates have been reported for selected patients by investigators employing careful mammographic evaluation, wide excisions, and painstaking examination of speciman margins histologically. Whether these results will worsen with time is not known.

14.8.3 Conservative Surgery and Radiotherapy

The results of treatment with conservative surgery and radiotherapy are summarized in Table 14.3. In most series the tumors were usually discovered by palpation and were fairly large. Again, patient numbers and follow-up intervals were limited. Crude local recurrence rates ranged from 4% to 18%.

In the past, physicians did not routinely pay careful attention to pre-operative mammographic evaluation and assessing the completeness of resection microscopically. The results of a collaborative study of patients treated by nine institutions illustrate the outcome of such a policy (SOLIN et al. 1991). A total of 259 patients with 261 breast cancers were

Table 14.3. Results of treatment with conservative surgery and radiotherapy

Country of institution	Dates Dates	Follow-up (months) Median	Range	Nonpalpable (%)	Breast recurrence %	*n*	Salvage (*n*)	Reference
Collaborative	1967–85	76	17–194	42	11	28/261	24/28	SOLIN et al. (1991)
Van Nuys CA	1979–90	?	?	?	6	6/98	?	SILVERSTEIN et al. (1991b)
Yale	1974–87	43	24–180	?	7	4/60	4/4	HAFFTY et al. (1990)
MSKCC[a]	1977–88	36	24–156	67	18	10/55	10/10	MCCORMICK et al. (1990)
Institut Curie[a]	1967–83	75	?	24	11	6/54	5/6	ZAFRANI et al. (1986) ZAFRANI (1988)
Penn[a]	1978–85	68	25–126	47	10	5/51	5/5	SOLIN et al. (1990)
France	1970–81	?	?	?	12	of 45	?	ASSELIAN et al. (1990)
Marseille/[a] Basel	1975–83	61	?	?	7	3/44	2/3	KURTZ et al. (1989)
MD Anderson[a]	1955–85	92	12–208	39	7	3/44	1/3	STOTTER et al. (1990)
JCRT-Penn[a]	1976–83	44	14–97	33	10	4/40	4/4	RECHT et al. (1985)
JCRT[a]	1976–85	81	35–115	53	21	8/38	7/8	BORNSTEIN et al. (1990)
Italy	1968–89	?	?	?	5	2/37	?	CIATTO et al. (1990)
Strasbourg	1982–87	37	?	53	6	2/32	2/2	CUTULI et al. (1989)
NSABP B-06	1976–84	?	50–141	?	7	2/27	2/2	FISHER et al. (1991)
Kaiser-LA	1978–85	42	?	95	4	1/25	?	RYOO et al. (1989)
Charlebourg	1956–79	132	?	?	5	1/22	?	DELOUCHE et al. (1987)
Cincinatti[a]	1969–84	Minimum 5 years		?	5	1/20	0/1	KUSKE et al. (1989)

?, no data
[a] Patients from this series included in collaborative study (SOLIN et al. 1991)

treated from 1967 to 1985. The tumor was palpable in 153 cases (58%). Median follow-up was 78 months (range, 11–197 months). There were 28 local failures (11%) with a median time to failure of 50 months (range, 17 to 129 months). The five- and ten-year actuarial local failure rates were 6% and 16%, respectively. Fourteen recurrences (50%) were invasive. Four patients with local failure developed distant metastases, as did two other patients (of whom one had already developed a contralateral invasive cancer). The 10-year cancer-specific survival rate was 97%. It is of note that the time course to recurrence in this series was prolonged. This also has been true of recurrences in patients treated with conservative surgery without radiotherapy (GALLAGHER et al. 1989). Hence, the short-term results of therapy may not fully reflect the long-term outcome.

It is not known what factors may be associated with an increased risk of local failure following treatment with conservative surgery and radiotherapy. In the collaborative study discussed above, no clinical or treatment factor was found to significantly affect the risk of failure (SOLIN et al. 1991). However, these small series have had very limited statistical power to reliably point out what may be clinically significant differences in outcome. One factor that may have accounted for some failures was incomplete resection of the primary tumor in patients with a subareolar primary, especially when nipple discharge was present. Three of the four breast failures in a combined series from the Joint Center for Radiation Therapy (JCRT) and the University of Pennsylvania occurred in such situations; the fourth failure occurred in a patient who had a central lesion but no nipple discharge (RECHT et al. 1985). However, this was not true in a larger study (SOLIN et al. 1991).

Patients with palpable lesions had a higher risk of breast recurrence than patients with nonpalpable lesions after treatment with breast-conserving surgery in one series, but the results were not divided according to whether radiotherapy was given postoperatively or not (CIATTO et al. 1990). Again, this finding has not been confirmed (SOLIN et al. 1991).

The influence of histology on the risk of recurrence is not clear. The 7-year actuarial risk of local failure in one series of patients treated with conservative surgery and radiotherapy for comedo DCIS was 20%, compared with 4% for patients with noncomedo DCIS treated with conservative surgery either with or without radiotherapy (SILVERSTEIN et al. 1991a).

Other investigators have suggested that recurrence rates were higher when tumor involved the resection margins or when the patient had a first-degree relative with breast cancer (MCCORMICK et al. 1991). However, the number of patients in this series was small and therefore the results may have been due to chance. Such findings must be confirmed by other studies before used routinely in the clinic.

These studies show that even though a late local failure may occur after treatment with conservative surgery and radiotherapy, a very high survival rate can be achieved. Improved methods of evaluation, patient selection, and surgery will likely decrease the risk of local failure in patients treated at present and in the future as compared to results achieved in the past.

14.9 Tamoxifen as Adjuvant Therapy and as Prophylactic Therapy Against Developing Contralateral Breast Cancers

The use of tamoxifen decreased the risk of local recurrence in patients with invasive cancers treated with conservative surgery and radiotherapy, at least in one randomized study with short follow-up (FISHER et al. 1989). The use of adjuvant tamoxifen also decreased the incidence of contralateral primary tumors in this and other series. The NSABP and British investigators recently began protocols that randomly assign patients with DCIS to receive tamoxifen or not. However, there is as yet no information on how effective tamoxifen ultimately will be in these roles, nor on the duration of use necessary to achieve a substantial reduction in these risks. Since tamoxifen may cause life-threatening complications (e.g., thrombosis or endometrial carcinoma), we do not recommend its use for patients with noninvasive disease not included in a study.

14.10 Management Recommendations

14.10.1 Pretreatment Evaluation

Careful physical examination should be performed; the presence of Paget's disease or nipple discharge, confirmed by history or examination, should especially be noted. All patients should undergo mammography before biopsy, and after biopsy when feasible in those patients who present with microcalcifications, in order to insure the completeness of resection. Film–screen mammography is generally preferred. Magnification views help delineate the presence and extent of microcalcifications as accurately as possible. Specimen radiography is extremely helpful and should be performed routinely, including for patients who present with a nonpalpable mass without microcalcifications.

Careful evaluation of the tumor specimen is mandatory, especially with regards to the margins of resection (see Chap. 10). When possible, tumor size should be assessed by clinical, radiologic, and pathologic techniques. The edges of the specimen should be inked or otherwise evaluated or marked before the specimen is sectioned. It is critical for the pathologist to note whether and how far tumor extends beyond the edges of any grossly apparent mass, and whether calcifications are associated with the tumor, benign tissue, both, or neither.

14.10.2 Selection of Treatment Options

Selecting the optimal treatment for patients with DCIS is difficult because of the wide spectrum of presentation and the poorly understood natural history of these lesions. Physicians treating patients with breast-conserving therapies must carefully consider and discuss with the patient the possibility of breast failure and salvage rates after this event. The following discussion is intended to serve as a guide. As always, individual circumstances may require modifications, and our limited knowledge of this disease allows for many plausible but different approaches to its management.

Mastectomy is always considered acceptable treatment for patients with DCIS. In addition, breast-conserving treatment in some patients appears to be associated with a substantial risk of local recurrence. This group includes patients who present with a subareolar primary or nipple discharge unless nipple–areola resection is performed. (Paget's disease, when not accompanied by invasion, also falls into this category.) Also, patients with evidence of tumor spread diffusely through one or more quadrants of the breast or with multiple tumors on physical exam, mammography, or pathologic evaluation are not considered good candidates for breast-conserving therapy, as poor results have been seen in such patients with invasive lesions (Kurtz et al. 1990; Leopold et al. 1989).

There are currently insufficient data to define exact limits on the size, histologic subtype, characteristics and size of margins, radiologic appearance, and other features of lesions that characterize patients who are likely to do well after wide excision alone versus those who need further treatment with radiation. A subgroup from the NSABP B-06 trial is currently the only reported group of patients randomly assigned to receive radiotherapy or not following excision with "negative" margins. As noted above, these patients were originally classified as having invasive disease (Fisher et al. 1986, 1991). Patients treated with conservative surgery alone had a breast failure rate of 43% (9 of 21). In contrast, patients who received radiotherapy had a breast failure rate of 7% (2 of 27). However, since most of these tumors were fairly large and palpable, the results may not apply to the majority of patients currently seen with DCIS. A number of trials specifically designed to compare conservative surgery with conservative surgery plus radiotherapy have been recently conducted or are in progress. Much more information should become available when these studies have matured.

In general, patients with 1- to 2-cm tumors or smaller well-localized lesions with wide, clearly negative, histologic margins may be considered for treatment with wide local excision only. Treatment with conservative surgery and radiotherapy is also likely to be very successful in this patient group. If negative margins cannot be obtained but the amount of disease at the margins appears small, then radiotherapy definitely should be used in patients desiring breast conservation.

Patients with lesions larger than 2 cm or palpable tumors (and perhaps some patients with smaller tumors) appear to have a higher likelihood of having residual disease left near the primary tumor site even when margins are histologically "negative". Radiotherapy should be used in these patients unless they are participating in a prospective study designed to test the need for such treatment. Although having histologically negative margins is probably desirable, as is true for invasive lesions (see Chaps. 10, 11), this is probably not necessary in all cases to ensure successful results when radiotherapy is used. Ideally, the correlation between tumor features, extent of margin involvement, and outcome will be closely examined in future series of patients managed with breast-conserving therapies.

14.10.3 Surgical Techniques

The details of breast-conserving surgical techniques were discussed in Chap. 12. Although the exact size of microscopically "adequate" negative margins currently cannot be defined, the aim should be for gross normal tissue margins of 1 cm. In practice, re-excision of the primary site is usually needed to accomplish this after an initial needle-localization biopsy.

Given the very low likelihood of nodal involvement, use of a level I–II axillary dissection probably should be reserved for patients with large lesions (i.e., in the range of 3–5 cm or greater) or where the pathologist finds equivocal evidence of invasion. Otherwise, axillary dissection should be performed only when patients develop clinically suspicious axillary adenopathy following primary therapy or for those who develop an invasive breast recurrence.

14.10.4 Radiotherapy Techniques

At the JCRT, patients selected to receive radiotherapy after excision receive a whole-breast dose of 45–46 Gy in 23–25 fractions over 4.5–5 weeks followed by a boost of 16 Gy in eight fractions with electrons of appropriate energy to treat the tumor bed. Further details of radiotherapy technique are discussed in Chap. 11.

14.10.5 Follow-Up and Management of Breast Recurrence

Follow-up and treatment of recurrences are critical issues for patients treated with conservative surgery. Patients should have a physical examination every 3–4 months for at least the first several years, and then at least every 6 months for an indefinite period. Mammograms should be obtained at least yearly. In those patients who presented with microcalcifications, it would also be reasonable (although of uncertain benefit) to obtain mammograms of the ipsilateral breast every 6 months.

About one-half of breast recurrences are invasive. Mastectomy salvage of breast failures following conservative surgery with or without radiation therapy produces high levels of further relapse-free survival, but the length of follow-up of such patients is still short.

The optimal management of patients who have breast recurrences following conservative treatment is unknown. If the lesion of patients not previously irradiated appears limited and there is no evidence of multicentric disease after careful clinical, radiologic, and pathologic evaluation, then further conservative surgery and radiotherapy can be considered rather than mastectomy. Mastectomy will be the usual treatment of choice for those patients who have received radiotherapy. Adjuvant systemic therapy may be recommended for patients with invasive tumors, using the guidelines employed for patients presenting de novo.

14.11 Conclusion

Limited information suggests that both mastectomy and breast-conserving treatment (combined with surgical salvage when necessary) provide a very high likelihood of preventing death due to breast cancer. However, results from mastectomy have the longest follow-up with cure rates approaching 100%. In order to better select patients for breast-conserving treatment, further research is necessary to identify clinicopathologic factors possibly related to outcome. For patients treated with conservative surgery, radiotherapy appears to reduce the chance of breast recurrence, especially for patients with large or palpable masses. Randomized prospective studies recently or currently being conducted may help determine which patients may be adequately treated with excision alone or with excision plus radiotherapy. Many of these issues will likely be clarified in time for the centennial of Roentgen's discovery of the X-ray.

References

Aasmundstad TA, Haugen OA (1990) DNA ploidy in intraductal breast carcinomas. Eur J Cancer 26: 956–959

Abbes M, Caruso F, Bourgeon Y (1988) Subcutaneous mastectomy: a review of 130 cases. Int Surg 73: 107–111

Allred DC, Clark GM, Molina R et al (1990) Immunocytochemical evaluation of HER-2/neu oncogene expression in different evolutionary stages of breast carcinoma and correlation with clinical-pathological characteristics. Proc Am Soc Clin Oncol 9: 23 (Abstract)

Arnesson L-G, Smeds S, Fagerberg G, Grontoft O (1989) Follow-up of two treatment modalities for ductal carcinoma in situ of the breast. Br J Surg 76: 672–675

Ashikari R, Hadju SI, Robbins GF (1971) Intraductal carcinoma of the breast (1960–1969). Cancer 28: 1182–1187

Ashikari R, Huvos AG, Snyder RE (1977) Prospective study of non-infiltrating carcinoma of the breast. Cancer 39: 435–439

Asselain B, Contesso G, Zafrani B et al (1990) Etude intercentre de 387 cas de carcinomes intracanalaires du sein: premieres conclusions. Bull Cancer (Paris) 77: 643–644 (Abstract)

Austin DF, Reynolds P, Boyd PT et al (1989) Progress in the war against cancer (letter). N Engl J Med 321: 1197–1198
Baird RM, Worth A, Hislop G (1990) Recurrence after lumpectomy for comedo-type intraductal carcinoma of the breast. Am J Surg 159: 479–481
Baker LH (1982) Breast cancer detection demonstration project: five-year summary report. CA 32: 194–225
Barnes DM, Meyer JS, Gonzalez JG et al (1991) Relationship between c-erbB-2 immunoreactivity and thymidine labelling index in breast carcinoma in situ. Breast Cancer Res Treat 18: 11–17
Bartkova J, Barnes DM, Millis RR, Gullick WJ (1990) Immunohistochemical demonstration of c-erbB-2 protein in mammary ductal carcinoma in situ. Hum Pathol 21: 1164–1167
Bedwani R, Vana J, Rosner D et al (1981) Management and survival of female patients with "minimal" breast cancer: as observed in the long-term and short-term surveys of the American College of Surgeons. Cancer 47: 2769–2778
Benz C, Thor A, Edgerton S, He M, Liu E (1991) HER2/neu overexpression and gene amplification in comedo-type in situ breast cancers. Proc Am Soc Clin Oncol 10: 46 (Abstract)
Bornstein BA, Recht A, Connolly JL et al (1991) Results of treating ductal carcinoma in situ of the breast with conservative surgery and radiation therapy. Cancer 67: 7–13
Brandon C, Raju U, Rebner M (1990) Mammographic and pathologic correlation in the appearance of subtypes of ductal carcinoma in situ. Radiology 177 (P): 137 (Abstract)
Brown PW, Silverman J, Owens E et al (1976) Intraductal "noninfiltrating" carcinoma of the breast. Archiv Surg 111: 1063–1067
Ciatto S, Bonardi R, Cataliotti L, Cardona G (1990) Intraductal breast carcinoma: review of a multicenter series of 350 cases. Tumori 76: 552–554
Cooke TG (1988) Prognostic value of cellular DNA content in the management of ductal carcinoma in situ of the female breast. EORTC In Situ Breast Cancer Workshop, Castle Marquete, the Netherlands, November 24–25, 1988
Cutuli BF, Teissier E, Methlin A et al (1989) Conservative treatment of in situ breast carcinoma: preliminary results. Proceedings of the 5th European Conference on Clinical Oncology P-0912 (Abstract)
Delouche G, Bachelot F, Premont M, Kurtz JM (1987) Conservation treatment of early breast cancer: long-term results and complications. Int J Radiat Oncol Biol Phys 13: 29–34
Farrow JH (1970) Current concepts in the detection and treatment of the earliest of the early breast cancers. Cancer 25: 468–477
Fentiman IS, Fagg N, Millis RR, Hayward JL (1986) In situ ductal carcinoma of the breast: implications of disease pattern and treatment. Eur J Surg Oncol 12: 261–266
Fisher B, Constantino J, Redmond C (1989) A randomized clinical trial evaluating tamoxifen in the treatment of patients with node-negative breast cancer who have estrogen-receptor positive tumors. N Engl J Med 320: 479–484
Fisher ER, Sass R, Fisher B (1986) Pathologic findings from the National Surgical Adjuvant Breast Project (Protocol 6). I. Intraductal carcinoma (DCIS). Cancer 57: 197–208
Fisher ER, Leeming RL, Anderson S et al (1991) Conservative management of intraductal carcinoma (DCIS) of the breast. J Surg Oncol 47: 139–147
Frykberg ER, Santiago F, Betsill WL, O'Brien PH (1987) Lobular carcinoma in situ of the breast. Surg Gynecol Obstet 164: 285–301
Gallagher WJ, Koerner FC, Wood WC (1989) Treatment of intraductal carcinoma with limited surgery: long-term follow-up. J Clin Oncol 7: 376–380
Goldschmidt RA, Prindiville S, Merkel DE et al (1990) Comparison of HER-2 expression, histology, and flow cytometry in ductal carcinoma-in-situ. Breast Cancer Res Treat 16: 191 (Abstract)
Goldwyn RM (1977) Subcutaneous mastectomy. N Engl J Med 297: 503–505
Graham MD, Lakhani S, Gazet J-C (1991) Breast conserving surgery in the management of in situ breast carcinoma. Eur J Surg Oncol 17: 258–264
Gump FE, Jicha DL, Ozello L (1987) Ductal carcinoma in situ (DCIS): a revised concept. Surgery 102: 790-795
Haffty BG, Peschel RE, Papadopoulos D, Pathare P (1990) Radiation therapy for ductal carcinoma in situ of the breast. Conn Med 54: 482–484
Holland R, Henricks JHCL, Verbeek ALM et al (1990) Extent, distribution, and mammographic/histological correlations of breast ductal carcinoma in situ. Lancet 335: 519–522
Kinne DW (1991) Clinical management of lobular carcinoma in situ. In: Harris JR, Hellman S, Henderson IC, Kinne DW (eds) Breast diseases, 2nd edn. Lippincott, Philadelphia, pp 239–244
Kinne DW, Petrek JA, Osborne MP et al (1989) Breast carcinoma in situ. Arch Surg 124: 33–36
Kurtz JM, Jacquemier J, Amalric R et al (1990) Breast-conserving therapy for macroscopically multiple cancers. Ann Surg 212: 38–44
Kuske R, Compaan P, Cross M et al (1989) Breast conservation therapy: 417 breast cancers with a minimum follow-up period of five years. Int J Radiat Oncol Biol Phys 17 [Suppl 1]: 235–236 (Abstract)
Lagios MD (1990) Duct carcinoma in situ: pathology and treatment. Surg Clin N Amer 70: 853–871
Lagios MD, Westdahl PR, Margolin FR, Rose MR (1982) Duct carcinoma in situ: relationship of occult invasion, multicentricity, lymph node metastases, and short-term treatment failures. Cancer 50: 1309–1314
Lagios MD, Margolin FR, Westdahl PR, Rose MR (1989) Mammographically detected duct carcinoma in situ: frequency of local recurrence following tylectomy and prognostic effect of nuclear grade on local recurrence. Cancer 63: 618–624
Lemanne D, Simon M, Martino S, Swanson M (1991) Breast carcinoma in situ (CIS): greater rise in ductal carcinoma in situ (DCIS) vs lobular carcinoma in situ (LCIS). Proc Am Soc Clin Oncol 10: 45 (Abstract)
Leopold KA, Recht A, Schnitt SJ et al (1989) Results of conservative surgery and radiation therapy for multiple synchronous cancers of one breast. Int J Radiat Oncol Biol Phys 16: 11–16
Locker AP, Ellis IO, Bell J et al (1991) Erb B2 expression in ductal carcinoma-in-situ (DCIS) of the breast. Eur J Surg Oncol 17: 106–107 (Abstract)
Lodato RF, Maguire HC, Greene MI et al (1990) Immunohistochemical evaluation of c-erbB-2 oncogene expression in ductal carcinoma in situ and atypical ductal hyperplasia of the breast. Mod Pathol 3: 449–454
Mayr NA, Staples JJ, Robinson RA et al (1991) Morphometric studies in intraductal breast carcinoma using computerized image analysis. Cancer 67: 2805–2812
McCormick B, Rossen PP, Kinne D et al (1991) Duct carcinoma in situ of the breast: an analysis of local control after conservative surgery and radiotherapy. Int J Radiat Oncol Biol Phys 21: 289–292

Meyer JS (1986) Cell kinetics of histologic varients of in situ breast carcinoma. Breast Cancer Res Treat 7: 171–180

National Institutes of Health Consensus Conference (1991) Treatment of early-stage breast cancer. JAMA 265: 391–395

Nielsen KV, Blichert-Toft M, Andersen J (1989) Chromosome analysis of in situ breast cancer. Acta Oncol 28: 919–922

Osteen RT (1991) Paget disease of the nipple. In: Harris JR, Hellman S, Henderson IC, Kinne DW (eds) Breast diseases, 2nd edn. Lippincott, Philadelphia, pp 797–804

Page DL, Dupont WD, Rogers LW, Landenberger M (1982) Intraductal carcinoma of the breast: follow-up after biopsy only. Cancer 46: 919–925

Price P, Sinnett HD, Gusterson B et al (1990) Ductal carcinoma in situ: predictors of local recurrence and progression in patients treated by surgery alone. Br J Cancer 61: 869–872

Recht A, Danoff BS, Solin LJ et al (1985) Intraductal carcinoma of the breast: results of treatment with excisional biopsy and irradiation. J Clin Oncol 3: 1339–1343

Recht A, Connolly JL, Schnitt SJ, Harris JR (1989) Therapy of in-situ cancer. Hematol/Oncol Clin N Am 3(4): 691–708

Ringberg A, Palmer B, Linell F et al (1991) Bilateral and multifocal breast carcinoma: a clinical and autopsy study with special emphasis on carcinoma in situ. Eur J Surg Oncol 17: 20–29

Rosen PP, Braun DW, Kinne DE (1980) The clinical significance of pre-invasive breast carcinoma. Cancer 46: 919–925

Rosner D, Bedwani RN, Vana J et al (1980) Noninvasive breast carcinoma: results of a national survey by the American College of Surgeons. Ann Surg 192: 139–147

Ryoo MC, Kagan AR, Wollin M et al (1989) Prognostic factors for recurrence and cosmesis in 393 patients after radiation therapy for early mammary carcinoma. Radiology 172: 555–559

Salvadori B (1988) Ductal carcinoma in situ: retrospective analysis of 50 cases, including 19 cases treated with breast conservation. EORTC In Situ Breast Cancer Workshop. Castle Marquete, the Netherlands, November 24–25, 1988

Schnitt SJ (1991) Pathology of in situ carcinoma. In: Harris JR, Hellman S, Henderson IC, Kinne DW (eds) Breast diseases, 2nd edn. Lippincott, Philadelphia, pp 229–232

Schnitt SJ, Silen W, Sadowsky NL et al (1988) Current concepts: ductal carcinoma in situ (intraductal carcinoma) of the breast. N Engl J Med 318: 898–903

Schwartz GF, Patchefsky AS, Feig SA et al (1980) Clinically occult breast cancer: muticentricity and implications for treatment. Ann Surg 191: 8–12

Schwartz GF, Patchefsky AS, Finklestein SD et al (1989) Nonpalpable in situ ductal carcinoma of the breast: predictors of multicentricity and microinvasion and implications for treatment. Arch Surg 124: 29–32

Silverstein MJ, Waisman JR, Gamagami P et al (1991a) Duct carcinoma in situ (DCIS): 224 consecutive cases without microinvasion. Proc Am Soc Clin Oncol 10: 53 (Abstract)

Silverstein MJ, Waisman JR, Gierson ED et al (1991b) Radiation therapy for intraductal carcinoma: is it an equal alternative? Arch Surg 126: 424–428

Silverstein MJ, Gierson ED, Colburn WJ et al (1991c) Axillary lymphadenectomy for intraductal carcinoma of the breast. Surg Gynecol Obstet 172: 211–214

Solin LJ, Fowble BL, Schultz DJ et al (1990) Definitive irradiation for intraductal carcinoma of the breast. Int J Radiat Oncol Biol Phys 19: 843–850

Solin LJ, Recht A, Fourquet A et al (1991) Ten-year results of breast-conserving surgery and definitive irradiation for intraductal carcinoma of the breast. Cancer 68: 2337–2344

Stotter AT, McNeese M, Oswald MJ et al (1990) The role of limited surgery with irradiation in primary treatment of ductal in situ breast cancer. Int J Radiat Oncol Biol Phys 18: 283–287

Sunshine JA, Moseley HS, Fletcher WS, Krippaehne WW (1985) Breast carcinoma in situ: a retrospective review of 112 cases with a minimum 10-year follow-up. Am J Surg 150: 44–51

Van de Vijver MJ, Peterse JL, Mooi WJ et al (1988a) Neu-protein overexpression in breast cancer: association with comedo-type ductal carcinoma in situ and limited prognostic value in stage II breast cancer. N Engl J Med 319: 1239–1245

Van de Vijver MJ, Peterse JL, Mooi WJ et al (1988b) Neu protein overexpression and neu gene amplification in comedo type ductal carcinoma in situ. EORTC In Situ Breast Cancer Workshop, Castle Marquete, the Netherlands, November 24–25, 1988

Von Rueden DG, Wilson RE (1984) Intraductal carcinoma of the breast. Surg Obstet Gynecol 158: 105–111

Wanebo HJ, Huvos AG, Urban JA (1974) Treatment of minimal breast cancer. Cancer 33: 349–357

Westbrook KC, Gallagher HS (1975) Intraductal carcinoma of the breast: a comparative study. Am J Surg 130: 667–670

Zafrani B (1988) Conservative management of intraductal breast carcinoma with tumorectomy and radiation therapy: updated results. EORTC In Situ Breast Cancer Workshop, Castle Marquete, the Netherlands, November 24–25, 1988

Zafrani B, Fourquet A, Vilcoq JR et al (1986) Conservative management of intraductal breast carcinoma with tumorectomy and radiation therapy. Cancer 57: 1299–1301

15 How Successful Is Breast Reconstruction?

ROBERT M. GOLDWYN

CONTENTS

15.1 Introduction 155
15.2 Controversies Associated with Breast Reconstruction 155
15.2.1 Does Breast Reconstruction Hide or Promote Recurrence or Metastasis? 155
15.2.2 Who Should Have Breast Reconstruction? . . 156
15.2.3 Should the Reconstruction Be Immediate or Delayed? 156
15.2.4 What Type of Reconstruction? 157
15.2.5 Can a Silicone Gel Implant Cause Cancer or Immunologically Related Disease? 157
15.2.6 Should the Reconstruction Be Done with a Flap? 158
15.2.7 What to Do About the Opposite Breast? . . . 159
15.2.8 Should One Reconstruct the Nipple and Areola; If So, How? 159
15.3 Conclusion 159
References 160

15.1 Introduction

Twenty years ago the controversy over breast reconstruction was not whether or not it was successful, but whether it should be done at all. The reluctance two decades ago to consider doing breast reconstruction was due to fear that breast reconstruction of any sort would either hide or promote recurrence. Another reason, seldom discussed and rarely mentioned, was the attitude that the patient should be thankful to be alive and should not put herself at hazard by undergoing unnecessary surgery motivated by vanity – a sentiment patently punitive and sexist.

With the advent of better breast reconstruction techniques and the availability of morc plastic surgeons capable of performing these procedures, breast reconstruction is now a common procedure (GOLDWYN 1987, 1991). Women are also more at ease with undergoing breast reconstruction because they feel there is more empathy and support, especially from the increased number of female physicians and surgeons who treat them and by the growing number of women who have undergone the operation. Increased media coverage has also helped women become better informed about breast reconstruction, and the feminist movement has helped them feel justified about requesting a treatment for a condition that causes them anguish. No longer do women believe that they should bear the deformity of mastectomy in shame or in silence (BERGER and BOSTWICK 1984; JAMISON et al. 1978; LEVINSON 1984).

A decade ago, the majority of patients who came for a consultation regarding breast reconstruction did so on their own, without referral and generally without support from the surgeon performing the mastectomy. The problem for the plastic surgeon and the patient was how to circumvent the surgeon without disrupting his or her relationship with the patient. Today many, although not all, surgeons who have advised mastectomy also recommend breast reconstruction to their patients either as an immediate or as a delayed procedure. In fact, there are patients now who inquire about breast rebuilding more in response to their surgeon's insistence than in response to their own desire. Some of these women are indeed relieved when told that reconstruction is totally elective and they do not have to undergo it.

Breast reconstruction today is facilitated by the silicone prosthesis whose development represents a great advance over past implants, such as those made of polyurethane in the 1940s.

15.2 Controversies Associated with Breast Reconstruction

15.2.1 Does Breast Reconstruction Hide or Promote Recurrence or Metastasis?

Accumulated evidence has thus far not shown that breast reconstruction is responsible for cancer recurrence or for its spread, nor that it interferes with

ROBERT M. GOLDWYN, M.D., Head, Division of Plastic Surgery, Beth Israel Hospital, Clinical Professor of Surgery, Harvard Medical School, 330 Brookline Avenue, Boston, MA 02215, USA detection (Watts et al. 1980). A small percentage of patients will have local recurrence (Crowe et al. 1991) and some will have systemic manifestations after a modified radical mastectomy. Recurrence depends upon many factors, including size of primary tumor, its biologic nature (degree of aggressiveness), and status of the axillary node. Thus far, no study has been published on women who have died of causes other than breast cancer after undergoing breast reconstruction and who have been autopsied with serial sections of their breast and chest to determine local recurrence that may be present microscopically, even if not evident clinically. Moreover, breast reconstruction is associated with almost no mortality and minimum morbidity (Matheson and Drever 1990). Until data accumulate to show that breast reconstruction is deleterious to patient survival, breast reconstruction will be done because patients request it and surgeons performing the mastectomy now favor it.

15.2.2 Who Should Have Breast Reconstruction?

Almost any woman wanting breast reconstruction after mastectomy can have it unless severe systemic disease such as serious lung or cardiovascular conditions, preclude it because of a high unacceptable risk. Theoretically, therefore, any woman having a mastectomy, regardless of the staging of her cancer, can be reconstructed if she desires it and the plastic surgeon approves. Reasonable chance of cure is not a precondition to breast reconstruction. In fact, plastic surgeons believe, as do patients, that if the prognosis is poor and the woman has only a few months to live, her remaining days may have a better quality if she undergoes breast reconstruction. One of my patients who had metastatic breast cancer undertook the reconstruction because she wanted "to die a woman." The availability of breast reconstruction, however, does not necessitate its use. Individualization of treatment applies to this area of medicine as it does to all others.

15.2.3 Should the Reconstruction Be Immediate or Delayed?

Initially many plastic surgeons opposed immediate reconstruction because they thought that patients who did not experience the deformity of mastectomy would not appreciate the reconstructive effort; the fear was that patients would deem the reconstruction poor. (In retrospect, many of the early reconstructions were poor.) Plastic surgeons thought it likely that patients would be ungrateful, hypercritical, and angry because of the deficiencies of the reconstructed breast. This gloomy prediction has not proven true; patients very much appreciate their immediate reconstructions since it lessens the trauma of their mastectomy (Dean et al. 1983). Many patients have said that they want to "wake up with a breast" and that they would "not go through a mastectomy" if they had to wait for a reconstruction. The reconstructed breast is an immediate restitution of the lost breast, and patients seem to suffer less depression associated with the mutilation that mastectomy represents to them when they undergo immediate breast reconstruction. Also, the operation is less difficult if the reconstruction is done immediately, since defects caused by reconstructive surgeons are minimized.

In addition to the psychological advantages of immediate reconstruction, the patient is spared an additional operation, an additional anesthesia, further hospitalization, and another separation from her family. In my experience, the patient undergoing immediate reconstruction after mastectomy is in the hospital about 2 days longer than if she had only a mastectomy. Depending upon the type of reconstruction, operating time is prolonged by 1 h with an expander or an implant, or by 3 h with transposition of a musculocutaneous flap from the back (latissimus dorsi) or from the abdomen (rectus abdominis); the operation takes 5–8 h if either the musculocutaneous flap from the back or the abdomen – or other flaps, such as a superior or inferior gluteal flap – is transplanted and attached by microsurgical anastomosis of its vessels to the recipient site.

Another reason plastic surgeons, like most surgeons, were initially reluctant to perform an immediate reconstruction was because they preferred to reconstruct the breast after the wound from the mastectomy healed. They feared that an open wound, especially with bleeding and with a foreign body such as an implant, would lead to an unacceptably high rate of infection resulting in the extrusion of the implant. From a technical viewpoint, having a healed wound when one is performing a delayed reconstruction offers the advantage of more skin since closure over time will stretch the skin; whereas in doing an immediate reconstruction, part of the musculocutaneous flap must be used to close the defect with less available tissue left for reconstruction of the breast itself. However, little difference exists between the complications encountered in immediate reconstruction and those seen with delayed reconstruction, unless the patient has had previous irradiation with atrophy and decreased vascularity of the skin associated with it. A woman who has had cancer recurrence following partial mastectomy and irradiation, along with perhaps chemotherapy, is the most difficult candidate for reconstruction. Not only has irradiation negatively affected her tissues, but the extent of surgical resection will be greater. The first objective in these instances is to cover the wound, which usually can be achieved along with reconstruction of the breast. If the patient is a smoker, the incidence of flap necrosis and subsequent infection is even greater because of the ischemic effect of the long-term use of nicotine.

15.2.4 What Type of Reconstruction?

Deciding upon the type of reconstruction has prompted the most controversy. In general, the following factors affect rebuilding a new breast: type of mastectomy (e.g., is the pectoral muscle intact?), whether the mastectomy is immediate or delayed, whether the patient had irradiation, the size, shape and oncologic status of the opposite breast, the extent of the defect and the nature and amount of available skin, the general health of the patient (e.g., smoking history, pulmonary and cardiovascular disease, obesity), and the preferences of the patient and plastic surgeon regarding the reconstruction.

In some patients the simple insertion of an implant may be all that is necessary if the skin is ample and if the opposite breast is small. The presence of an implant, however, may lead to abnormal firmness as a result of spherical, capsular contracture. Expansion techniques have evolved to decrease the incidence of capsular contracture (Bayet et al. 1991). Serial expansion of the skin definitely lessens capsular contracture and produces a more pleasing breast. The patient must be committed, however, to returning every week or so to have the expander filled with 100–300 cm^3 saline, the amount depending upon the nature of the skin and how quickly and painlessly it can be expanded. The usual objective is to achieve a volume two to three times the eventual size of the breast when the expander is replaced by a permanent prosthesis. Expanders have a higher rate of complications, such as infection and implant loss resulting from skin breakdown, in patients who have had previous irradiation. In addition, leakage and mechanical failure can occur (Pira and Olbrisch 1991).

To further decrease capsular contracture the textured implant was developed. Its rough surface may be made either of silicone or of polyurethane, which has been under recent close inspection by the Federal Drug Administration because of the findings in animals, not humans, that some of its degradation products may cause cancer. This has not been seen with the silicone textured implant, which is made of silicone outside and silicone gel inside. The polyurethane implant of today is a coating of polyurethane over a silicone implant and is not to be confused with the implants made of a different form of polyurethane a half century ago. The Federal Drug Agency has recently ordered all polyurethane implants off the market.

To avoid the expander and the necessity of replacing it with a permanent silicone gel or saline filled implant, one may now choose the so-called "permanent expander" which, after being overfilled, can be deflated to the desired volume and left in place (Berrino and Santi 1991). This implant is being employed more because it avoids another procedure and it contains only saline and not silicone, which many patients prefer because of misleading reports in the media of the dangers of silicone. Herein lies another controversy discussed in the following section.

15.2.5 Can a Silicone Gel Implant Cause Cancer or Immunologically Related Disease?

Other than a few reported anecdotal cases, no causal relationship as has yet been demonstrated in humans between the presence of a silicone implant and the subsequent development of autoimmune disease, such as scleroderma, rheumatoid arthritis, and lupus erythematosus. Silicone itself is supposedly not an adjuvant, and by itself has not been shown thus far to induce adjuvant disease. Although silicone can induce granulomas, these are not synonymous with autoimmune disease.

However, due to the controversy over silicone gel implants, the Food and Drug Administration (FDA) requested a moratorium on 6 January 1992 on the further use of all silicone gel implants until its advisory panel of outside experts (which in November 1991 had recommended not withdrawing the silicone gel implants) could consider new information on the safety of these devices. According to the FDA Medical Alert (MDA 92-1), the focus of the panel is to address the question of autoimmune disorders and the implications for the future availability of the implants. The FDA recommended that, during the moratorium, surgeons abandon silicone gel breast implants and use saline-filled implants (which nevertheless have a silicone envelope), without mentioning that saline implants can deflate – a fact that led the manufacturers to previously concentrate their efforts on the silicone gel prosthesis. The FDA did not state that women with silicone gel implants should have them removed. The recommendation was that any women having symptoms that "may be related" to implants should have periodic evaluations for "problems such as rupture", which mammography and ultrasound can detect with high accuracy and reliability.

The American Society for Plastic and Reconstructive Surgeons has asked the FDA to make public the new data that prompted its decision for a moratorium. Most practicing plastic surgeons who have used silicone gel implants for breast augmentation and breast reconstruction have not had patients whose connective tissue disease could be ascribed to silicone.

In view of the controversy surrounding the silicone gel implant, a reasonable alternative would seem to be the use of only saline-filled implants, especially because they are associated with a lower rate of capsular contracture. They do have the problem, however, of deflation. Patients must understand that their implant may deflate for various reasons: trauma, valve malfunction, ingrowth of tissue into the valve, underfilling, damage from surgical instruments, close capsulotomies (external pressure put on the patient's breast in an attempt to restrict the scar and lessen capsular contraction), and shearing forces that are accentuated when the implant has been underfilled. While it is true that the implant can be replaced if leakage occurs, the patient and surgeon will certainly be inconvenienced and the patient will have the additional problem of paying for a second procedure as well as for a new implant.

The enormous variety of implants available of varying shapes and of differing material attests to the uncertainty and the unpredictability of results. The type of implant, if any, that will be used for breast reconstruction must await further investigation.

15.2.6 Should the Reconstruction Be Done with a Flap?

The principal reason for using a flap for breast reconstruction is that it is not a foreign body and it provides added tissue; therefore, it may serve as a new breast, as a supplement to an implant or to a breast that has been partially removed, or as a covering of a defect in patients who have had recurrent breast cancer after partial mastectomy and irradiation. In patients with recurrence after radiation therapy, the flap functions primarily to cover the defect that cannot be easily resurfaced by a skin graft because of the poor vascularity of the base. The flap, which brings good tissue and its own blood supply, can resurface the wound.

The type of flap used is determined by the size of the opposite breast, the preferences of the patient and plastic surgeon, and the experience of the surgeon. The two musculocutaneous flaps most commonly used are the latissimus dorsi and the rectus abdominis. The latissimus dorsi flap has little morbidity except for about a 5% decrease in shoulder function (retroversion) for which patients readily compensate (Tschopp 1991). Some may complain of stiffness in their shoulder or tightness in their back, but these symptoms generally subside after a year or sooner. Since the latissimus dorsi flap can furnish only a moderate volume, an implant is usually added. The major disadvantage that may result is capsular contracture. To decrease the incidence of capsular contracture and abnormal firmness and to increase the volume of the latissimus dorsi flap, expansion can be used either prior to transferring the flap or afterwards, before a permanent silicone implant is placed.

The rectus abdominis musculocutaneous flap can furnish a larger volume of tissue than the latissimus dorsi flap and may eliminate the need for an implant, thereby also eliminating capsular contracture and abnormal firmness. Both the latissimus dorsi and rectus abdominis flaps can be transposed on their vascular pedicles or transplanted by microsurgical techniques to recipient vessels (so-called free flap). Other free flaps are the superior gluteal or the less often used inferior gluteal flap. Because these flaps come from the buttocks, the donor site scar is well-hidden, especially with the superior gluteal flap. A specific drawback of the rectus abdominis musculocutaneous flap is that it may produce abdominal weakness or a hernia. This is more likely to happen (with an incidence of about 3%–15%, varying with the reported series) if the flap is transposed and not transplanted (free flap). Under the latter circumstance less muscle and fascia have to be taken, thereby facilitating tight closure of the abdomen.

15.2.7 What to Do About the Opposite Breast?

A woman who has had cancer in one breast has a higher risk of developing cancer in the opposite breast than a woman who has never had breast cancer. If the patient has precancerous changes, as evidenced by biopsy or mammography, she may be a candidate for a prophylactic mastectomy. Subcutaneous mastectomy for this purpose was once popular but is less so now because cancer may later arise from the nipple and areola, which are generally spared in a subcutaneous mastectomy. Therefore, a "simple" or "total" mastectomy is the alternative. It should be pointed out, however, that even a modified radical mastectomy does not remove *all* breast tissue and neither will a "simple" or "total" mastectomy (Temple et al. 1991). Nevertheless, women develop breast cancer less frequently after a total or simple mastectomy done for prophylactic reasons or for precancerous disease than after a subcutaneous mastectomy.

In patients who have had a bilateral mastectomy, reconstruction of both breasts by means of flaps is more cumbersome and less desirable than reconstruction by expanders with subsequent implants. In some patients who are very large breasted, even a rectus abdominis flap, which may have been expanded and to which a prosthesis has been added, may fail to achieve the desired size. A breast reduction of the opposite breast may be an easier alternative.

15.2.8 Should One Reconstruct the Nipple and Areola; If So, How?

It is the patient's decision whether or not to reconstruct the nipple and areola. Some do not choose to do so because they wish to avoid another procedure, even one that is relatively minimal. Some of these patients may prefer a stick-on artificial nipple–areola.

When the nipple is reconstructed, it is usually done from the patient's own tissues – from her chest or from the flap that was used to reconstruct the breast. Controversy exists about whether to simulate the areola by grafting the skin or by a tattoo. The latter is becoming more popular because it can be done easily in the office and avoids morbidity and scarring of a donor site. Tattooing also can be used to give the appearance of a nipple, but it fails to provide the nipple with projection. When the new breast has a nipple, the psychological benefits to the patient are significant (Wellisch et al. 1987). The nipple–areola, in one patient's words, "makes the breast a real breast."

15.3 Conclusion

The current controversy over breast reconstruction focuses on questions regarding the best way to achieve successful reconstruction. There is no controversy over the positive psychological value breast reconstruction has for the patient and her family as well as for her intimates (Schain et al. 1984, 1985; Stevens 1987; Wellisch 1978). Women after reconstruction experience an improvement in self-image, confidence, and psychological wellbeing, enabling them to function better socially, sexually, and professionally (Schain et al. 1984, 1985; Stevens 1987; Teimourian and Adhan 1982). Sometimes these benefits are disproportionate to the objective result of reconstruction (Goin and Goin 1987). No matter how good the reconstructed breast appears, it remains an imitation. It also lacks erotic sensation (Lehmann et al. 1991). Yet, reconstructed breasts bring reassurance and may enhance physical intimacy for women who choose this procedure. Despite its obvious imperfections, a reconstructed breast does more to rehabilitate the patient than does an external prosthesis with all its inconveniences. There are no fears with the reconstructed breast that it will slip, nor does it need to be removed at night and put on again in the morning. The reconstruction soon becomes internalized.

In most studies, women who have had a breast reconstruction overwhelmingly report it as successful and as meeting their expectations (Filiberti et al. 1989; Gildoa et al. 1990), even though "successful" is by no means synonymous with "optimal" or "excellent." A minority of patients, however, experience complications and unfavorable results and therefore consider reconstruction unsuccessful.

These patients remain an important, albeit distressing, segment of the reconstructive surgeon's practice. Since techniques for breast reconstruction continue to evolve, better methods will undoubtedly be available in the future that will be successful for an increasing number of patients. Governmental decisions about implants and insurance coverage also will influence the type of reconstruction patients have and surgeons recommend.

References

Bayet B, Mathieu G, Lavand'Homme P, Vanwijck RC (1991) Primary and secondary breast reconstruction with a permanent expander. Eur J Plast Surg 14: 73–79

Berger KJ, Bostwick J III (1984) A woman's decision: breast care, treatment, and reconstruction. Mosby, St. Louis, pp 90–291

Berrino P, Santi PL (1991) The permanent expandable implant in breast aesthetic, corrective and reconstructive surgery. Eur J Plast Surg 14: 63–68

Crowe JP, Jr., Gordon NA, Antonez MD et al (1991) Local-regional breast cancer recurrence following mastectomy. Arch Surg 126: 429–432

Dean C, Chetty U, Forrest APU (1983) Effects of immediate breast reconstruction on psychosocial morbidity after mastectomy. Lancet i: 459–462

Filiberti A, Rimoldi A, Tamburini MC et al (1989) Breast reconstruction: a psychological survey. Eur J Plast Surg 12: 214–219

Gildoa D, Borenstein A, Floro S et al (1990) Emotional and psychosocial adjustment of women to breast reconstruction and detection of subgroups at risk for psychological morbidity. Ann Plast Surg 25: 397–401

Goin JM, Goin MK (1987) Psychological understanding and management of the plastic surgical patient. In: Geogiad NC (ed) Essentials of plastic, maxillofacial, and reconstructive surgery. Williams and Wilkins, Baltimore, pp 1127–1143

Goldwyn RM (1987) Breast reconstruction after mastectomy. N Engl J Med 317: 1711–1714

Goldwyn RM (1991) The patient and the plastic surgeon. 2nd edn. Little Brown, Boston, pp 190–207

Jamison KR, Wellisch DK, Pasnau RO (1978) Psychological aspects of mastectomy: I. The woman's perspective. Am J Psych 135: 432–436

Lehmann C, Gumener R, Montandon D (1991) Sensibility and cutaneous reinnervation after breast reconstruction with musculocutaneous flaps. Ann Plast Surg 26: 325–327

Levinson J (1984) Breast reconstruction: a patient's view. Plast Reconstr Surg 73: 703

Matheson G, Drever JM (1990) Psychological preparation of the patient for breast reconstruction. Ann Plast Surg 24: 238–247

Pira L, Olbrisch RR (1991) Complications in more than 250 uses or expanders in breast reconstruction. Eur J Plast Surg 14: 15–16

Schain WS, Jacobs E, Wellisch DK (1984) Psychosocial issues in breast reconstruction: intrapsychosocial, interpersonal, and practical concerns. Clin Plast Surg 11: 237–256

Schain WS, Wellisch DK, Pasnau RO, Landsverk J (1985) The sooner the better: a study of psychological factors in women undergoing immediate versus delayed breast reconstruction. Am J Psych 142: 40–46

Stevens LA (1987) The psychological aspects of breast surgery. In: Blacher RS (ed) The psychological experience of surgery. Wiley, New York, pp 87–98

Teimourian B, Adhan MN (1982) Survey of patients' responses to breast, reconstruction. Ann Plast Surg 9: 321–325

Temple WJ, Lindsay RL, Magi E, Urganski SL (1991) Technical considerations for prophylactic mastectomy in patients at high risk for breast cancer. Am J Surg 161: 413–415

Tschopp HC (1991) Evaluation of long-term results in breast reconstruction using the latissimus dorsi flap. Ann Plast Surg 26: 328–340

Watts GT, Caruso F, Waterhouse A (1980) Mastectomy with primary reconstruction. Lancet ii: 967

Wellisch DK, Jamison KR, Pasnau RO (1978) Psychosocial aspects of mastectomy: II. The man's perspective. Am J Psych 135: 543–546

Wellisch DK, Shain WS, Noone RB, Little JW III (1987) The psychological contribution of nipple addition in breast reconstruction. Plast Reconstr Surg 80: 699–704

Subject Index

Adriamycin (see chemotherapy, doxorubicin)
Amenorrhoea, chemotherapy induced
- age and 35–38, 42, 49
- negative results from 38–39
- positive results from 35–38
American College of Surgeons, survey on invasive carcinomas 14
American Joint Committee on Cander (AJCC) 49
American Society for Plastic and Reconstructive Surgeons 158
Australian and New Zealand Breast Cancer Trials Group 47
Autoimmune disease 157
Axillary dissection
- benefits of 111–112, 126–127
- complications from 32–33, 111
- distant metastases and 12, 13
- edema 32–33, 111
- future of 51–52
- lumpectomy and 31
- mastectomy and 7, 12, 13, 20, 59, 62, 118, 126–127
- morbidity from 29, 33
- pathologic assessment of axillary status 29–30, 33, 111, 126–127
- pectoral node biopsy 29–30
- prophylactic 29, 30
- recommendations for 27, 126–127, 152
- sampling 29–30
- staging and 28
Axillary lymph nodes
- adenopathy 111, 152
- anatomy of 29, 58
- chemotherapy and 8, 23, 118, 120
-- recurrence and 31–32, 45–46
- chest wall recurrence and 59, 61, 68
- ductal carcinoma in situ 27, 28, 32, 33
- false-negative rate 29, 30
- histologically positive 1–3, 13, 19–22, 61, 64, 65, 69, 126
- internal mammary nodes and 19–20, 59
- JCRT studies 30, 31, 111, 126
- Level I–III 29, 111, 112, 152
- metastases 28, 44
- mortality rates and 16
- negative
-- survival rates and 28
- NSABP studies 29, 30, 31, 44
- occult involvement 13, 44, 45, 62
- prognostic factor status 14, 27–28, 33, 111
- radiotherapy and 20, 22, 30–32, 61–70, 84, 111–113, 126
- recurrence and 20, 30–31, 45–46, 58, 59, 68, 111, 126–127
- removal of 12, 13, 27
- staging 27, 28
- tumor involvement and 16–19, 117
- tumor location and 18, 19, 58
- tumor size and 16–18, 28, 52, 58, 101, 147

Biopsy
- excisional 118–119, 123
- incisional 123
Bowman Grady Study 77
Brachial plexopathy 111, 112
Breast Adjuvant Chemotherapy study of the Anti-Cancer Council of Victoria 29
Breast cancer
- adjuvant therapy (see Chemotherapy, Hormonal therapy, Radiotherapy)
- advanced stage 6, 57, 61, 65, 69
- as systemic disease 12, 43, 61, 62
- axillary lymph node involvement and (see Axillary lymph nodes)
- biology of spread 9, 61, 95, 146
- Cathepsin D and 50
- chemotherapeutic resistance 50
- conservative surgery for
-- ductal carcinoma in situ 143, 146
-- cosmesis and 94, 117, 120–121
-- psychological effects of 117
-- radiotherapy and 68–69
--- pathologic features 93–102
--- technique 105–114
- contralateral 98, 122, 147, 150, 159
-- radiogenic 108
- cost-effective intervention 48
- criteria of inoperability 5, 7–9
- cure rates 3, 28
- death from 1–3, 12, 44, 147, 152
- development of prognostic index 49
- early diagnosis of 12, 45
- early metastasis and 12
- extensive intraductal component (EIC) 97–100, 123–127
- growth pattern of 95
- invasive
-- infiltrating ductal carcinomas 100
- late distant dissemination and 12
- limited stage 6, 57
- metastatic 46
- multimodality therapy 8, 9
- natural history of 13–19, 22, 23
- nipple-areola complex and 122, 147, 151, 159
- node-negative 13, 19, 23, 118, 126
-- as occult node-positive 45–46
-- chemotherapy for 43–52, 140
-- definition of 44
-- prognostic factors in 49–51
-- recurrence and 45–46
-- tumor size and 45, 52
- node-positive
-- chemotherapy and 89, 101, 129–130, 134–136, 139–141
-- definition of 43–44
- premenopausal 20, 23
- prognostic indicators 14, 17, 19, 27–28, 33, 50–51, 92, 97, 99
- radiotherapy for (see Radiotherapy)
- recurrence
-- axillary nodes and 20, 30–31, 58, 59, 68, 126–127
-- extensive intraductal component (EIC) 97–100, 102, 110, 123–124
-- fear of 117
-- high risk treatments 68–69
-- internal mammary chain and 20

Breast cancer (cont.)
-- invasive 152
-- local 11, 12, 14, 23
--- chemosensitivity of 24, 45
--- distant metastases and 12, 20, 117
--- lymph node involvement and 3, 18, 61
--- radiotherapy and 24, 110, 119
--- survival rates and 2-3, 7-8, 12, 13, 93, 118, 119
-- mastectomy and 30, 59, 117-120, 145
-- microcalcifications and 97-98, 122
-- mediastinal 18
-- pleural 18
-- rates of 2-3, 60, 117-118
-- tumor excision and 94-97
-- tumor size and 59, 101, 123
-- type of biopsy and 123
-- wide excision and 94, 97, 99, 100, 110, 149, 151
- residual 99
- salvage treatment 86, 90, 148, 151, 152
- screening for 12
- secondary 21
- surgery (see Mastectomy)
- TNM staging system and 6, 27, 29
Breast Cancer Detection Demonstration Project 143
Breast Intergroup Trial 139
Breast reconstruction 155-160

Cancer and Leukemia Group B (CALGB)
- radiotherapy doses 109
- chemotherapy and tamoxifen 139
Cancer computerized registries 14
Cancer Research Campaign (CRC) Trial 30, 107
Carcinogenesis 121-122
Carcinoma
- ductal in situ (DCIS)
-- axillary lymph nodes and 27, 28, 32
-- characteristics of 125, 144-146
-- comedo 32, 144-145, 146, 147, 148, 150
-- conservative surgery and 147-149, 151
-- conservative surgery and radiotherapy 149-152
-- cribiform 144, 145, 148
-- distribution in breast 146
-- estrogen receptors (ER) and 146
-- excisional margins and 97, 148, 151
-- increase in 143
-- lobular carcinoma in situ and 144
-- mammography and 143, 144, 147
-- micropapillary 144
-- *neu* oncogene and 144-145
-- noncomedo 32, 33, 144, 146, 150
-- occult invasion and 146-147
-- Paget's disease and 143, 150
-- papillary 144, 145, 147, 148
-- presentation of 144
-- pretreatment evaluation 150-151
-- progesterone receptors and 146
-- radiotherapy boost and 110
-- recurrence and 144
-- selecting treatment for 151-152
-- solid 144
- infiltrating ductal 99-100
- infiltrating lobular
-- local recurrence and 100
- invasive 143, 145, 150
- lobular in situ (LCIS) 32, 97, 143, 144, 145
- medullary 100
- noninvasive 143, 145
- presentation 144
- mucinous (colloid) 100
Case Western Reserve Group
- postmenopausal patient trials 137-138
Cathepsin D 50
Chemohormonal therapy
- node-negative patients 47
- postmenopausal patients and 136-139
- versus tamoxifen 136-139
Chemotherapy
- adjuvant 9, 14, 18
-- controversy over 73
-- long-term toxicity of 48-49
-- patient benefit from 46
-- second malignancies and 49
- age and 36-39, 41, 92
- axillary lymph node and 8, 23, 118, 120
-- recurrence 31-32, 45-46
- 5-fluorouracil (CAF) 49, 77
- chemotherapeutic resistance 50
- chlorambucil 46
- CMF 23, 35, 49, 63-65
-- effect on hormones 36-39
-- side-effects of 48, 108
-- versus radiation therapy 89-90
-- versus tamoxifen 134
- CMFP 36, 38, 51, 139, 140
- CMFPT 36
- CMFVP 136, 138
- conservative surgery and 8
-- cosmetic results and 121
- costs of 48
- criteria for inoperability and 8
- DNA and 44
- doxorubicin (Adriamycin) 47, 49, 65, 70, 136
-- side-effects of 48, 107-108
- epirubicin 134, 137
- Guy's Hospital study and 36, 37, 38
- high-dose treatment 46-47
- hormone manipulation and 35-39, 50-51
- L-phenylalanine mustard 49, 77
- length of 47
-- psychiatric effects from 47, 48
- low-dose treatment 46-47
- mechanisms of 44-45
- melphalan 38, 49
- node-negative cancer and 43-52, 140
-- survival 46
-- estrogen receptors and 50-51
- node-positive cancer and 89, 101, 129-130, 134-136, 139-141
- oophoretomy and 47
- polychemotherapy 47
-- postmenopausal patients and 131, 134, 138
-- vensus tamoxifen 134-136
-- premenopausal patients and 131, 139
- postmenopausal patients and 23-24, 36-39, 41, 63-65, 89, 129-141
- prednisone 36, 136
- premenopausal patients and 23-24, 27, 35-39, 41, 63-65, 78, 89, 139
- preoperative 28
- radiotherapy and 8-9, 23-24, 65, 67, 70, 89-90, 93
-- brachial plexopathy 112
-- pneumonitis 107, 112
-- toxicity of 24, 107
- randomized clinical trials
-- meta-analysis of 77-78
- side-effects of 48-49
- single-agent 47
- survival and 35-42
- systemic 8
- tamoxifen and 24, 35, 36, 46, 47, 89-90, 92, 136-138
- triethylthiophosphamide (TSPA) 62
- vincristine 65, 136
Chemotherapy-induced amenorrhoea (see Amenorrhoea)
Chest wall
- radiotherapy and 1, 3, 61-63, 68, 87, 89

- recurrence and 3, 59, 61, 68, 147
Children's and Adults' Hospital of San Francisco recurrence study 148
Clinical trials (see also individual trial name)
- Australian and New Zealand Breast Cancer Trials Group 47
- Bowman Gray Study 77
- Breast Adjuvant Chemotherapy study of the Anti-Cancer Council of Victoria 29
- Breast Cancer Detection Demonstration Project 143
- Breast Intergroup Trial 139
- Cancer and Leukemia Group B (CALGB) 109, 139
- Cancer Research Campaign (CRC) Trial 30, 107
- Case Western Reserve Group 137-138
- Children's Adults' Hospital of San Francisco 148
- Danish Breast Cancer Cooperative Group Trials 23, 65, 67, 120
- difficulties of 52
- Early Breast Cancer Trialists' Collaborative Group (EBCTCG) 76, 78, 86
- Eastern Cooperative Oncology Group (ECOG) 31-32, 36, 65
- effects of errors in statistical technique 74-74, 78
- European Organization for Research on Treatment of Cancer (EORTC) quality control and 78-79
- flaws in 61, 74
- GABG Trial 1, 134
- Glasgow Study 77
- GROCTA study 134, 137
- Guy's Hospital Study 12, 13, 36-38, 119-120
- Haagensen study 59
- Helsinki study 65
- importance of 73, 79
- Institut Curie 99, 119, 123
- Institut Gustave-Roussy (Villejuif) studies 12, 14, 19, 20, 22, 24, 30, 64, 89, 123
- Instituto Nazionale Tumori study 61
- "intent to treat" classification 74-75
- Joint Center for Radiation Therapy (JCRT) 105-107, 109, 110-113, 152
- Ludwig Breast Cancer Study Group 36×39, 46, 136
- Manchester clinical trials 74, 107
- Marseilles Cancer Institute 98, 99, 119
- Mayo Clinic trial 139
- Medical College of Virginia (MCV) 7, 8
- Memorial Sloan-Kettering Center 3, 8
- meta-analysis of 11, 22-23
- multi-institutional studies 78
- National Cancer Institute in Bethesda 120
- National Cancer Institute of Milan 29, 31, 65, 73, 77, 89, 111, 120, 129, 131, 139
- National Surgical Adjuvant Breast and Bowel Project (NSABP)
-- trial B-02 22, 62-63
-- trial B-04 29, 30, 44, 63
-- trial B-05 77
-- trial B-06 31, 95, 96, 98, 110, 111, 118, 120, 123, 148, 151
-- trial B-13 140
-- trial B-16 74, 77, 79, 136
- North Central Cancer Treatment Group (NCCTG) 137, 139, 140
- Oslo-II clinical trials 22, 23, 77, 85, 86, 89, 107
- Princess Margaret Hospital 119
- problems in 78-79, 93
- prognostic factors 74
- risk factors in 75
- Royal Marsden Hospital study 109-110
- Southwest Oncology Group Study (SWOG) 77, 134-136, 139
- Stockholm Breast Cancer Study Group 22-24, 63-64, 73, 83-92
- subset anaylses 78
- "treatment received" classification 74-75
- University of Pennsylvania 98
- University of Texas M.D. Anderson Cancer Center 1-3, 7, 8, 61-62
- value of 49, 52
Cosmetic concerns
- breast-conserving therapy and 94, 105, 117, 120-121, 122, 126
- chemotherapy and 121
- radiotherapy and 105, 108, 120-121

Danish Breast Cancer Cooperative Group Trials 23, 65, 67, 120
- chemotherapy and amenorrhoea 37, 38-39
- postmenopausal patients 137
Death
- breast cancer and 1-3, 12, 44
- cause-specific 87-88
- distant metastases and 12, 16
Deoxyribonucleic acid (DNA) 44, 50
- flow cytometry 145
Disease-specific relapse-free survival rate (DSRFS) 62, 67

Early Breast Cancer Trialists' Collaborative Group (EBCTCG) 78, 86
- meta-analysis of adjuvant trials 130-131, 138
- chemotherapy 37-38, 43, 47, 76, 130-131
- survival 44-48
Eastern Cooperative Oncology Group (ECOG) 65
- chemotherapy and amenorrhoea 36-37
- chemotherapy and tamoxifen 139
- chemotherapy of axillary nodes 31-32
- node-negative cancer 140
Edema, arm
- axillary dissection and 32-33, 111
- contraindication for surgery 5, 7, 9
Edema, breast
- axillary dissection and 32-33
Electronic portal imaging devices (EPID) 106-107, 114
Enzyme production
- axillary metastases and 28
Estrogen receptor (ER) (see Hormone receptors)
European Organization for Research on Treatment of Cancer (EORTC)
- quality control and 78-79
Extensive intraductal component (EIC)
- breast-conserving surgery and 123-127
- JCRT study 97-99
- lymphatic vessel invasion (LVI) and 101
- mammography and 97-98, 100, 102
- negative 97-99
- positive 97-100
- radioresistant 99
- recurrence and 97-100, 102, 110, 123-124
- survival rates and 97

False-negative rates 29, 30
Flow cytometry
- node-negative disease and 49-50
- DNA
-- oncogenes and 145
Fluroscopy
- radiotherapy set-up and 106
Food and Drug Administration (FDA)
- breast implants and 157-158

GABG Trial 1, 134
Gene overexpression
- axillary metastases and 28
Glasgow Study 77
GROCTA trials 134, 137
Guy's Hospital studies 12, 13, 36-38, 119-120

Haagensen study 59
Heart disease
- breast reconstruction and 157
- ischemic, radiation therapy and 68, 70, 87-89, 91, 107-108
Helsinki clinical trials 65
Hematogenous spread 16, 17, 18
Hormonal therapy
- chemotherapy and 47-48
-- postmenopausal patients and 37-41, 76, 130-131, 134-139, 141
-- premenopausal patients and 36-41, 76, 130
- manipulation 35, 79
- tamoxifen 24, 35, 36, 46, 47, 65, 89-90, 129
- tamoxifen and fluoxymesterone 140
Hormone receptors
- estrogen receptor (ER)
-- axillary metastases and 28
-- cathpsin D and 50
-- ductal carcinoma in situ and 146
-- negative 123
--- amenorrhoea and 37, 39
--- chemohormonal therapy 136
--- node-negative
---- survival and 50-51
--- postive nodes and 139-140
--- tamoxifen and 130, 131, 136, 137
-- positive 123
--- amenorrhoea and 39
--- chemohormonal therapy 136-139
--- node-negative
---- survival and 50-51
--- tamoxifen and 129-131, 136
- progesterone receptors 136, 146
- prognostic factors 14, 28, 51
Hormones
- chemotherapy's effect on 36-39
- estrogens 36
- follicle-stimulating (FSH) 36
- luteinizing (LH) 36, 42
- plasma androstenedione 36
- plasma dehydroepiandrosterone sulphate 36
Hypoxic tumor cells 144

Immunodepression
- radiotherapy and 11-12
Imprint cytology 94
Inked margins of excision 94, 151
Institut Curie studies 99, 119, 123
Insttiut Gustave-Roussy (Villejuif) studies
- axillary recurrences 30, 31
- distant metastases 12, 14, 22, 120
- extensive intraductal component (EIC) 124
- internal mammary node treatment 19, 20, 24, 64, 89
- radiotherapy 20, 123
Instituto Nazionale Tumori study 61
Internal mammary chain (IMC)
- mastectomy and 5, 20-22, 64
- postoperative radiotherapy and 1-2, 20-24, 61, 64, 68-71
- tumors and 18-20
Internal mammary nodes
- anatomy of 58, 88
- axillary node involvement and 19, 59
- difficulty of detection 20
- dissection of 88-89
-- survival rates and 19, 20, 89
- distant dissemination and 20
- lymphoscintigraphy and 2, 11, 29, 106
- metastases in 89
- radiotherapy and 84, 87-89, 112, 113
- tumor location and 20, 59, 89
- tumor size and 19

Joint Center for Radiation Therapy (JCRT)
- axillary dissection 111, 126
- axillary recurrence 30, 31, 111
- boost of radiotherapy 110-111, 114
- cosmetic results and radiotherapy 120-121
- excisional biopsy and radiotherapy 118-119
- extensive intraductal component (EIC) 97-99, 123
- infiltrating lobular carcinomas 100
- local recurrence study 110, 123, 150
- lung volume and radiotherapy study 109
- radiotherapy complications 120-121
- radiotherapy policies 105-107, 109, 110-113, 152

Leukemia
- chemotherapy and 49
- radiotherapy and 121-122
Ludwig Breast Cancer Study Group
- chemotherapy studies 36-39, 46, 136
Lumpectomy (wide excision)
- axillary dissection and 31
- cosmetic results 94, 122, 126
- Guy's Hospital study and 12, 13, 119
- radiotherapy and 12, 117, 120
Lymph nodes
- anatomy of 57-58
- apical 123
- axillary (see Axillary Lymph Nodes)
- internal mammary (see Internal Mammary Nodes)
- interpectoral 57
- intramammary 57
- metastatic dissemination and 12-14, 17, 63
- negative 13, 19, 23, 61, 118, 126
-- definition of 44
-- false-negative 45
-- metastases and 44
-- true-negative 44
- parasternal 68
- peripheral lymphatic system
-- radiotherapy and 1-2, 61, 68
- positive 19-20, 22, 23, 63, 118, 126
-- definition of 43-44
- prognostic significance and 17, 19, 51
- radiotherapy and 11
-- techniques 112-113
- regional management of 117
- Rotter's nodes 29, 57
- subpectoral 57
Lymphatic vessel invasion (LVI) 101
Lymphoscintigraphy 2, 11, 29, 106
- radionuclide 113

Macrometastases
- survival rates and 28
Mammography
- breast implants and 158
- ductal carcinoma in situ 143, 144, 147, 150
- extensive intraductal component (EIC) and 97-98, 100, 102
- importance of 123
- microcalcifications and 122, 144, 150-151, 152
- occult invasion and 147
- postbiopsy 123, 124
- prebiopsy 123, 124, 150-151
- preoperative 97-98, 149
- recurrence and 144
- screening 28, 114, 143
Manchester clinical trials 74, 107
Marseilles Cancer Institute studies 98, 99, 119

Mastectomy
- axillary dissection 7, 12, 13, 20, 27, 59, 62, 118, 126-127
- bilateral 159
- breast reconstruction and 122-123, 157
-- techniques 122, 156-160
- chemotherapy and 8
- compared to primary radiotherapy 86-87, 119-120, 127
- comparison of types 120
- conservative
-- amount of tissue removed 123, 152
-- cosmetic concerns and 94, 105, 117, 120-121, 126
-- ductal carcinoma in situ 147-149
-- evaluation of patients for 113, 124-125
-- follow-up of 152
-- hemostatis and 126
-- local excisions and recurrence 97, 110
-- nipple and 95, 113, 122, 125-126, 147, 151
-- pathologic features and 93-102, 123
-- poor candidates for 122, 124-125, 151
-- principle for 125-126
-- radiotherapy and 8, 30, 93, 100-101, 105, 117-120
--- complications from 121
--- ductal carcinoma in situ 149-152
-- recurrence rates and 93, 117-119
-- types of 117
-- wide excisions 93, 119, 122, 124
- contraindications for 5-6, 59
- delayed 12
- diffuse disease and 122
- ductal carcinoma in situ 143, 147, 151
-- recurrence and 145, 147
- extended 19, 20, 62
- Halsted (see Mastectomy, radical)
- indications for 7-9, 122-123
internal mammary chain (IMC) and 5, 20-22,64
- margins of excision
-- close 95
-- inked 94, 151
-- negative 95-96, 151
--- recurrence and 96, 110, 148
-- positive 95-96
--- recurrence and 96
- modified radical 73, 120
-- versus radiotherapy 83
- occult invasion and 146
- partial 117
- patient preference and 122
- postoperative radiotherapy and 7-8
- preoperative radiotherapy and 7, 83
- prophylactic 159
- quadrantectomy 31, 93, 94, 117, 120, 123, 124, 149
-- radiotherapy boost and 110
- radical
-- as old-fashioned treatment 73
-- Guy's Hospital study and 12, 13, 119-120
-- Institut Gustave-Roussy study 20-21, 22, 120, 123
-- internal mammary nodes and 59
-- psychological effects of 105, 117
-- recurrence rates and 117-118, 120
-- removal of lymph nodes 29
-- survival rates and 19-22, 61-63
-- survival rates and 5
- radiotherapy and 20, 61-63
- segmental 117, 120
- simple 22, 110
- stage III patients and 6, 7
- stage IV patients and 6
- subcutaneous 147, 159
- superradical 88
- supraclavicular metastases and 5, 9
- total 13, 119, 120
-- salvage rates and 86, 119
Mayo Clinic trial 139
Medical College of Virginia (MCV) studies 7, 8
Memorial Sloan-Kettering Center studies 3, 8
Metastases
- blood-borne 12
- brain 12, 21
- disease definition 43
- distant
-- cause of death and 12, 16
-- extensive intraductal component (EIC) and 98
inoperability and 5, 9
-- local control and 12, 13, 14, 23
-- local recurrence and 12, 20, 117, 119
-- radiotherapy and 2-3, 12-13, 23, 62-63, 84, 89-90, 119
-- tumor location and 20, 21, 84
-- tumor size and 17, 18, 19, 23, 101
- lymph nodes and 17, 18, 22, 28, 30, 44, 58, 59, 119, 126, 147
- micrometastases 28
- occult 14, 17, 23, 62, 68
- pleural 20
- pulmonary 20
- skip 30, 44, 69
- subclinical 22
Metastatic dissemination 12, 13
- lymph nodes and 14, 17, 63
- tumor size and 14
Microcalcifications
- mammograms and 144, 150-151, 162
- recurrence and 97-98, 122

National Cancer Institute in Bethesda
- Clinical Alert 28, 51
- studies done at 120
National Cancer Institute of Milan studies
- chemotherapy meta-analysis 65, 73, 77, 89, 129, 131, 139
- mastectomy vs conservative surgery and radiotherapy 29, 31, 111, 120
- opphorectomy 38
National Institutes of Health (NIH) Consensus Conference 93, 117, 120, 139, 140
National Surgical Adjuvant Breast and Bowel Project (NSABP)
- axillary lymph nodes and 29, 30, 31, 44
- chemotherapy
-- adjuvant 77, 89
-- amenorrhoea and 38
- distant metastases and radiotherapy 12-13
- ductal carcinoma in situ 148, 150
- radiotherapy doses 109
- re-evaluation of trials 74, 77
- recurrence rates 96, 110, 123, 148, 151
- tamoxifen and ductal carcinoma in situ 150
- trial B-02
-- mastectomy and radiotherapy vs mastectomy and observation 22, 62-63
- trial B-04
- axillary node assessment 29, 30, 44, 63
- trial B-05
-- chemotherapy 77
- trial B-06
-- conservative surgery vs conservative surgery and radiotherapy vs
-- mastectomy 31, 111, 118, 120
-- margins of excision 95, 96, 98, 110, 151
-- recurrence 123, 148, 151

NSABP (cont.)
- trial B-13
-- chemotherapy and postmenopausal patients 140
- trial B-16
-- tamoxifen and chemotherapy 136
Netherlands Cancer Institute
- electronic portal imaging devices (EPID) 106-107
- oncogene study 144-145
- radiotherapy and lung homogeneity 108-109
- radiotherapy two-dimensional planning system 109
Nipple-areola complex
- reconstruction and 159
- tumor involvement and 122, 147, 151
North Central Cancer Treatment Group (NCCTG) 140
- chemotherapy and tamoxifen 137, 139

Oncogenes, c-*erb*B-2 (*neu*, HER-2)
- node-negative cancer and 51
- node-positive cancer and 51
- ductal carcinoma in situ and 144-145
Oophorectomy 38, 39, 42, 47
Oslo-II clinical trials
- flaws in study 77, 86
- postoperative radiation 22, 23, 85, 86, 89, 107
Ovarian ablation 35, 36, 76, 78
- relapse-free survival and 38, 39, 42

Paget's disease 32, 143, 150
Pathologic features
- conservative surgery and 123
- conservative surgery and radiation and 93-102
- local recurrence and
-- extensive intraductal component (EIC) 97-100, 102
-- histologic features 100-101
-- microscopic margins of excision 94-97, 110
Ploidy
- as prognostic factor 28, 50
- recurrence and 145
Polyurethane prosthesis 155, 157
Pregnancy
- surgery and 5, 122
Princess Margaret Hospital studies 119
Progesterone receptors (see Hormone receptors)
Prognostic factors
- axillary involvement 14, 17-19, 33, 49, 111
- cathepsin D 50
- C-*erb*B-2 51
- enzyme production 38
- epidermal growth factor receptors 50
- extensive intraductal component (EIC) 97, 99
- factor VII innunocytochemistry 50
- flow cytometry 50
- hormone receptors 14, 28, 51
- laminin receptors 50
- need to develop index for 49
- ploidy 28, 50
- proteins 50
- s-phase fraction 28, 50
- thymidine incorporation 28, 50
- tumor glycosylation 50
- tumor size 14, 27-28, 52
- tumor grade 14, 28, 52
- use in randomized clinical trials 74

Quality of life
- length of chemotherapy and 47
- locoregional control and 6-9, 57, 83
- quality-adjusted life year (QALY)

Radiotherapy
- adjuvant
-- controversy over 73
-- local control and 86-87, 89-90
-- versus CMF chemotherapy 89-90
-- versus surgery alone 83-84
- axillary recurrence and 30-32
- boost of 7, 96, 97, 102, 117, 118, 123
-- tumor bed 110-111
- breast reconstruction and 157
- breast-preserving therapy and 68, 70, 93, 100, 105-114
- carcinogenesis from 121-122
- cardiac damage and 68, 70, 87-89, 91, 107-108
- cause-specific mortality and 87-88, 107
- chemotherapy and 8-9, 23-24, 65, 67, 70, 89-90, 93
-- brachial plexopathy 112
-- pneumonitis 107, 112
-- toxicity of 24, 107
- chest wall and 1, 3, 61, 62, 63, 68, 87, 89
- cold spots 112
- compared to mastectomy 86-87, 111, 114, 119-120, 127
- conservative surgery and 8, 30, 68-69, 93, 100, 105-114
-- ductal carcinoma in situ 110, 149-152
- cosmetic concerns and 105, 108, 120-121
- cumulative radiation effect (CRE) 87
- distant metastases and 2-3, 23, 62-63, 84, 89-90, 119
- dose homogeneity 108-110
- en face axillary boost (EAB) 113
- excisional biopsy and 118-119
- extensive intraductal component (EIC) and 99
- fibrosis 106
- high dosage effects 3
- hot spots 108-109, 112
- implants 110, 117, 118
- internal mammary nodes and 84, 87-89, 112, 113
- isodose level 108, 110
- JCRT policies on 105-107, 109, 110-113, 152
- limiting heart and lung exposure 105-108, 113
- lung volume influences on 108-109
- lymph nodes and 111-112
- morbidity and 108, 111
- new primary malignancies and 49
- node-positive patients and 84, 85, 90
- peripheral lymphatic system and 1-2, 61, 68
- posterior axillary boost (PAB) 113
- postmenopausal patients and 23-24, 65, 67, 89-90
- postoperative
-- axillary nodes and 20, 22, 30-31, 61-70, 84, 111-113, 126
-- doses of 11, 12, 69, 70
-- duration of 11
-- immunodepression and 11-12
-- indications for 69
-- internal mammary chain (IMC) and 1-2, 20-24, 61, 64, 68-71
-- local recurrence and 11, 12, 23, 63, 110, 119
-- mastectomy and 7-8, 20, 30, 61-63, 93, 100-101, 105, 117-121
-- metastatic spread and 13-14, 63
-- node-negative tumors and 13, 23, 61
-- randomized clinical trials
--- meta-analyses of 11, 23, 67-68, 76-77
-- rationale for 57, 61, 63, 70
-- Stage I patients and 13, 117-119

-- Stage II patients and 13, 69, 117-119
-- survival and 11-13, 62-63, 67, 70-71, 85
- premenopausal patients and 20, 23, 65, 67, 89-90
- preoperative 7, 21, 63, 69, 83
- primary 123, 127
-- conservative surgery and 117-120
--- complications from 121
-- mammography and 123
-- recurrence rates and 118-120
- radiologic castration 85
- recurrence rates and 62-65, 84
- reproducting daily set-up 106, 112
- side effects of 87, 91, 107, 111, 112, 157
- stage I and II patients
-- homogeneous tumoricidal dose 105-106
- supraclavicular area and 1-2, 7, 9, 31, 61, 69, 84, 89, 111-113
- tamoxifen and 24, 65, 89-90, 92
- tangential field irradiation 107
- target volume 106
- techniques
-- breast-conserving therapy and 105-114
-- cobalt
--- postoperative treatment 22, 85
--- preoperative treatment 87, 88, 107
--- electron beam 1-2, 61, 68-70, 87-88, 92, 107, 111
--- equipment 105
--- lymph nodes and 112-113
--- megavoltage 22, 83, 84, 86, 89, 108, 109
--- orthovoltage 61, 62, 68, 85, 86, 107
--- outmoded 68
--- overdosages 77, 88
--- photons 62, 69, 70, 108, 109
--- refinement of 92
--- underdosages 77
- three-dimensional planning system 109, 114
- three-field irradiation 112
- tomography scan 106, 107, 108, 113
- two-dimensional planning system 109
- ultrasonography 111
- whole breast 119, 152
Recurrence
- breast reconstruction and 155-156, 158
- conservative surgery and 148-149, 151
- conservative surgery and radiotherapy 149-152
- ductal carcinoma in situ (DCIS) and 144, 145, 147, 148
- local
-- age and 93
-- extensive intraductal component (EIC) and 97-100, 102, 110
-- histologic grade and 101, 148
-- histologic tumor type and 100
-- lymphatic vessel invasion (LVI) 101
-- mononuclear cell reaction and 101
-- radiation and chemotherapy and 93
-- tumor excision and 93-97, 110
-- tumor necrosis and 101
-- tumor size and axillary nodel status 101
-- wide reaction and 93, 94, 97, 99, 100, 110, 149
Rotter's nodes (see Lymph nodes, Rotter's nodes)
Royal Marsden Hospital study 109-110

S-phase fraction
- as prognostic indicator 28, 50
Scleroderma 122, 157
Silicone prosthesis 155, 157-158
Southwest Oncology Group Study (SWOG) 77, 134-136, 139
Specimen radiography 151
Stockholm Breast Cancer Study Group 22-24, 63-64, 73
- radiation versus CMF chemotherapy 89-92
- radiation versus surgery alone 83-91
Supraclavicular area
- fossa 57, 69, 70 84
- nodes
-- adenopathy 58
-- anatomy of 57
-- recurrence in 111
-- resudual tumor sites 59
- radiotherapy and 1-2, 7, 9, 31, 61, 69, 89, 89, 111-113
Surgery (see Mastetomy
Survival
- chemohormonal therapy and 136-139
- disease-free 2-3, 7, 19, 20, 23, 28, 61-63, 118
-- node-negative chemotherapy and 46, 140
-- tamoxifen and 134
- Early Breast Cancer Trialists' Collaborative Group 44
- extended mastectomy and 19-20, 62
- five-year index 1
- local recurrence and 12, 13
- metastasis-free 19, 23, 85
- occult nodal metastases and 44
- ovarian ablation and 35, 36, 76, 78
- overall 73
- radical mastectomy and 19-22, 61-63
- radiotherapy and 11-13, 62-63, 70-71, 85
- relapse-free (RFS) 20
-- chemotherapy and amenorrhoea 36-39, 41-42
-- radiotherapy and 89-92
- whole breast irradiation and 119
Systemic subclinical disease 35, 118
Systemic therapy 8, 12, 28, 65, 111, 114

Tamoxifen
- chemotherapy and 24, 35, 36, 46, 47, 89-90, 136-138
- ductal carinoma in situ 150
- fluoxymesterone and 140
- postmenopausal patients and 27, 130-141
-- versus polychemotherapy 134-136
- radiotherapy and 24, 65, 89-90, 92
- versus chemohormonal therapy 136-139
Thiotepa 119
Thymidine
- as prognostic factor 28, 50
- labelling index 145
TNM staging system 6
Tomography scan 106, 107, 108, 113
Tumors
- analysis of
-- prognostic factors 14, 17, 19, 27-28, 50, 52, 97
- anaplastic 28
- aneuploid 50, 145
- biology of 43
- contiguous spread 146
- diploid 50, 145
- distribution in breast 146
- early diagnosis of 16, 45
- early metastasis 12
- estrogen receptors (ER) and 123
- extensive intraductal component (EIC) 123-127
-- negative 97-99
-- positive 97-100
- growth pattern of 95
- hematogenous spread 16, 17, 18
- histologic grades 14, 28, 52, 101

Tumors (cont.)
– – dissemination and 13 – 15, 22
– – high-grade 14, 15, 148
– – low-grade 15, 18, 148
– histologic type 100
– hypoxic cells 144
– in situ 96
– inner quadrant 18, 19, 58
– – survival rates and 20, 22
– – treatment of 1, 20, 61, 68
– internal mammary chain (IMC) and 18, 19, 20
– invasive 96, 143
– ipsilateral 146
– lateral
– – survival rates and 19
– – treatment of 21, 22, 85
– local treatment of 12, 14
– medial quadrants
– – survival rates and 19 – 21, 89
– – treatment of 21, 22, 24, 64, 70, 85, 89
– metastatic dissemination 14
– multicentric disease 146, 152
– N0 survival rates 119
– N1 survival rates 120
– necrotic 101, 144
– node-negative 13, 19, 23, 61, 118, 126
– node-positive 19 – 20, 22, 23, 63, 118, 126
– nuclear grade 52, 148
– occult node-positive 45
– outer quadrant 18, 20, 21, 58
– palliative tumor responses 45
– palpable lesions 143, 144, 147, 151, 152
– – recurrence and 147 – 150
– pathologic characteristics
– – recurrence and 93 – 102
– progression 15
– re-excisions 99, 124
– residual 59, 95, 99
– – markers for 94 – 96
– S-phase fractions and 50, 145
– screening for 12, 14
– size of
– – occult invasion and 146 – 147
– – assessment of 151
– – axillary involvement and 16 – 19, 28, 52, 58, 101, 147
– – inner quadrant and 18
– – metastastic dissemination and 14 – 15, 147
– – node-negative patients and 45
– – node-positive patients and 45, 52, 147
– – outer quadrant and 18
– – prognostic factors 14, 17, 19, 27 – 28, 52
– staging system 6
– T1
– – EIC and 123
– – mastectomy and 19
– – survival rates 28, 52, 119
– – wide resections and 99
– T2
– – EIC and 123
– – mastectomy and 19
– – survival rates 28, 52, 119
– – wide resections and 99

Ultrasonography 111
University of Pennsylvania 98, 113, 150
University of Texas M.D. Anderson Cancer Center 1 – 3, 7, 8, 61 – 62

Villejuif studies (see Gustave-Roussy)

Springer-Verlag and the Environment

We at Springer-Verlag firmly believe that an international science publisher has a special obligation to the environment, and our corporate policies consistently reflect this conviction.

We also expect our business partners – paper mills, printers, packaging manufacturers, etc. – to commit themselves to using environmentally friendly materials and production processes.

The paper in this book is made from low- or no-chlorine pulp and is acid free, in conformance with international standards for paper permanency.

MIX
Papier aus verantwortungsvollen Quellen
Paper from responsible sources
FSC® C105338

If you have any concerns about our products,
you can contact us on
ProductSafety@springernature.com

In case Publisher is established outside the EU,
the EU authorized representative is:
Springer Nature Customer Service Center GmbH
Europaplatz 3, 69115 Heidelberg, Germany

Printed by Libri Plureos GmbH
in Hamburg, Germany